AF181325

ALLE ZEIT WACH 1842

Gerontology

4th International Symposium

Present State and Research Perspectives
in the Experimental and Clinical Gerontology

Edited by Dieter Platt

With 75 Figures and 65 Tables

Springer-Verlag Berlin Heidelberg New York
London Paris Tokyo Hong Kong

Professor Dr. med. DIETER PLATT
Lehrstuhl für Innere Medizin – Gerontologie
der Universität Erlangen-Nürnberg
Heimerichstr. 58
D-8500 Nürnberg, FRG

ISBN-13: 978-3-642-74998-8 e-ISBN-13: 978-3-642-74996-4
DOI: 10.1007/978-3-642-74996-4

This work is subject to copyright. All rights are reserved, whether the whole or part of the material is concerned, specifically the rights of translation, reprinting, reuse of illustrations, recitation, broadcasting, reproduction on microfilms or in other ways, and storage in data banks. Duplication of this publication or parts thereof is only permitted under the provisions of the German Copyright Law of September 9, 1965, in its version of June 24, 1985, and a copyright fee must always be paid. Violations fall under the prosecution act of the German Copyright Law.

© Springer-Verlag Berlin Heidelberg 1989
Softcover reprint of the hardcover 1st edition 1989

The use of registered names, trademarks, etc. in this publication does not imply, even in the absence of a specific statement, that such names are exempt from the relevant protective laws and regulations and therefore free for general use.

Product Liability: The publisher can give no guarantee for information about drug dosage and application thereof contained in this book. In every individual case the respective user must check its accuracy by consulting other pharmaceutical literature.

2122/3130-543210 – Printed on acid-free paper

List of Contributors

You will find the addresses at the beginning of the respective contribution

Preface

At the beginning of the century the average life span in developed societies was less than 50 years. It is now more than 70 years and will continue to increase in the near future.

Aging is a challenge to science and society. There are several theories of aging. The programmed aging hypothesis suggests that aging cannot be altered by any external influence, that aging is programmed from the beginning of life until the end of senescence. Another theory is based on genetic instability, with repair processes correcting errors in the cells that cause aging. Aging processes manifest themselves at the molecular and cellular level, in different organs, and in the whole organism. Most older persons acquire multiple diseases, primarily chronic ones. The multimorbidity of the elderly raises many questions as to nutrition, metabolism, immunity, drug therapy, and rehabilitation. Nutrition may be able to intervene in the aging process. Aging is associated with declining immunity and reduced resistance to many diseases, and it is possible that nutritional changes in old age contribute to the declining immunity in the elderly. The elderly take 40% of the prescription drugs in Germany and adverse drug reactions are more frequent in geriatric patients. There are not only problems in drug therapy for elderly patients, but also in their rehabilitation. The aim of rehabilitation is the restoration of geriatric patients to their former functional and environmental status.

In 1971 I organized the first Giessen symposium on experimental gerontology, with the title molecular and cellular aspects of aging. Three further meetings were held in 1973, 1975, and 1978 at the Justus-Liebig University in Giessen, where I used to do my experimental gerontological research and dealt with aging theories, drugs and aging, and the central nervous system and liver.

Since 1979, when I accepted the chair of gerontology at the University of Erlangen-Nuremberg, I have continued the series with international workshops on cardiology, drug therapy, blood cells and rheology. All of these meetings were sponsored by the pharmaceutical industry.

This 4th international symposium at the University of Erlangen-Nuremberg was intended to deal with physiological and pathological aging processes at the molecular, cellular, organ, and organism level, and was the first meeting sponsored by a state grant. The *Ministry of*

Research and Technology intends to concentrate efforts and resources in gerontological research. The development of an acknowledged geriatric science is only possible on the basis of improved experimental gerontology. The participants at this international meetings came from different disciplines, including biology, biochemistry, pathology, clinical gerontology, clinical pharmacology, and immunology.

The symposium serves as the basis for future topics in experimental and clinical research in gerontology. The interdisciplinary character of the workshop demonstrates the necessity of personal contact between basic research scientists and those working in geriatrics. Both the present state and future perspectives are discussed. This gives an indication of future research directions and of the fields for which grants are likely to be given by the Ministry of Research and Technology.

Erlangen-Nuremberg DIETER PLATT

Words of Welcome at the Opening of the Symposium Present State and Research Perspectives in Experimental and Clinical Gerontology

Ladies and Gentlemen,

The Federal Minister for Research and Technology, Dr. Riesenhuber, has asked me to convey to you his greetings and his best wishes for the success of the Symposium. He hopes that this meeting will help us to establish research funding in the field of gerontology. At the same time, I would like to give you some indications on the aims pursued by the Federal Minister for Research and Technology in making gerontological research an area of priority funding, and to point out some of the tasks to be tackled in this field.

The German scientists assembled here will probably all be familiar with the Federal Government's funding programme entitled "Research and Development in the Service of Health". This programme was first launched ten years ago; the latest version covering the period from 1988 to 1991 was adopted by the Federal Cabinet early this year. The programme is implemented jointly by the Federal Ministry for Research and Technology and the two Ministries responsible for health care policy, i.e. the Federal Ministry of Labour and Social Affairs and the Federal Ministry for Youth, Family Affairs, Women and Health. As the programme is intended to contribute by research results to improving health policy and our health care system, it focuses on those diseases which most frequently result in death, invalidity or inability to work. Federal Government support for research within the programme only supplements the activities of other organizations already supporting medical research, and it is therefore performed in close cooperation with the other major research funding organizations in the Federal Republic of Germany. The key issues of health care policy which lend themselves to innovative research were selected for the programme in joint discussions with the scientific community. Estimates of future demographic development both on the worldwide average and in the Federal Republic of Germany lead us to expect that the treatment and care of the elderly will form an increasingly large part of health care. This is why one chapter of the health research programme is devoted exclusively to gerontological and geriatric research. The chapter entitled »Health in Old Age« sets a dual task for research: One is for clinical research to develop and test therapeutic concepts effective for elderly patients, who often suffer from several diseases at the same time, and the other for medical research applicable to disease prevention, i.e. the study of the biological processes of aging, the physical and emotional stress originating from social environment and the interaction of these stress factors and the aging processes in producing symptoms of disease. Intervention models to prevent diseases of old age are necessarily of a long-term nature and therefore require a sound scientific basis if they are to be successful. Gerontological research has to cover biological, clinical and psychological as well as social aspects. This symposium will discuss the present status and identify the future needs of the biological and clinical aspects of gerontology. The psychological and social aspects are to be dealt with at a later date.

Demographic trends in industrialized countries are comparable with those in the Federal Republic of Germany; hence the problems of health care for elderly people are also similar. The results of this symposium should therefore be of interest not only in the FRG. International cooperation is, I think, also required for another reason: Long-term prevention models and methods of long-term therapy and care for the elderly affect the structure of the health care system. A comparison with the differently structured health care systems of other countries may provide useful hints as to the structural conditions required to enable public health care to effectively apply research results in order to better cope with old-age diseases.

Let me finally add a few words to explain the procedure of determining a research priority area for public announcement: As a result of this symposium, a research concept for experimental and clinical gerontology in the FRG will be drawn up. This together with a concept in the field of social gerontology will then be discussed with other research-funding institutions such as the Max Planck Society and the German Research Association in order to avoid overlaps with established or planned funding programmes. The concept will then be discussed again by a small interdisciplinary panel of experts before being published together with a call for research proposals. It is hoped that the concept will provide a basis not only for national research support but also for joint international research projects.

In conclusion I should like to thank all experts for their cooperation at the present symposium, which will help in developing a concept for gerontological research. I am especially grateful to Professor Platt for the excellent preparation and the subsequent evaluation of the symposium, for which I wish you all my best.

G. FRANK

Contents

Metabolism and Nutrition in the Elderly

Molecular Aspects of Aging

DNA – Information and Aging: The Balance Between Alteration and Repair

Z. A. Medvedev[1]

Introduction

The unique role of DNA in transfering genetic information from cell to cell and from generation to generation in evolution means that it is necessary to preserve the integrity of DNA molecules and their nucleotide sequences throughout millions of years and billions of replications. The complementarity of nucleotide base pairs in a double helix provides the main mechanism of the high accuracy of replication, but the potential of the hydrogen-bonded base pair complementarity alone would never be enough for this "thread of life" to preserve life on Earth in conditions where numerous environmental hazards, UV radiation, ionising radiation, free radicals, chemicals, and variations in temperature permanently produce changes in functional DNA molecules and errors during their replication. The highly efficient correction of DNA sequence errors is, therefore, absolutely essential and very many biochemical systems exist in cells and their nuclei for this purpose. The DNA repair system in prokaryotes and in germ cells of eukaryotes needs to preserve the integrity of genetic information over long evolutionary periods. However, somatic cells which function for only days, months or years and leave no progeny after the death of individual organisms do not need the same level of efficiency of correction of DNA sequence errors. Kirkwood and Holliday (1979) have suggested that a lower level of accuracy in synthesis and repair of macromolecules in somatic cells is (as compared with germ cells) an adaptation which saves energy; they postulate that aging occurs as a consequence (Kirkwood 1977; Kirkwood and Holliday 1979). It is attractive to link the DNA repair capability in somatic cells with evolutionary variation of life span (Hart and Setlow 1974). However, the possibility of immortalization of clones of somatic cells in culture, experiments which replace the nuclei in fertilized eggs with nuclei from somatic cells, and the use of somatic cells for reproduction in many plants in experimental and natural conditions, indicates that the *potential* for the "germ cell quality" of DNA repair does exist is somatic cells as well, particularly in proliferating tissues. Probably only terminally differentiated and non-dividing cells do not need some DNA repair systems which are specifically attached to the DNA replication processes.

[1] Genetics Division, National Institute for Medical Research, Mill Hill, London NW7 1AA, UK

Gerontology
Ed. by D. Platt
© Springer-Verlag Berlin Heidelberg 1989

The primary role of DNA not only in transfer of genetic information between generations but also in the use of this information for constant expression of cellular functions has made it possible to consider aging in tissues to be linked to age-associated changes in DNA. Any changes in DNA which can be found in old cells or old tissues most likely represent only a minor fraction of these much more numerous and common changes of DNA which for one reason or another remained uncorrected and unrepaired. Among many different factors of aging, the proper balance between DNA alteration and repair is likely to play an important role in the rate of aging. The existence of many forms of change in DNA creates many forms of repair of different complexity, and it is possible that some changes in DNA are irreversible or irreparable and might therefore play a more important role in accumulation of age changes. On the other hand the DNA repair systems may also change with age, and aging therefore might reflect a decline in the DNA repair capability. I do not plan to analyse all aspects of this very complex problem in this review, but I will try to make at least brief outlines of both problems; DNA age-related alterations and DNA repair. The last comprehensive reviews on the role of DNA damage in aging processes were published several years ago (Gensler and Bernstein 1981; Williams and Dearfield 1981; Rothstein 1982) and I will therefore try to analyse the most recent studies and some problems which were not analysed in these reviews.

Age Changes in the Integrity of DNA Molecules. Double- and Single-Stranded Breaks

Even very mild methods of extraction of DNA from animal tissues show an age-related decrease in its molecular weight (Struchkov 1962; Massie et al. 1972; Turner et al. 1981; Zahn 1983; Chen and Srivastava 1986). However, these changes are tissue and species specific and sometimes seem to occur only during the first half of life and not during senescence (Massie et al. 1975; Polson and Webster 1982; Zahn et al. 1987) Detectible reduction in molecular weight might occur only as a result of the accumulation of double-stranded breaks and single-stranded breaks in single-stranded sections of DNA molecules. Single-stranded breaks, which represent a more common form of the DNA damage, might not be reflected in the molecular weight, but can reduce the accuracy of transcription. The systems of repair of double- and single-stranded breaks are also different.

Age-related accumulation of single-stranded breaks in DNA was demonstrated as a more universal phenomenon in different species and tissues and was studied by very different methods (Price et al. 1971; Price and Makinodan 1973; Makinodan et al. 1977).

It seems that there is also an age-related increase in single-stranded sections of DNA, particularly in highly differentiated cells. DNA in old tissues was shown to have an increased susceptibility to endonuclease SI, which specifically attacks only single-stranded gaps (Chestanga et al. 1977). These results, however, were not confirmed by other authors (Ono and Okada 1976; Dean and Cutler 1978; Finch 1979; Nakanishi et al. 1979).

Accumulation of single-stranded gaps can occur only in non-dividing cells. In the cells of proliferating tissues, harmful DNA alterations should not accumulate because they are eliminated by cellular selection. The proportion of single-stranded sections reported by Chestanga et al. (1975, 1976, 1977) in the liver, heart and brain of old mice seemed, at 25%, 15% and 14% respectively, to be too high, and this contradiction between results of two groups of studies stimulated new experiments in which different methods of extraction and nuclease SI digestion were used (Mori and Goto 1982). Breaks in DNA strands could be artefacts and linked to methods of DNA isolation. The new study showed that brain DNA from old mice contained 3% single-stranded regions while that from younger animals contained 2% – these figures are more realistic. The DNA from liver, kidney, heart and spleen did not show significant age-associated changes. In liver only between 3.8%–4.8% of DNA was single stranded.

However, the age-related accumulation of single-stranded breaks is more universal. In nematodes, in which no cell division occurs in adult forms and in which normal life span is measured only in days, a fourfold increase in single-stranded breaks in DNA was observed between the 5th and 15th days of life (Klass et al. 1983). Very careful investigation of the age-related changes in the molecular weight of DNA in different tissues (brain, liver and kidney) of mice from different families (short-lived *Mus musculus* and longer-lived *Peromyscus leucopus*) showed no change in the molecular weight of DNA between young and old in brain cells and a detectible change in liver (Su et al. 1984). At the same time the rate of accumulation of DNA damage (breaks) in liver and kidney cells with age was greater in the shorter-lived species (*M. musculus*) and was inversely proportional to maximum achievable life span. The authors suggested that a similar threshold might exist for tolerance of DNA damage in the two species in specific organs, and that these species differ in the rate at which this threshold is reached as a function of maximum achievable life span.

Lawson and Stohs (1985) found an accumulation of DNA damage (as single-stranded breaks) in livers of female Swiss-Webster mice between 6 and 24 months of age. At any time the amount of damage was a balance between formation of breaks and their repair. Administration of some antioxidants was able to reduce the level of hepatic DNA damage.

Age-Related Increase in Deleterious Adducts to DNA

Many normal functions of DNA as an informational macromolecule are regulated by specific DNA-binding proteins. Conformational changes of DNA in different cells, particullarly in some unique cases, like very compact packaging of DNA during spermatogenesis and inactivation of transcription in nuclei of avian erythrocytes, need synthesis of unique DNA-binding proteins (e.g. protamines, sperm-specific HI histones and H5 histone). However, this capability of the DNA molecule to interact specifically with certain proteins and polypeptides makes it also possible that some non-chromatin proteins or some other substances could also react with DNA chemically and produce a deleterious mutagenic effect or inhibition of certain DNA functions. Age-related and tissue-specific accumulation of metal ions in DNA was at first reported by Goldstein et al. (1966) as a repair process in which ions, like Fe^{3+}, might be able to restore single-stranded breaks. However, it was reported later that many metal ions (Mg^{2+}, Fe^{3+}, Mn^{2+}, Cu^{2+}, Zn^{2+}), when binding the opposite strands in DNA, can form cross-links between these and other strands, intramolecular and intermolecular, and produce degradation or unwinding of polynucleotides. Increases in the concentration of some ions can induce the mispairing of the nucleotide bases. This deleterious effect of metal ions on DNA was suggested as one of the main causes of aging (Eichorn 1979). Some other possible DNA adducts were also expected to cause the cross-linkage between nucleotides and inactivation of transcription. These observations made it possible to suggest that accumulation of the DNA adducts in chromatin represents one of the primary causes of aging and support the relevance of the cross-linkage theory of aging (Cutler 1976). Numerous carcinogenic chemicals also form DNA adducts as a key part of their action (Swenberg and Fennell 1987). The capability of repair of DNA adducts was studied mostly for liver and in relation to hepatocarcinogenesis, not aging. The repair was found to be tissue specific and it varied widely among healthy human individuals (Oesch et al. 1987).

DNA Methylation and Aging

DNA methylation or the formation of 5-methylcytosine is the most common postsynthetic enzymatic modification of polynucleotides, which involves transfer of methyl group from *S*-adenosylmethionine. The pattern of DNA methylation is normally reproduced during DNA replication. The first hypothesis which tried to link sequential methylation of repeated DNA sequences with aging (a kind of genetic clock) was suggested by Holliday and Pugh (1975). I do not plan to discuss here the possible role of DNA methylation in the control of gene expression – which has been well reviewed (Razin and Cedar 1984; Adams and Burdon 1985). Age-related changes in DNA methylation in different tissues have been studied by several authors (Vanyushin et al. 1973; Romanov and Vanyushin 1981; Ono et al. 1986; Singhal et al. 1987) who in general have registered a modest and tissue-specific decrease in 5-methylcytosine in DNA of aged animals. However, the differences between young, adult and old animals were not significant and it was suggested that these changes might be related to an age-associated increase in cancer incidence rather than to some basic mechanisms of aging (Ono et al. 1986), In some lower eukaryotes, like nematodes, an exponential increase was found in the amount of 5-methylcytosine in DNA with maturation and aging (Klass et al. 1983).

In vitro aging of fibroblasts of different origin (mice, hamsters and human) was shown to be linked with progressive loss of 5-methylcytosine whereas immortal cell lines in culture have stable rates of DNA methylation (Wilson and Jones 1983; Holliday 1985). 5-Azacytidine-induced demethylation shortens the in vitro life span of fibroblasts in culture (Fairweather et al. 1987).

Methylation of DNA is commonly associated with a reduction in transcriptional activity. The loss of methyl groups indicates that the relevant gene is switched on. There are several models of mechanism of this regulation. The presence of 5-methylcytosine preferentially in repeated DNA sequences, a very high level of 5-methylcytosine in plant DNA (from 5 to 10 mol% against about 1 mol% in rats' DNA) and the practically total absence of DNA methylation in *Drosophila* and some other lower vertebrates represent some evidence that methylation is not a universal mechanism of gene regulation. DNA methylation is now considered one among many mechanisms of gene control in the development of mammals and to be of "secondary" importance and the "bottom level of control" (Kolata 1985).

Methylation is closely linked with DNA replication. The pattern of methylation is heritable. Methylation in vertebrates occurs at sequences where a cytosine is followed by a 3′ guanine. This means that opposing DNA strands are symmetrically methylated. The cytosine of the newly synthesised DNA strand is methylated as soon as the sequence is made. These features of methylation make it clear that the decrease in the level of methylation could be a result of either reduced activity of enzymes involved in methylation in aged cells or failure of methylation of cytosine during DNA repair synthesis, or a combination of these two factors. But in both cases demethylation is the secondary, not the primary process.

Aging and Depurination of DNA

Depurination or the loss of purine bases from double-stranded DNA is quite common and it has been suggested that it might be linked with the mutations and carcinogenesis (Lindahl and Nyberg 1972; Lindahl 1976). Apurinic sites were shown to be a stable form of DNA lesion and they may not be repaired for weeks and months. It was also found that depurination decreases the fidelity of DNA synthesis in vitro, either by the insertion of an incorrect nucleotide opposite the apurinic site or by a deletion at that point during DNA replication or repair. The error rate was proportional to the percentage of depurination (Shearman and Loeb 1977).

Depurination of DNA results from the breakage of the glycosidic bond between the purine base and the deoxyribose moiety of the purine nucleodies without disrupting the structural integrity of the phosphodiester backbone. It was shown that some chemical carcinogens (particularly alkylation agents which act in conjunction with specific glycosylases) sharply increase the rate of depurination (Shearman and Loeb 1977).

It is likely that the number of depurinated sites increases during aging, particularly in non-dividing cells. Depurination also might be partly responsible for the age-related decrease in the fidelity of DNA synthesis in proliferating tissues.

However, the problem of depurination of DNA has not yet been studied by molecular gerontology.

Age-Related Changes in the Fidelity of the DNA Synthesis

In proliferating tissues DNA synthesis is normally well synchronized with the S phase of the cell division cycle. In non-dividing cells DNA synthesis could be linked to polyploidization, polytenyzation, synthesis of DNA in mitochondria and the DNA repair processes. There are some other forms of possible increase of DNA in non-dividing cells (like amplification of some DNA sequences), but they have never been included in experiments on the accuracy of DNA synthesis. In most proliferating tissues the rate of DNA synthesis declines with age proportionally to the reduction in mitotic activity.

Older animals could be more prone to the errors of DNA synthesis simply because of the age-related increase in the duration of the S phase of mitosis. DNA in known to be most sensitive to damage during the S phase. It was shown that in young clones of *Paramecium* the duration of the S phase is half that in the old clones (3.5 vs 7.5 h), whereas the duration of the G_I phase does not change (Smith-Sonneborn and Klass 1974). The duration of the S phase in embryos is shorter than in proliferating tissues in adults (Wegener et al. 1964). In mammals the duration of the S phase in different proliferating tissues varies from 6–8 h to 10–20 h (Cleaver 1967; Mitchinson 1971). However, the duration of the S phase did not change during human fibroblast aging in culture (Hasegawa et al. 1985).

DNA synthesis of different types (replication, repair, etc.) needs very many enzymes and other proteins and co-factors. However, DNA polymerases play a central role in accuracy. There are four main DNA polymerases, α, β, γ and δ, in mammalian cells. DNA polymerase-α plays a major role in S phase DNA replication and is often named the "replicase". DNA polymerase-β is a repair enzyme. DNA polymerase-γ is present in mitochondria, but it has also been found in nuclei, where its functions are not yet clear. It is involved in intranuclear viral replication, which also suggests that it might be responsible for amplification of DNA sequences and recombination events (for review see Hübscher 1983). DNA polymerase-δ is associated with 3′- to 5′-exonuclease activity and is linked with the proofreading capacity during DNA synthesis (So and Downey 1988). DNA polymerase-α activity decreases in bone marrow cells of senescent mice (Müller et al. 1980), which the authors link to a possible loss of stem cells. Activity of this enzyme also declines in aging human fibroblast cultures (Collins and Chu 1985).

Fidelity of DNA synthesis depends upon very many factors, accuracy of nucleotide selection, proofreading and error correction. Each step in this multistep process has its own rate of errors. Error rates vary widely when tested in vitro for purified eukaryotic polymerases. Polymerases of the α and γ groups show a much higher accuracy than polymerase-β (for review see Loeb and Reyland 1987). However, even the highest figures of fidelity estimated in vitro are several orders of magnitude less than the real fidelity of DNA synthesis, which is estimated on the basis of spontaneous mutation rates (Drake 1969; Loeb and Kunkel 1982). The base substitution rate for polymerase-α from several sources varies from 10^{-3} to 10^{-5} per base pair, whereas mistakes in DNA replication in animal cells in culture occur at a frequency of 10^{-9}–10^{-11} per nucleotide per cell generation. We do not need to review here a very large volume of information about the fidelity of DNA synthesis in general, or studies of the accuracy of individual DNA polymerases. However, it is necessary to consider at least two relevant problems: age-related changes in the fidelity of DNA synthesis in somatic cells and the possible mechanisms of the higher fidelity of DNA synthesis in germ cells.

Barton and Yang (1975) reported that the DNA polymerases (mixed group) purified from spleen nuclei of old mice incorporate nucleotides into the wrong position at about a two times higher rate than polymerases extracted from liver nuclei of young animals. Agarwal et al. (1978), who studied the accuracy of polymerase-α from human lymphocytes stimulated by phytohemagglutinin, did not find a change in accuracy for polymerase obtained from healthy individuals of various ages (from 22 to 77 years old). Tests were carried out in vitro with synthetic polynucleotide templates (in some experiments the fidelity was higher in "old" lymphocytes). However, the DNA polymerase isolated from old lymphocytes was clearly more sensitive to heat inactivation. The increase in heat lability normally indicates some conformational changes of protein molecules. This can be linked to post-translation modifications or some alterations in the enzymes during their synthesis. However, the observed level of accuracy of the DNA polymerase in these experiments was too low for both groups (young and old), only between 1.5×10^{-3} and 3×10^{-3} substitutions per base pair. It was very far from the real "biological" level of accuracy. There are some purely technical problems with regard to such in vitro tests when labelled phosphorylated nucleotides (dATP or dGTP) are used together with synthetic template (poly dC or poly dG, etc.). Both labelled nucleotides and templates usually contain contaminations with other nucleotides; this creates a certain "error background", which for DNA is nearly always higher than the accuracy of the DNA synthesis in vivo.

Murray and Holliday (1981), who tested crude extracts of polymerase-α from young and old human fibroblast cultures, demonstrated age-related changes and a higher level of accuracy (4×10^{-4} for young cells and 1.8×10^{-3} for old cells). It is possible that the crude enzyme extracts show higher accuracy than purified enzymes because of the presence of different cofactors. When Murray (1981) tried to repeat the same experiments with better purified DNA polymerase-α he found that it showed lower accuracy.

It is known that the mammalian polymerase-α exists in the form of a mixture of three or more subspecies. There is still some doubt about the origin of the molecular heterogeneity of DNA polymerase-α. Some authors consider the smaller molecules to be possible products of degradation of larger ones (Loeb and Reyland 1987).

Brosius et al. (1983) were able to isolate from calf thymus DNA polymerase-α at 9 S (molecular weight about 500000 daltons) which showed even higher accuracy in vitro. The error rate for this enzyme was about 10^{-5}. 7S polymerase-α from thymus was seven times less accurate, while the smallest 5.7S polymerase-

α molecules had an error rate at the level of 3×10^{-3} and were classified as "error-prone".

It is possible that the 7S and 5.7S enzyme subspecies arise from proteolysis (uncontrolled or genetically programmed) of 9S molecules. There was some speculation that some error-prone polymerases could be "mutator enzymes" responsible for programmed senescence (Linn et al. 1976; Murray 1981). Brosius et al. (1983) suggested that 5.7S polymerase-α might be a suitable candidate for such "programmed suicide", which is typical in thymus.

There is still only one known study in which the accuracy of DNA polymerase-β was tested in relation to aging and evolutionary variations of life span (Fry et al. 1981). This polymerase is relevant to DNA repair and in general has lower fidelity of in vitro DNA synthesis. The authors tested DNA polymerase-β isolated from liver chromatin of two murine species with contrasting maximum life spans, short-lived *Mus musculus* and long-lived *Peromyscus leucopus*. In each case enzyme was isolated from young, adult and old animals. The idea of the experiment was related to the earlier findings of much higher efficiency of DNA excision repair in longer-lived species (Hart and Setlow 1974).

The authors tested the fidelity of DNA synthesis using poly[d(A-T)] as an external template and [^{3}H]dGTP to determine errors of incorporation. Substrates for complementary synthesis contained a mixture of dATP and [^{32}P]-dTTP. The fidelity of chromatin-directed poly [d(A-T)] synthesis was similar for the comparatively short-lived *M. musculus* and the relatively long-lived *P. leucopus* and remained unaltered in old animals. At all ages in both species examined, the murine liver DNA polymerase-β, both chromatin associated and solubilized, exhibited high error frequencies; approximately one dGMP was incorporated for every 500–1000 complementary nucleotides polymerized.

The authors did not try, however, to generalise their results. They stressed that these results are relevant only for polymerase-β from liver. This polymerase had very low accuracy anyway. For other somatic cell types and for other more accurate DNA polymerases the results could be different, particularly if natural DNA templates are used. The main problem of in vitro tests of accuracy of synthesis (DNA, RNA or proteins) still remains. The experimental conditions reduce the level of accuracy so much from normal biological accuracy that one cannot be entirely certain that the differences of very fine nature which are relevant for in vivo systems, remain relevant for in vitro tests as well.

Differences in the Accuracy of DNA Synthesis and Repair in Germ and Somatic Cells

An error frequency of one incorrect base pair in 10^4–10^5 internucleotide linkages, which was shown in most experiments in vitro with eukaryotic DNA polymerase-α, is certainly much higher than the in vivo accuracy of DNA synthesis, when many co-factors, repair systems and "proofreading" exonuclease activity performed by DNA polymerase-δ provide a level of accuracy comparable with the mutation rates. It is possible that some highly differentiated non-dividing cells which do not have active replication of DNA involving polymerases-α and -δ are able to survive limited periods of time with comparatively high levels of error during DNA repair synthesis directed by DNA polymerase-β. But for actively dividing cells, for germ cells and for prokaryotes there is a threshold of accuracy below which the survival of the cell lineage is impossible. If the in vivo accuracy of DNA synthesis was the same as shown for DNA polymerase-α in the template experiments, too many genes would undergo harmful mutations at each replication and the cell line might die out after two to three generations. Evolution and selection of mutations are possible only if the level of mutations is several magnitudes lower. The more genes are in the genomes, the higher the accuracy needed to preserve their viability. On the other hand the smaller genomes (viruses and phages) have lower accuracy of replication which increases their variability and potential rate of adaptation and evolution. Both very high accuracy and very low accuracy of DNA synthesis create problems for survival and evolution, and a certain intermediate optimal mutation rate is adopted by each genetic system. Measured rates of mutation vary between 10^{-4} and 10^{-5} mutations per gene per generation in viruses and phages and between 10^{-5} and 10^{-6} in bacteria (which corresponds to about 10^{-10} mutations per base pair); they are about 10^{-9} in low eukaryotes and animal cells in culture (Drake 1969; Loeb and Kunkel 1982). Because of different sizes of the genomes, the total mutation rate (per genome/generation) varies between 10^{-3} and 10^{-4} in phages and bacteria and is about 10^{-5} in low eukaryotes. In mammals it is probably two orders of magnitude lower.

It is necessary to mention that the error rates of certain DNA polymerases of bacterial and viral origin in vitro are close to the rate of spontaneous mutations of these organisms in vivo (Fersht and Knill-Jones 1983). The high accuracy of these polymerases is due to their dual capability, base pairing and proofreading. The first step has an error rate of about 10^{-5} per base pair, and the second step is responsible for further increases in accuracy by a factor of 10–100. In eukaryotes the main replication polymerase – polymerase-α – does not possess proofreading capacity and this was the main cause of its lower accuracy when it was compared with polymerase of bacterial origin. However, proofreading does take place during DNA synthesis and is linked with polymerase-δ, which was isolated only recently (Lee et al. 1980). The accuracy of DNA polymerase-δ has not yet been tested in relation to aging and nobody has tried to test the accuracy of DNA synthesis in vitro by using both the enzymes as a system.

However, it is possible that the above-mentioned high accuracy of DNA synthesis in eukaryotes is necessary only for germ cells, rapidly dividing embryonic cells and non-differentiated stem cells in proliferating tissues. Specialized cells, like neurons, muscle cells and polyploid liver cells, do not need highly efficient systems of DNA replication, proofreading and repair because these cells are designed for limited periods of function. The accumulation of changes at the DNA level might, therefore, represent the main mechanism of their tissue-or species-specific aging rate.

Kirkwood (1977) was the first to try to explain the immortality of germ cells by the higher accuracy of the DNA synthesis. He thought that the same level of accuracy in somatic cells "may be a luxury our genes do better to forego". Kirkwood and Holliday (1979) suggested that the frequency of mutations may be much higher in somatic than in germ cells. However, rapidly dividing somatic cells, particularly embryonic cells and stem cells in proliferating tissues, also need high accuracy of DNA replication. It seems possible that some co-factors of DNA replication and repair which make high accuracy of DNA synthesis possible in germ cells, embryonic cells, stem cells etc. are repressed during terminal differentiation of specialised functional cells. But this repression is not irreversible and could be restored if these cells were dedifferentiated in cell cultures or during regeneration processes. It is very unlikely that the immortality of germ cells is due only to the high fidelity of the DNA replication. Several more mechnisms of the unique DNA repair are only possible in germ cells during meiosis. The most important of them has a form of genetic recombination during crossing-over, which may repair errors in codons which cannot be repaired in somatic cells. DNA recombination which needs several new enzymes (recombinase) and co-factors makes possible the replacement of large portions of double-stranded DNA between pairing chromosomes. Somatic DNA repair systems can easily eliminate a lesion which occurs in one of the strands of the double DNA helix. They are less efficient when damage affects both strands in close proximity, or if the change in sequence during replication has resulted in the formation of the complementary change in coding (stable mutation). Recombination together with selection can remove DNA mutations in some of the progeny.

Johnson et al. (1972) suggested that some forms of DNA repair are also possible during somatic crossing-over. However, somatic recombination, although possible in some cells, is rather rare and does not include specialized non-dividing cells.

It is well known that aging processes are tissue specific and that the age changes in highly differentiated tissues and organs, like brain, lungs, liver, kidney, and heart, are more important for life span than are the age changes in proliferating tissues, like bone marrow and intestine. Some organs with active cell divisions, like the thymus, have clear morphogenetic, programmed aging. However, functional processes in specialised and highly differentiated cells are still dependent on transcription of genetic information. This made it attractive to consider the accumulation of changes in DNA as the main factor in cellular aging (Hart and Turturro 1981; Gensler and Bernstein 1981), with independent changes at the level of proteins (like cross-linkage, or errors of translation) being of only supplementary importance, not the primary cause. But if DNA damage is considered as the primary cause of cellular aging, it makes DNA repair the most important factor which may regulate the aging rates. Germ cells have four (or even more) options for preserving their genetic information integrity as accurately as possible: genetic recombination during meiosis, DNA replication, proofreading and the repair of postsynthetic damages. Actively dividing somatic cells have three options and simple selection also eliminates some defective cells from progeny. [This difference between germ and somatic cells may explain why a sexual population can tolerate and resist a much higher genetic load of harmful mutations than an asexual population (Kondrashov 1988)].

Non-dividing highly specialised somatic cells have only one option – DNA repair – and the accuracy of the DNA polymerase-β which is responsible for such repair is not high. It is, therefore, natural that the attempts to find correlations between the efficiency of DNA repair and evolutionary variations in life span could emerge as one of the most attractive trends in molecular gerontology.

Some Other Age-Related Changes in DNA in Somatic Cells

It is difficult in a short review to indicate all age-related changes in DNA and to analyse the differences in the capability of dividing or non-dividing cells to repair them. However, it is possible that the most common changes, like single-stranded breaks or mismatched base pairs, are less relevant for aging just because they are more easily reparable. On the other hand, some less well studied changes in DNA could be more relevant for aging of somatic cells because they represent difficulties for DNA repair systems which remain operational in somatic cells. The age-related changes in DNA which were discussed earlier (breaks, methylation, adducts, errors of synthesis, etc.) have been better studied not because they are more important for aging but because the same changes are also most common as mutagenic or carcinogenic, which led many geneticists, molecular biologists and biochemical oncologists to study them. However, there are several types of possible DNA change which were studied or suggested only by gerontologists. It was found, for example, that the highly differentiated somatic cells could experience the excision or inactivation of tandemly reiterated portions of the genome and loss of part of tandemly repeated general-purpose or "house-keeping" genes, like rDNA (Strehler et al. 1979). Most highly reiterated genes (like genes for histones or rRNA) are active during embryonic and fetal stages of development, when rapid cell divisions make it necessary to support the synthesis of large amounts of certain proteins and rRNA over some very short periods, like the S phase of mitosis. In non-dividing cells the turnover of histones depends on a new set of genes, which are not reiterated (Zweidler 1984). The loss of a portion of the reiterated genes is not mutagenic, but it could reduce functional activity and the capacity for adaptive or induced changes. The age-related decrease in adaptive synthesis of DNA and some enzymes (Adelman 1971; Piantanelli et al. 1978) in specialised tissues could be linked to this decrease in the number of reserve genes available for this purpose. Amplification of some DNA sequences as an age-related change is also possible. Such amplification could be neutral, but also could be deleterious.

There have been several suggestions and studies regarding age-related structural changes in DNA, either specific for the DNA molecules only (Cutler 1976; Glaser and Luchnik 1982) or for protein – DNA complexes in chromatin (von Hahn 1970; Medvedev 1984).

The Role of the DNA Repair Processes in the Control of the Rate of Aging

The capability to repair damage is a universal phenomenon for biostructures of different complexities. However, in most cases the processes of repair are designed in a form of regeneration and replacement and the capability of such repair is often under genetic control. At the level of RNA and proteins the repair also means replacement of faulty molecules. Repair processes represent evolutionary adaptation to environmental damage and errors of internal processes. Biological systems with large numbers of different irreplaceable structures and molecules as a rule belong only to the short-lived species (nematodes, insects, etc.).

DNA repair processes have been particularly well studied because of their crucial role in the biological effect of different forms of radiation. As soon as the postradiation recovery was associated with the DNA repair, many thousand of studies in this field were carried out for different organisms and biological systems (cell cultures), molecular and enzymatic mechanisms of repair, different forms of radiation and chemical damage and in relation to aging as well (the repair capabilities in tissues and cells of different age). I do not plan to discuss too many aspects of this problem, which has already been extensively analysed in many recent reviews (Kirkwood 1981; Grossman 1981: Strauss 1985; Modrich 1987).

It is obvious that the level of mutations which is optimal for evolution is created by the balance between DNA damage and DNA repair and this balance operates not only at the level of species and organisms but also at the level of individual tissues and cells. It is natural, for example, that skin cells need most efficient systems of repair from UV radiation damage, whereas liver cells should be protected from toxic agents, external and internal. The development of the genetic system in evolution also creates new requirements for repair processes. If in prokaryotes the DNA repair systems are sufficient to reach a certain balance for the mutation rates, the eukaryotic systems need more complex repair capabilities making it possible to restore the integrity of chromosomal structures as well. The repair is apparently only the second line of defence. The first line is presented by biological protectors, which include naturally occurring antioxidants and free-radical scavenger enzymes.

In eukaryotic somatic cells there are four main DNA repair processes which are most common and have been widely discussed in relation to aging: excision repair, strand breakage rejoining, postreplication repair and photoreactivation (Hart and Trosko 1976). Each of these repair systems is very complex and consists of several stages, which are linked with certain enzymes. Different repair systems remove different lesions. *Excision repair* is apparently a dominant DNA repair system in eukaryotic cells. It normally consists of removal of a faulty part of one of the DNA strands: mismatched base pairs, intrastrand cross-links, thymidine dimers, or apurine sites. Repair normally includes cleaving of either the base-sugar bond or the phospoester bond between nucleotides by means of an endonucleolytic incision, excision of the damaged base and several adjacent bases and insertion of new bases to fill the excised region. The process could have some variations and needs several specific enzymes (endonuclease, DNA polymerase and ligase) and some co-factors.

Excision repair is easy to test in age-related studies when the DNA damage is induced by UV radiation (formation of dimers is the most common lesion after UV damage). The efficiency of repair can be judged by the activity of so-called unscheduled DNA synthesis after irradiation, which reflects the increased incorporation of labelled nucleotides into DNA.

Photoreactivation is normally accelerated by the energy of visible light. *Strand breakage rejoining* depends on combination of enzymes, some of which are also active during excision repair. Double-stranded breaks are usually the most difficult lesions to repair in somatic cells: it needs at least two homologous DNA molecules (i.e. a pair of chromosomes) and recombination. *Postreplication repair* is a process of mismatch correction (base replacement). Mismatches might arise as a consequence of genetic recombination, as a result of DNA biosynthetic errors, or after the deamination of 5-methylcytosine (Modrich 1987).

The importance of DNA repair for somatic cells was obvious, and many studies in molecular gerontology tried to identify the age-related changes of the repair processes. Incorporation of labelled thymidine into nuclear DNA in cells which do not have mitotic activity was considered to be a reflection of DNA repair processes, and young and old cells were compared in this respect. Surprisingly, it was found in several studies that the incorporation of [^{3}H]thymidine into DNA (or the volume of "unscheduled DNA synthesis") increases in aging liver tissues (Samis et al. 1966). This was interpreted as showing the existence of a higher level of DNA damage in old tissues. Later a similar increase was registered for aging brain, on kidney and muscle cells (Falzone et al. 1967). The authors (Falzone et al. 1967) formulated this as a theory of aging in which an increased level of primary processes of DNA damage provokes a series of imperfect homeostatic compensations which eventually fail. The theoretical part of this picture is valid, because it is necessary to consider age changes of DNA as an interaction between the DNA damage and incomplete repair.

The other theory which tried to link the aging rate to DNA repair was suggested by Alexander (1967) in his criticism of the somatic mutation theory of aging. He argued that small doses of radiation do not shorten life span because induced DNA damage is easily repaired. Higher (but sublethal) doses of radiation reduce life span, because they damage not only the DNA but the DNA repair systems as well. This effect is more explicit in dividing cells; specialised non-dividing cells can tolerate much higher doses of radiation due to the absence of radiation-sensitive DNA replication processes. The author suggests that the level of DNA repair in differentiated cells may correlate with their rate of aging and that "programmed cell death" may operate via the system of reduced repair.

Strand breakage rejoining was also studied in a few experiments. Neurones of young and old dogs did not show clear age-associated differences (Wheeler and Lett 1972, 1974). Similar results were reported for DNA repair in ganglia in fish (Ishikawa et al. 1978). The muscle cells of old rats were not as efficient as those of young rats in repairing X-ray induced breaks in DNA (Karron and Ormerod 1973). Dell'orco and Anderson (1981) compared the activity of excision repair of

DNA in human fibroblasts taken from donors of different age. No differences were reported. Fibroblasts from embryonic tissues and from old donors maintained the same ability to perform the unscheduled DNA synthesis throughout their life span in culture. The absence of decline in DNA repair in cultured human fibroblasts from young and old human donors was confirmed by Hall et al. (1982), who not only tested DNA repair by meens of the chemical manifestation of repair processes (unscheduled synthesis of DNA), but also studied the real restoration of biological competence after UV or chemical damage. However, if DNA repair in human fibroblasts did not show any clear dependence on the age of the donor, the results might be different in different species and in different tissues (Kempf et al. 1984). The actual type of repair process also matters. The repair of damage produced by radiation does not have the same age-dependence picture as the repair of damage from chemical substances. There are many studies of DNA repair in different systems and some of them report a possible reduction in the repair synthesis in older cells: in hepatocytes and other rat cells (Niedermüller et al. 1985; Kennah et al. 1985; Plesko and Richardson 1984) and nematodes (Targovnik et al. 1984). However, other studies which included a rather wide range of cellular systems and damaging agents yielded negative results (Hennis et al. 1981; Turner et al. 1982; Gensler 1981) and suggested that the decline in the DNA repair capacity is not an important factor in normal aging. It was also reported that the activity of DNA polymerase-β, which is a repair polymerase, does not vary significantly with the age of tissue (Ove and Goetzee 1978; Hanaoka et al. 1983).

Despite some contradictory results which are unavoidable in studies which include different species, different tissues, different tissue cultures and different forms of repair process, the overall picture still indicates that the decline in repair of DNA damage is certainly not a primary cause of cellular aging. DNA repair emerged in evolution as a function related to different forms of radiation and chemical damage. It is efficient with the range of radiation which is hazardous for DNA only. If radiation is too high and starts to damage the repair systems themselves, the efficiency of DNA repair also declines. Similar relations probably exist in aging. Because the DNA repair systems are designed to deal with external factors, they have enough reserve repair capacity to remove lesions which originate from weaker internal factors. But eventually the aging processes should reduce the efficiency of complex repair systems and influence the activity and quality of repair enzymes. Aging in tissues is not caused by the progressive decline in DNA repair, but it eventually leads to the decline in DNA repair along with many other deleterious changes.

It is, however, important to study the age-related changes in the accuracy of repair. It was mentioned earlier that the DNA polymerase-β is an error-prone enzyme. This means that the repaired sequences contain more errors than the DNA strands which are formed during replication. Tests of the age-related accuracy of DNA repair have been carried out in only one study to date (Hall et al. 1982). The authors tested the repair of herpes simplex virus type I incorporated into DNA of human fibroblasts from young and old donors. They also used different DNA damaging factors. UV irradiation and chemical agents. They did not find a decline in the quality of repair of viral DNA which was inside the host genome. Their conclusion, that DNA repair levels do not decline with age but that aging itself may result from accumulation of damage which is not repaired, is logical. This conclusion can be supported by findings in respect of some faults in the DNA repair systems in humans and animals suffering from genetic syndromes associated with premature aging and very high sensitivity to radiation.

DNA Repair Deficiencies and the Premature Aging Syndromes

A number of rare human inherited syndromes are clearly associated with defects in different DNA repair systems. In most cases these syndromes are also associated with an increased frequency of cancer. The relations between these DNA genetic repair defects and aging are much more complex. The most frequent and better studied DNA repair deficiency syndrome, *xeroderma pigmentosum* (XP), is normally expressed in an inability to repair UV damage. This is a recessive inherited disease. Patients with XP are hypersensitive to sunlight. Their skin fibroblasts in culture show reduced levels of unscheduled DNA synthesis after UV irradiation (Robbins 1978; Tice 1978). However, if protected from exposure to UV radiation, individuals do not show accelerated aging. In vitro senescence of skin fibroblasts from normal individuals and from XP patients is also identical and occurs after an equal numer of cell passages (Cleaver 1984). This makes it clear that the efficiency of DNA repair of this particular form of DNA damage is not linked directly with the aging rate. XP fibroblasts have an increased sensitivity not only to UV light but also to many chemical carcinogens.

There are several other pathological syndromes in which different parts of the complex DNA repair systems have been shown to be defective: Cockayne's syndrome, Fanconi's anemia, Bloom's syndrome and some others (Lindahl 1987). They are linked to increased frequency of cancer but are not associated with the acceleration of tissue-specific age changes.

If attempts to link specific DNA repair deficiency syndromes with accelerated aging have so far proven negative, attempts to link specific premature aging syndromes, like progeria and Werner's syndrome, with possible deficiencies of the DNA repair systems in their cells have also failed. DNA repair systems in cells from patients with these syndromes seem to be grossly normal following UV and other types of irradiation (Fujiwara et al. 1977; Bradley et al. 1976; Brown et al. 1980). Progeria fibroblasts do show some heterogeneity for DNA repair, but it is now thought that the decreased DNA repair capacity does not belong to the basic genetic defects in progeria. Premature aging syndrome in BB Wistar rats has no effect on excision repair capacity in fibroblasts (Wright et al. 1986).

Correlation Between Longevity and DNA Repair in Evolution

The finding of a clear correlation between the efficiency (or activity) of DNA excision repair of UV damage and the maximal life span in seven mammalian species with very different longevity potentials (Hart and Setlow 1974) resulted in the most stimulating single hypothesis in molecular gerontology during the last 15 years. However, as is now obvious, the main importance of this study was the interest which it generated in the role of DNA and DNA repair in aging processes, and not, as was initially expected, the fact that it laid down the first foundations for the understanding of the mechanism of aging and the evolution of longevity.

The experimental design of these experiments was very simple. The authors obtained fibroblasts for culture from biopsies of the superficial dermis from the right hind limb of animals that dad completed about 1/20th of their maximal life span (indicated in parentheses): shrew (1.5 years), mouse (2 years), rat (3.5 years), hamster (4 years), cow (30 years), elephant (70 years) and man (100 years). The ability of fibroblasts to perform unscheduled DNA synthesis (a measure of excision repair) after UV radiation (initial rate and maximum incorporation of [^{3}H]thymidine) increased nearly proportionaly to the logarithm of the life span of these species. However, despite the clear correlation, this experiment was not conclusive. In the seven species tested there was also a positive correlation between the number of genes in the genome and life span. In a normal environment human skin, which is not protected with hairs, needs a much higher level of repair from UV damage than does skin of cows or rodents. Hamsters are not normally exposed to sun in their habitats as much as elephants. It was clear that the relation between life span and capacity for DNA repair may arise from their correlations with many other variables.

In order to answer such obvious objections the authors decided to compare the efficiency of DNA repair among species that differ significantly in longevity, while at the same time differing as little as possible in physiology, ecological adaptation and taxonomic position (Hart et al. 1979b).

Their first pair for comparison consisted of two small rodent species, the house mouse *Mus musculus* (maximum life span 1250 days) and a field mouse native in the north-eastern United States, *Peromyscus leucopus* (maximum life span about 3000 days). Both species were kept in captivity for several generations with inbreeding in the collection of different mice species. The authors decided to compare not only the excision repair after UV irradiation but also the repair of single-stranded breaks produced by gamma rays in fibroblasts of both species.

The unscheduled DNA synthesis (excision repair) showed very good correlation with life span potentials. However, there were no detectable differences between the two species in terms of the efficiency of rejoining of single-stranded breaks in fibroblasts induced by gamma radiation. The authors therefore concluded that DNA repair probably represents a part of "the longevity-assurance systems", but that there is no clear cause-effect relationship for any single form of DNA repair or for DNA repair in general in the process of aging.

Comparison of the activity of excision repair in skin fibroblasts between several species of primates also showed a near linear correlation, with the highest efficiency of DNA repair in skin fibroblasts taken from man (Hart et al. 1979a; Cutler 1979). However, one can argue that human skin needs a higher level of protection from UV damage anyway. It is known that, for example, amphibian skin cells have a very high capacity for DNA excision repair of UV lesions (Regan et al. 1968).

Later studies of the correlation between the activity of DNA excision repair and longevity carried out in different laboratories, which included more species, yielded contradictory results. Kato et al. (1980) compared the activity of DNA repair in fibroblasts and life span potentials in 34 species from 11 orders of mammals and found no correlation. There was also no correlation between longevity and DNA repair in different tissues among cold-blooded vertebrates (Woodhead et al. 1980). Such controversial results in attempts to test a very interesting hypothesis predictably stimulated many new experiments with the use of more sophisticated methods. Francis et al. (1981), who prepared cell line cultures from 21 mammalian species, also used UV irradiation damage, but in addition they treated cells with 5-bromodeoxyuridine (BrdU), which was incorporated into DNA during repair synthesis and later cleaved the DNA by photolysis at the points of BrdU insertion. This assay allows more direct measurement of the excision repair system than unscheduled synthesis of DNA. The authors found an approximately linear correlation between the life span of the majority of mammals and the number of DNA excision repair sites measured 20–22 h following ultraviolet irradiation of the cell cultures. However, there were several exceptions; the most striking were the whale, Prezewalski's horse and the polar bear, all of which showed an efficiency of DNA repair at the level of rat and mouse. These results underline the limitations of an approach in which the test of DNA repair is made in a system which consists of UV damage and skin fibroblasts. The observed differences could be linked with evironmental and evolutionary requirements. It is obvious that the longer-lived mammals also have longer exposure to the natural ultraviolet irradiation. But neither polar bear nor whale should have selective advantages in evolution if they possess a high level of protection from sunlight.

It was, therefore, natural that similar tests were carried out later with DNA repair in cells of different origin. In lens epithelial cells the correlation between UV postirradiated DNA repair activity and life span was positive when tested for five species (rat, rabbit, cat, dog and horse) (Treton and Courtois 1982). For primates (six species) the same correlation was confirmed not only for skin fibroblasts but also for non-stimulated lymphocytes (Hall et al. 1984). UV-induced DNA repair synthesis in hepatocyte cultures of different rodents correlated positively with their life span only if UV radiation doses were comparatively low (between 0.5 $J/m^2/s$ and 5 $J/m^2/s$. At higher intensity levels, however, there were no differences in the amount of induced repair (Maslansky and Williams 1985). Thus the maximal repair potential of hepatocytes derived from the rat, mouse, hamster, guinea pig and rabbit were the same. The implications of these results are unclear, but the authors suggest that the species that are more responsive to a minimal amount of DNA damage may also delay the accumulation of age changes in DNA.

The intention to overcome the environment or evolutionary factors of adaptation in the UV damage tests when different species were selected for comparison lead to attempts to compare longer and shorter lived strains within the same species. The results of the first study in this direction, carried out by Paffenholz (1978), who found a positive correlation between life span and DNA repair for three strains of inbred mice, were later criticised as unreliable. Several years later Collier et al. (1982) compared the rate of UV-induced DNA excision repair in embryonic cells derived from a congeneic pair of short-lived (C57BL/10.F) and long-lived (C57BL/10) mice. Excision repair was measured by both BrdU photolysis and arabinofuranosyl cytosine inhibition. No difference in rate of repair was observed between the two cell lines.

However, there could be very many genetic and non-genetic factors which could explain the difference of life span in such cases. Negative results found with excision repair indicate only that this form of DNA repair is not one of them.

Conclusion

The key role of DNA in the transfer of information from generation to generation in evolution and in cell lineages requires such a high level of accuracy of DNA reproduction and repair that it is difficult to suggest that the same system of DNA synthesis and repair could also be primary in the countless variations of manifestation of aging and aging rates that are observed in different organisms, tissues and cells. On the other hand, the aging rates in all their variations are genetically controlled and therefore depend in one way or another on information stored in DNA. We also know that aging expresses itself in very many ways and is reflected in practically all structures and functions which have direct or indirect links with information stored in DNA, because structural proteins and enzymes which play a major role in every cellular function are being formed via transcription of genes and translation of their nucleotide sequences. However, between these two major functions of DNA, transfer of genetic information from generation to generation and operational control of transcription of this information in every cell, there is the third – the control of development, morphogenesis and differentiation according to the programme stored in DNA.

This central role of DNA in all major manifestations of life makes it understandable that so many attempts are made to link DNA in one or other way to aging phenomena as well. The disposable soma theory (Kirkwood 1977) and its specific application to the problem of reproduction and repair in different species (Kirkwood 1981) attempted in a general form to explain aging by selection of the quality of somatic repair in iteroparous species (in which reproduction occurs repeatedly during adulthood) at an optimal level which would always be less than the germ cell repair. In this case "the senescence is the result of a progressive accumulation of unrepaired damage". In general theoretical form this is certainly a valid conclusion, but can it be valid if only DNA damage and DNA repair are taken into account? Immortality of germ lines is supported by the maximal number of DNA repair systems, some of which are specifically linked to meiotic crossing-over and recombination and are not available for somatic cells. A very high level of accuracy in reproduction of the integrity of the developmental programme in DNA is also absolutely vital for the continuation of life. Non-differentiated and actively dividing somatic cells also could provide some nearly ageless systems (like in the case of vegetative reproduction of plants) because they are able to supplement their less perfect DNA repair (absence of meiotic rejuvenation) by selection of undamaged genomes during cell divisions and growth. But as soon as cells differentiate and are prepared for specialised functions, they also lose most of their efficient DNA repair systems (essentially linked to DNA polymerase-α and -γ and DNA proofreading and co-factors) and have to maintain the integrity of DNA with repair enzymes only, which, like DNA polymerase-β, have comparatively low accuracy. This model makes efficiency of DNA repair and accuracy of repair enzymes very likely candidates for a universal role as modulators of longevity of non-dividing somatic cells.

But I still think that such a model, despite its attractive simplicity, does not explain real aging, which in its natural manifestations is much more complex and random and involves more processes, some of which are not linked directly to DNA or reparable changes in DNA. Aging and mortality of individuals are so essential for the evolutionary process that it is unlikely that there could be only one option as a cause for cellular aging – imperfect, inaccurate or faulty repair of DNA. Many irreversible and irreparable changes can occur at the level of RNA, proteins and different cellular structures. They might represent either reserve or primary routes of aging. I think it possible that the role of DNA and DNA repair in the aging rate is important in long-living systems and proliferating tissues, whereas the aging and life span of short-lived and very short-lived species (like nematodes, insects and many low eukaryotes) and of highly differentiated non-dividing cells are not dependent on accumulation of changes in DNA of their somatic cells. This is reflected in the fact that such DNA damaging factors as radiation do not reduce the life span of many lower eukaryotes, like insects, and do not kill differentiated cells, like neurones, within the range of doses which are already damaging for DNA. Radiation starts to have a life-shortening effect in these systems at a much higher "protein synthesis damage" level. Evolution did perfect the system of DNA reproduction and repair to serve life forever. The countless forms and rates of species- and tissue-specific aging and other methods of mortality of individual organisms, tissues and cells have to use very many different options to fulfil their evolutionary role.

In conclusion I would like to summarize the material discussed in this review in Table 1, which shows the possible differences in DNA repair in different cellular systems. The table makes it clear that somatic cells in differentiated tissues have fewer repair capabilities. It is natural to expect that precisely those DNA lesions which are not capable of repair play a more important role in the accumulation of age changes.

Table 1. DNA alteration and repair in different cellular systems

DNA alterations and lesions	Type of repair	Factors of repair in cellular systems[a]		
		Germ cells *(Immortality)*	Dividing cells (embryonic, proliferating tissues, cell cultures) *(Clonal aging)*	Non-dividing specialised somatic cells *(Functional aging)*
Pyrimidine dimers Single-stranded breaks Single-stranded gaps Missing bases	Excision repair Strand-breakage rejoining Postreplication repair	DNA polymerase-β DNA photolyase	DNA polymerase-β DNA photolyase	DNA polymerase-β DNA photolyase
Errors of replication Mismatched base pairs Demethylation Deamination	Replication repair Replication proofreading	DNA polymerase-α DNA polymerase-δ DNA methyltransferase	DNA polymerase-α DNA polymerase-δ DNA methyltransferase	
Adducts Double-stranded breaks Loss of sequences	Cell selection Mitotic recombination	Meiotic diploidization Survival of viable genomes	Survival of viable genomes	
Cross-links Errors of repair Amplification of sequence	Genetic recombination	Crossing-over Recombination enzymes DNA polymerase-γ		

[a] Relevant to nuclear DNA. Age changes and repair of mitochondrial DNA represent a separate specific problem.

Acknowledgements. The author wishes to thank T. B. L. Kirkwood and G. R. Banks for discussion and comments, J. E. Pugh and Miss H. M. Crowne for reading the manuscript and making linguistic and editorial corrections and Miss D. Moss for typing the manuscript.

Discussion

Frenzel

Could you please comment on the relation between DNA disturbances and the increased frequency of cancer in old age.

Medvedev

A connection certainly exists between the development of cancer and damage to DNA, but it could have a very complex nature. Some suggestions have linked carcinogenesis not only with deleterious mutations of somatic cells, but with changes in the expression of genes, alterations in regulation which may depend on modifications of DNA, expression of some early embryonic genes, and so on. All carcinogens can interact with DNA and produce some damage, but there is no direct correlation between the amount of DNA breaks and the incidence of cancer. Some specific changes could be more important than gross damage.

Klotz

Is there any new treatment involving a kind of special inducing system or inducing agent for polymerases to stimulate repair mechanisms?

Medvedev

Certainly it will be possible in the future to use some methods or factors which may influence DNA repair processes. Probably different co-factors for DNA polymerases or stimulation of molecular transfer of energy will be used to stimulate repair. Current knowledge of molecular repair processes is not comprehensive. It has not yet been established how the syndromes of premature aging, like Down syndrome, progeria, and Werner syndrome, are related to the repair processes. Only in the case of xeroderma pigmentosum has the mechanism which links it with DNA repair been identified – the deficiency of excision repair. People who have this syndrome are vulnerable to UV damage and suffer from skin cancer. But a cure has not yet been found, and the only way to protect people with this syndrome is to prevent the UV exposure.

Hofecker

Several years ago another form of DNA repair was described in bacteria, photoreactivation. This means that an enzyme is activated by visible light in order to repair DNA damage caused by UV light. What's an enigma is that this enzyme is also found in mammalian tissue, e.g., in liver tissue. What could be the function of this mechanism in liver tissue, where no visible light appears?

Medvedev

Yes, this system is a puzzle. Photoreactivation repair does exist in mammalian cells and there is no visible light involved in its activity. However, this system was discovered in studies in prokaryotes and simple eukaryotes, like yeasts. It is possible that in evolution some other factors became involved and able to activate repair enzymes, like free radicals. I do not think that this enzymatic system is just an evolutionary residue without proper functions in higher eukaryotes.

Hofecker

Could it be that a small light quant is delivered in biochemical reactions and acts in the cell to activate this enzyme?

Medvedev

Biochemical reactions, particularly those which involve transfer of energy or oxidation, produce quants of energy and photons and may activate this repair system. Activation by free radicals is the other possibility. They are known to damage DNA and it is likely that in evolution simultaneous induction of the DNA repair system has emerged as a form of adaptation or as the second line of defence. The first line of defence against free radicals is represented by antioxidants which are present in tissues and cells.

Barrows

Is it possible that genetic damage can result from the use of the code and therefore limitations of its use may minimize age changes?

Medvedev

Yes, damage to DNA as a result of reproduction and transcription is possible. Many authors have tried to find the explanation for the age changes in the fidelity of DNA polymerases and to identify how their functions suffer with age. There were some reports about negative changes in DNA polymerase accuracy with age. However, most studies in this field were carried out with in vitro systems in which the accuracy of DNA reproduction or transcription is very low, several orders of magnitude lower than in real cells. Therefore researchers who work with in vitro systems were not able to assess many additional factors relating to the accuracy of DNA functions. There are studies which show an accumulation of breaks in DNA with age. This is natural because some damage to DNA is irreversible and DNA repair systems are also probably less effective in old tissues.

References

Adams RLP, Burdon RH (1985) The molecular biology of DNA methylation. Springer, New York Berlin

Adelman RC (1971) Age-dependent effects in enzyme induction – a biochemical expression of aging. Exp Gerontol 6: 75–87

Agarwal SS, Tuffner M, Loeb LA (1978) DNA replication in human lymphocytes during aging. J Cell Physiol 96: 235–243

Alexander P (1967) The role of DNA lesions in the process leading to ageing in mice. In: Woolhouse HW (ed) Aspects of the biology of ageing. Cambridge University Press, Cambridge, pp 29–50

Barton RW, Yank WK (1975) Low molecular weight DNA polymerase: decreased activity in spleens of old mice. Mech Ageing Dev 4: 123–136

Bradley MO, Erickson LC, Kohn KW (1976) Normal DNA strand rejoining and absence of DNA cross-linking in progeroid and aging human cells. Mutat Res 37: 279–292

Brosius S, Grosse F, Krauss G (1983) Subspecies of DNA polymerase-α from calf thymus with different fidelity in copying synthetic template primers. Nucleic Acids Res II: 193–202

Brown WT, Ford JP, Gershey EL (1980) Variations of DNA repair capacity in progeria cells unrelated to growth conditions. Biochem Biophys Res Commun 97: 347–353

Chen S, Srivastava BIS (1986) Fragmentation of DNA and chromatin during senescence in barley leaves. Mech Ageing Dev 34: 57–61

Chestanga CJ, Boyd V, Peterson L, Rusholow K (1975) Single-stranded regions in DNA of old mice. Nature 253: 130–131

Chestanga CJ, Tuttle M, Jacoboni A (1976) Changes in structural integrity of heart DNA from aging mice. Life Sci 18: 1405–1412

Chestanga CJ, Tuttle M, Jacoboni A, Johnson C (1977) Age-associated structural alterations in senescent mouse brain DNA. Biochim Biophys Acta 474: 180–187

Cleaver JE (1967) Thymidine metabolism and cell kinetics. North Holland, Amsterdam

Cleaver JE (1984) DNA repair deficiencies and cellular senescence are unrelated in *Xeroderma pigmentosum* cell lines. Mech Ageing Dev 27: 189–196

Collier JE, Popp DM, Lee WH, Regan JD (1982) DNA repair in a congeneic pair of mice with different longevities. Mech Ageing Dev 19: 141–156

Collins JM, Chu AK (1985) Reduction of DNA synthesis in aging but still proliferating cells. J Cell Physiol 124: 165–173

Cutler RG (1976) Cross-linkage hypothesis of aging; DNA adducts in chromatin as a primary aging process. In: Smith KC (ed) Proteins and other adducts to DNA. Their significance to ageing, carcinogenesis and radiation biology. Plenum, New York, pp 443–493

Cutler RG (1979) Evolution of human longevity: a critical overview. Mech Ageing Dev 9: 337–354

Dean RG, Cutler RG (1978) Absence of significant age-dependent increase of single-stranded DNA extracted from mouse liver nuclei. Exp Gerontol 13: 287–292

Dell'Orco RT, Anderson LE (1981) Unscheduled DNA synthesis in human diploid cells of different donor ages. Cell Biol Intern Rep 5: 359–364

Drake JW (1969) Comparative rates of spontaneous mutations. Nature 221: 1132

Eichorn GL (1979) Aging, genetics and the environment.Potential of errors introduced into genetic information transfer by metal ions. Mech Ageing Dev 9: 291–301

Fairweather DS, Fox M, Margison GP (1987) The in vitro lifespan of MRC-5 cells is shortened by 5-azacytidine-induced demethylation. Exp Cell Res 168: 153–159

Falzone JA, Samids HV, Wulff VJ (1967) Cellular compensations and controls in the aging process. J Gerontol 22: 4 (part II) 42–51

Fersht AR, Knill-Jones JW (1983) Fidelity of replication of bacteriophage ∅X174 DNA in vitro and in vivo. J Mol Biol 165: 633–654

Finch CE (1979) Susceptibility of mouse liver DNA to digestion by SI nuclease: absence of age-related change. Age 2: 45–46

Francis AA, Lee WH, Regan JD (1981) The relationship of DNA excision repair of ultraviolet-induced lesions to the maximum lifespan of mammals. Mech Ageing Dev 16: 181–189

Fry M, Loeb LA, Martin GM (1981) On the activity and fidelity of chromatin-associated hepatic DNA polymerase-α in aging murine species of different life span. J Cell Physiol 106: 435–444

Fujiwara Y, Higashikawa T, Tatsumi M (1977) A retarded rate of DNA replication and normal level of DNA repair in Werner's syndrome fibroblasts in culture. J Cell Physiol 92: 365–374

Gensler HL (1981) The effect of hamster age on UV-induced unscheduled DNA synthesis in freshly isolated lung and kidney cells. Exp Gerontol 16: 59–68

Gensler HL, Bernstein H (1981) DNA damage as the primary cause of aging. Q Rev Biol 56: 279–303

Glaser VM, Luchnik AN (1982) Decrease in the density of DNA topological turns during in vitro ageing of Syrian hamster cells. Exp Cell Res 139: 249–255

Goldstein BI, Rud SG, Polyakova LL (1966) Age changes of iron content in tissues and DNA of white rats. Vopr Med Khim 12: 618–621

Grossman L (1981) Enzymes involved in the repair of damaged DNA. Arch Biochem Biophys 211: 511–522

Hall JD, Almy RE, Scherer KL (1982) DNA repair in cultured human fibroblasts does not decline with donor age. Exp Cell res 139: 351–359

Hall K, Hart RW, Benirschke AK, Walford RL (1984) Correlation between ultraviolet-induced DNA repair in primate lymphocytes and fibroblasts and species' maximum achievable life span. Mech Ageing Dev 24: 163–173

Hanaoka F, Sayato J, Arai H, Hasegawa N, Inui N, Mitsui Y, Yamada MA (1983) Changes in DNA polymerase-α, β, δ in mouse liver as a function of age. Mech Ageing Dev 23: 315–327

Hart RW, Setlow RB (1974) Correlation between deoxyribonucleic acid excision repair and life-span in a number of mammalian species. Proc Natl Acad Sci USA 71: 2169–2173

Hart RW, Trosko JE (1976) DNA repair processes in mammals. Interdiscipl Topics Gerontol 9: 134–167 (Karger, Basel)

Hart RW, Turturro A (1981) Evolution and longevity-assurance processes. Naturwissenschaften 68: 552–557

Hart RW, D'Ambrosio SM, Ng KJ, Modak SP (1979a) Longevity, stability and DNA repair. Mech Ageing Dev 9: 203–223

Hart RW, Sacher GA, Hoskins TL (1979b) DNA repair in short- and long-lived rodent species. J Gerontol 34: 808–817

Hasegawa N, Hanaoka F, Yamada M (1985) Does capacity of DNA replication change during in vitro ageing? Exp Cell Res 156: 478–486

Hennis HL III, Braid HL, Vincent RA Jr (1981) Unscheduled DNA synthesis in cells of different shape in fibroblast cultures from donors of various ages. Mech Ageing Dev 16: 355–361

Henson P (1978) The presence of single stranded regions in mammalian DNA. J Mol Biol 119: 487–506

Holliday R (1985) The significance of DNA methylation in cellular aging. In: Woodhead AO, Blackett AD, Hollaender A (eds) Molecular biology of aging. Plenum, New York, pp 269–283

Holliday R, Pugh JE (1975) DNA modification mechanisms and gene activity during development. Science 187: 226–232

Hübscher U (1983) DNA polymerases in prokaryotes and eukaryotes: mode of action and biological implications. Experientia 39: 1–25

Ishikawa T, Tadayama S, Kitagawa T (1978) Autoradiographic demonstration of DNA repair synthesis in ganglion cells of aquarium fish at various age in vivo. Virchows Arch [Cell Pathol] 28: 235–242

Johnson R, Chrisp C, Strehler BL (1972) Selective loss of ribosomal RNA genes during the aging of post mitotic tissues. Mech Ageing Dev 1: 183–198

Karron P, Ormerod MG (1973) Is the ability to repair damage to DNA related to the proliferative capacity of the cell? Biochim Biophys Acta 299: 54–64

Kato H, Harada M, Tsuchiya K, Moriwaki K (1980) Absence of correlation between DNA repair in ultraviolet irradiated mammalian cells and the life span of the donor species. Jpn J Genet 55: 99–108

Kempf CH, Schmitt M, Danse JM, Kempf J (1984) Correlation of DNA repair synthesis with ageing in mice, evidenced by quantitative autoradiography. Mech Ageing Dev 26: 183–194

Kennah HE, Coetzee ML, Ove P (1985) A comparison of DNA repair synthesis in primary hepatocytes from young and old rats. Mech Ageing Dev 29: 283–298

Kirkwood TBL (1977) Evolution of ageing. Nature 270: 301–304

Kirkwood TBL (1981) Repair and its evolution: survival versus reproduction. In: Townsend CR, Calow P (eds) Physiological ecology: an evolutionary approach to resource use. Blackwell, Oxford, pp 165–194

Kirkwood TBL, Holliday R (1979) The evolution of ageing and longevity. Proc R Soc Lond [Biol] 205: 531–546

Klass M, Nguyen PN, Dechavingny A (1983) Age-correlated changes in the DNA template in the nematode *Caenorhabatis elegans*. Mech Ageing Dev 22: 253–263

Kolata C (1985) Fitting methylation into development. Science 228: 1183–1184

Kondrashov AS (1988) Deleterious mutations and the evolution of reproduction. *Nature,* 336: 435–440

Lawson T, Stohs S (1985) Changes in endogenous DNA damage in aging mice in response to butylated hydroxyanisole and oltipraz. Mech Ageing Dev 30: 179–185

Lee MYWT, Tan CK, So AG, Downey KM (1980) Purification of deoxyribonucleic acid polymerase-δ from calf thymus: partical characterization of physical properties. Biochemistry 19: 2096–2101

Lindahl T (1976) New class of enzymes acting on damaged DNA. Nature 259: 64–66

Lindahl T (1987) Regulation and deficiencies in DNA repair. Br J Cancer 56: 91–95

Lindahl T, Nyberg B (1972) Rate of depurination of native deoxyribonucleic acid. Biochemistry 11: 3610–3618

Linn S, Kairis M, Holliday R (1976) Decreased fidelity of DNA polymerase activity isolated from human fibroblasts. Proc Natl Acad Sci USA 73: 2818–2822

Loeb LA, Kunkel TA (1982) Fidelity of DNA synthesis. Ann Rev Biochem 52: 429–457

Loeb LA, Reyland ME (1987) Fidelity of DNA synthesis. In: Eckstein F, Lilley DMJ (eds) Nucleic acids and molecular biology, vol. I. Springer, Berlin Heidelberg New York, pp 156–173
Makinodan T, Peterson WJ, Baumgartner W, Kay MM (1977) Accumulation of DNA strand breaks with age in the liver and related organs. In: Platt D (ed) Liver and ageing. Schattauer, Stuttgart, pp 153–159
Maslansky CJ, Williams GM (1985) Ultraviolet light-induced DNA repair synthesis in hepatocytes from species of different longevities. Mech Ageing Dev 29: 191–203
Massie HR, Baird MB, Nicolosi BJ, Samis HV (1972) Changes in the structure of rat liver DNA in relation to age. Arch Biochem Biophys 153: 733–741
Massie HR, Baird MB, McMahon MM (1975) Changes in the structure of the DNA of *Drosophila melanogaster* during development and aging. Mech Ageing Dev 4: 113–122
Medvedev ZA (1984) Age changes of chromatin. A review. Mech Ageing Dev 28: 139–154
Mitchinson JM (1971) The biology of the cell cycle. Cambridge University Press, Cambridge
Modrich P (1987) DNA mismatch correction. Ann Rev Biochem 56: 435–466
Mori N, Goto S (1982) Estimation of the single-stranded region in the nuclear DNA of mouse tissues during aging with special reference to the brain. Arch Geront Geriatr I: 143–150
Müller WEG, Zahn RK, Geurtsen W, Munsch N (1980) Age dependent aterations of DNA synthesis. Terminal deoxynucleotidyl transferase and DNA polymerase activities in bone marrow subpopulations from mice. Mech Ageing Dev 13: 119–126
Murray V (1981) Properties of DNA polymerases from young and ageing human fibroblasts. Mech Ageing Dev 16: 327–343
Murray V, Holliday R (1981) Increased error frequency of DNA polymerases from senescent human fibroblasts. J Mol Biol 146: 55–76
Nakanishi K, Shima A, Fukuda M, Fujita S (1979) Age-associated increase of single-stranded regions in the DNA of mouse brain and liver cells. Mech Ageing Dev 10: 273–281
Niedermüller H, Hoffecker G, Skalicky M (1985) Changes of DNA repair mechanisms during the aging of the rat. Mech Ageing Dev 29: 221–238
Oesch F, Aulmann W, Platt KL, Doerjer G (1987) Individual differences in DNA repair capacities in man. Arch Toxicol [Suppl] 10: 172–179
Ono T, Okada S (1976) Comparative studies of DNA size in various tissues of mice during the aging process. Exp Gerantol II: 127–132
Ono T, Tawa R, Shinya K (1986) Methylation of the C-myc gene changes during aging process of mice. Biochem Biophys Res Comm 139: 1299–1304
Ove P, Goetzee ML (1978) A difference in bleomycin-induced DNA synthesis between liver nuclei from mature and old rats. Mech Ageing Dev 8: 363–375
Paffenholz V (1978) Correlation between DNA repair of embryonic fibroblasts and different life span of 3 inbred mouse strains. Mech Ageing Dev 7: 131–150
Piantanelli L, Brogli R, Bevilacqua P, Fabris N (1978) Age-dependance of isoproterenol-induced DNA synthesis in sumandibular glands of BALB/c mice. Mech Ageing Dev 7: 162–169
Plesko M, Richardson A (1984) Age-related changes in unscheduled DNA synthesis by rat hepatocytes. Biochem Biophys Res Comm 118: 730–735
Polson CDA, Webster GC (1982) Age-related DNA fragmentation in two varieties of *Drosophila melanogaster,* Phaseolus (coteledons) and three tissues of the mouse. Exp Gerontol 17: 11–17
Price GB, Makinodan T (1973) Aging: alteration of DNA-protein information. Gerontologia 19: 58–70
Price GB, Modak SP, Makinodan T (1971) Age-associated changes in the DNA of mouse tissues. Science 171: 917–920
Razin A, Cedar H (1984) DNA methylation in eukayotic cells. Int Rev Cytol 92: 159–187
Regan JD, Cook JS, Lee WH (1968) Photoreactivation of amphibian cells in culture. J Cell Physiol 71: 173–176
Rothstein M (1982) DNA. In: Biochemical Approaches to Aging. pp 132–173. Academic Press. New York
Robbins JH (1978) Significance of repair of human DNA: evidence from studies *Xeroderma pigmentosum.* J Natl Cancer Inst 61: 645–655

Romanov GA, Vanyushin BF (1981) Methylation of reiterated sequences in mammalian DNAs. Effect of the tissue type, age, malignancy and hormonal induction. Biochim Biophys Acta 653: 204–218

Samis HV, Falzone JA, Wulff VJ (1966) H^3-Thymidine incorporation and mitotic activity in liver of rats various ages. Gerontologia 12: 79–88

Shearman CW, Loeb LA (1977) Depurination decreases fidelity of DNA synthesis in vitro. Nature 270: 337–338

Singhal RP, Mays-Hoopes LL, Eichhorn GL (1987) DNA methylation in aging of mice. Mech Ageing Dev 41: 199–210

Smith-Sonneborn J, Klass M (1974) Changes in the DNA synthesis pattern of paramecium with increased clonal age and interfission time. J Cell Biol 61: 591–598

So AG, Downey KM (1988) Mammalian DNA polymerases α and δ: current status in DNA replication. Biochemistry 27: 4991–4995

Strauss BS (1985) Cellular aspects of DNA repair. Adv Cancer Res 45: 45–101

Strehler BL, Chang MP, Johnson LK (1979) Loss of hybridizable ribosomal DNA from human post-mitotic tissues during aging: I. Age-dependent loss in human myocardium. Mech Ageing Dev 11: 371–378

Struchkov VA (1962) On nature of superpolymer DNA. Biophysica (Moscow) 7: 538–550

Su CHM, Brash DE, Turturo A, Hart RW (1984) Longevity-dependent organ-specific accumulation of DNA damage in two closely related murine species. Mech Ageing Dev 27: 239–247

Swenberg SA, Fennell TR (1987) DNA damage and repair in mouse liver. Arch Toxicol [Suppl] 10: 162–171

Targovnik HS, Locher SE, Hart TF, Hariharan PV (1984) Age-related changes in the excision repair capacity of *Turbatrix aceti.* Mech Ageing Dev 27: 73–81

Tice RR (1978) Aging and DNA repair capability. In: Schneider EL (ed) The genetics of aging. Plenum, New York, pp 53–89

Treton JA, Courtois Y (1982) Correlation between DNA excision repair and mammalian lifespan in lens epithelial cells. Cell Biol Int Rep 6: 253–260

Turner DR, Morley AA, Seshadri RS, Sorrell JR (1981) Age-related variations in human lymphocyte DNA. Mech Ageing Dev 17: 305–309

Turner DR, Griffith VC, Morley AA (1982) Ageing in vivo does not alter the kinetics of DNA strand break repair. Mech Ageing Dev 19: 325–331

Vanyushin BF, Nemirovsky LE, Belozersky AN (1973) The 5-methylcytosine in DNA of rats: tissue and age specificity. Gerontologia 19: 138–152

von Hahn HP (1970) Structural and functional changes in nucleoprotein during ageing of the cell. Gerontologia 16: 116–128

Wegener K, Hollweg S, Maurer W (1964) Autoradiographische Bestimmung der DNA-Verdopplungszeit und anderer Teil-phasen des Zell-zyklus bei fetalen Zellarten der Ratte. Z Zellforsch Mikrosk Anat 63: 309–326

Wheeler KT, Lett JT (1972) Formation and rejoining of DNA strand breaks in irradiated neurons in vivo. Radiat Res 52: 59–67

Wheeler KT, Lett JT (1974) On the possibility that DNA repair is related to age in non-dividing cells. Proc Natl Acad Sci USA 71: 1862–1865

Williams JR, Dearfield KL (1981) DNA damage and repair in aging mammals. In: Florini JR (ed) CRC handbook of biochemistry in aging. CRC, Boca Raton, Florida, pp 25–48

Wilson VL, Jones PA (1983) DNA methylation decreases in ageing but not in immortal cells. Science 220: 1055–1057

Woodhead AD, Setlow RB, Grist E (1980) DNA repair and longevity in three species of cold blooded vertebrates. Exp Gerontol 15: 301–304

Wright JR, Stephens RE, Ford KC, Thibert P, Yates AJ (1986) DNA excision repair in spontaneously diabetic BB Wistar rats. Mech Ageing Dev 36: 109–116

Zahn RK (1983) Measurement of the molecular weight distributions in human muscular deoxyribonucleic acid. Mech Ageing Dev 22: 355–379

Zahn RK, Reinmüller J, Beyer R, Poneljak V (1987) Age-correlated DNA damage in human muscle tissue. Mech Ageing Dev 41: 73–114

Zweidler A (1984) Core histone variants of the mouse; primary structure and differential expression. In: Stein GS (ed) Histone genes and histone gene expression. Wiley, New York, pp 373–395

Nonenzymatic Glycosylation of Collagen as a Model of Posttranslational Aging

G. HOFECKER, S. VELETZKY, H. NIEDERMÜLLER, and M. SKALICKY[1]

Introduction

At the very beginning of experimental gerontology, Verzár (1957) put forward the idea that macromolecules with no or a slow turnover are altered irreversibly with time and, consequently, age. His favorite model of this posttranslational age-related change was the aging of the tail tendon collagen of the rat. Throughout life, tail tendon collagen shows a progressive increase in rigidity, accompanied by a rising resistance to thermal and chemical degradation.

For a long time it had been well-known that thermal and chemical denaturation causes collagen to shrink (so-called thermal and chemical contraction). However, Verzár was the first to observe that the extent of contraction, or the force necessary to prevent it, increases with age and provides an excellent measure of the animal's age. In accordance with the crosslinking hypothesis of aging, which was formulated for the first time by Bjorksten (1958), Verzár interpreted his findings as a result of progressive covalent crosslinking of the metabolically inert protein.

Verzár's theory of collagen stabilization by covalent crosslinking has since been confirmed by many authors. However, the lifelong increase in resistance to thermal and chemical degradation and the continuous rise in thermal and chemical contraction do not parallel the change in functionality, i.e., the tendon's ability to resist mechanical stress: Vogel (1980) showed that in rat tendons mechanical strength, measured as ultimate load, increase only up to an age of 12 months and thereafter decreases slightly. This suggest that different processes might be involved in the lifelong change in tendon collagen, one process related to maturation and the other to aging (for review see Bailey and Light 1985).

The increase in resistance to stress during maturation has been shown to be brought about by two processes:

1. The lysyl-oxidase-induced formation of reducible crosslinks of the aldimine and ketomine type.
2. The transformation of reducible crosslinks into more stable, multivalent bonds (Barnard et al. 1987). At the attainment of maturity, this process has been completed in most types of collagen.

[1] Institut für Physiologie der Veterinärmedizinischen Universität Wien, Linke Bahngasse 11, A-1030 Wien, Austria

Gerontology
Ed. by D. Platt
© Springer-Verlag Berlin Heidelberg 1989

The processes causing the changes of collagen fibers *after the attainment of maturity* are still unknown. A stabilizing process which might be closely related to aging is found in diabetes: the nonenzymatic glycosylation of proteins, which eventually leads to irreversible changes of the macromolecules. Andreassen et al. (1981) found an increase in the thermal contraction of the tendons of streptozotocin-diabetic rats, accompanied by a retarded relaxation, both changes being indicative of a higher biological age. Accelerated collagen aging was also suggested by steeper stress-strain curves in mechanical tests. Both changes were effectively prevented by insulin treatment of the diabetic animals. Chemical analysis of the "diabetic tendons" failed to show any change in the density of reducible crosslinks. However, the amount of glucose attached to lysyl and hydroxylysyl residues was considerably higher. Obviously, nonenzymatic glycosylation had stabilized the collagen molecule in a way which did not involve the lysyl-oxidase-derived crosslinks.

Kohn et al. (1984) suggested that the random (or stochastic) crosslinking of collagen and other long-lived proteins in diabetes and probably in senescence was identical with the Maillard reaction (browning reaction), well-known in food chemistry. This reaction starts when the aldehyde group of glucose reacts with a free amino group of a protein to form a Schiff base. This compound quickly undergoes an Amadori rearrangement, resulting in a stabler but still reversible ketoimine. After some rearrangement and dehydration processes, Amadori products from advanced glycosylation end products (AGEs), which can bind to free amino groups of adjacent proteins to form irreversible covalent crosslinks. Nonenzymatic glycosylation has been postulated to allow for interhelical crosslinks in collagen, a type of bond which cannot be induced by lysyl oxidase. In addition, glycosylation of collagen in diabetes is held responsible for the trapping of various plasma proteins in the wall of blood vessels, promoting renal disease and atherosclerosis. The formation of AGEs is prevented by a lowered pH and also by the drug aminoguanidine (Brownlee et al. 1986).

In order to decide whether nonenzymatic glycosylation may be a true aging process of tendon collagen, we investigated whether in vitro glycosylated tendons behaved like naturally aged fibers. As a test criterion we used the dynamics of the isometric contraction-relaxation during chemical denaturation (Hofecker et al. 1972, 1979; Hofecker 1975).

Materials and Methods

The present study is based on the above-mentioned investigations, which served to establish the contraction-relaxation model. In all studies tail tendons of male Sprague-Dawley rats (OFA 17, Institut für Versuchstierzucht der Universität Wien) were prepared as follows:

The animals were sacrificed under general anesthesia by bleeding, the tail was severed from the body, and tendon fibers were pulled out of the tip of the tail. The fibers were air-dried and cut to a length of 10 cm. For the chemical contraction-

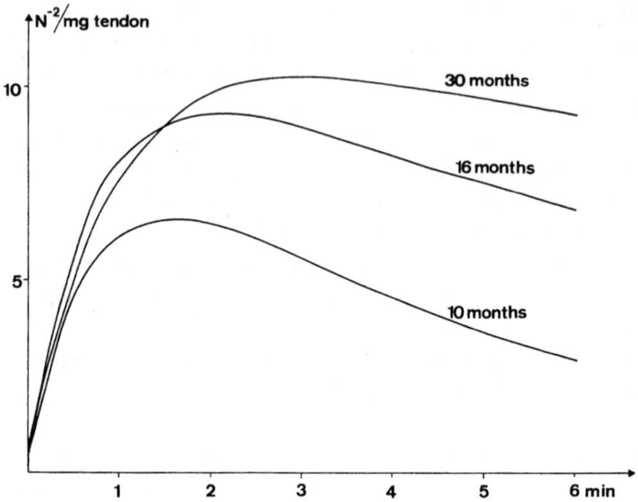

Fig. 1. Effect of age on the contraction-relaxation curves of rat tail tendons at various ages

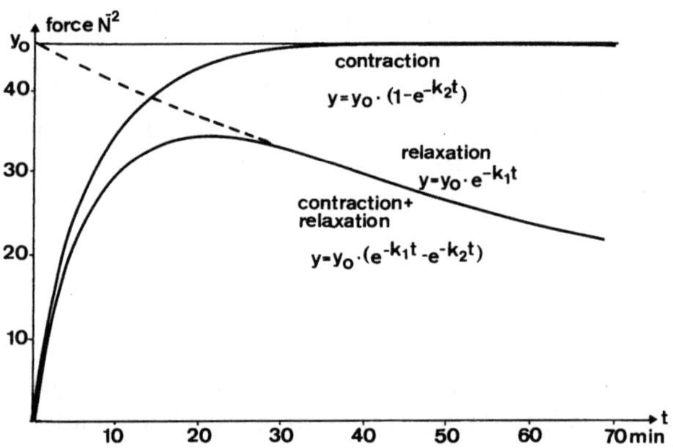

Fig. 2. Analysis of contraction-relaxation curves

relaxation procedure, fibers of 4–6 mg/10 cm were knotted between stainless steel wire hooks at a free length of 5 cm and fixed in a heatable glass tube in such a way that one end of the tendon was linked with an inductive power transducer. After 10 min of rehydration in Ringer's solution, the tendon was immersed in 5 M sodium perchlorate solution at 40 °C.

The Contraction-Relaxation Model (Hofecker et al. 1979)

Immediately after immersion the tendon rapidly develops an isometric tension which attains a maximum after approximately 2 min, followed by a slower relaxation (Fig. 1). During senescence, kinetics change in a characteristic manner: the maximum of isometric tension increases whereas the speed of the contraction and relaxation slows down. Since this behavior reflects the structural changes in the molecule, we analyzed the curve to provide a mathematical model of the processes involved.

All curves could be analyzed as being the result of two simultaneous processes, both induced by the perchlorate solution, but with different time constants (Fig. 2):

1. The rapid diffusion of perchlorate into the fiber, destroying intermolecular water bridges and bringing the contracting force of crosslinks into effect.
2. The slower dissolution of the fiber by the concentrated salt solution, which leads to the relaxation.

According to this model, the contraction-relaxation curves could be fitted exactly to a *two-term exponential function* of the form

$$y = y_o (e^{-k_1 t} - e^{-k_2 t})$$

y_o is the maximum of the isolated contraction function and the extrapolated starting point of the relaxation. It is interpreted as a measure of the stable crosslinks involved in the contraction process. y_o increases with age.

k_2 is the time constant of the contraction process, apparently determined by the diffusion speed of perchlorate into the fiber. It decreases in senescence and, in so doing, seems to reflect the lowering of the content of water and glycosaminoglycans in the fiber.

k_1 is the constant of the destruction of the fibers by the perchlorate solution and provides an inverse measure of fiber stability. During senescence, k_1 decreases steadily. If we extrapolate this decline to zero, we obtain the isolated contraction function

$$y = y_o (1 - e^{-k_2 t}),$$

the predictable endpoint of the stabilization of the tendon during collagen aging.

This model describes accurately the contraction-relaxation curves over the whole period of senescence and, therefore, reflects the molecular changes, especially those concerning the number, type, and location of crosslinks. Consequently we may postulate that an in vitro change of collagen fibers reflects in vivo aging only if (a) the model is still valid for the treated tendon, and (b) the parameters change in the predicted direction.

This presupposition is not met, for instance, by the $NaBH_4$ reduction of the reducible crosslinks. This procedure seems to mimic aging as it makes the fibers resistant to thermal and chemical degradation, increases the thermal and chemical contraction, and prevents the relaxation. However, the contraction curves of $NaBH_4$-treated tendons could not be fitted to the predicted model, confirming that this kind of stabilization was an artifact (Hofecker 1975).

In Vitro Glycosylation

In keeping with our hypothesis that nonenzymatic glycosylation is responsible for the molecular changes of collagen *after* the attainment of maturity, we used tail tendons of 12-month-old rats, an age at which a larger number of parameters indicate the progress of senescence. Tendon fibers were incubated for 10 days in 0.5 M phosphate buffer (pH 7.4) containing 1, 2, 4, or 100 mmol/l glucose. Control tendons from rats aged 12, 17, 24, and 30 months were incubated simultaneously in phosphate buffer without glucose. After incubation, the tendons were washed in Ringer's solution, dried, and submitted to the chemical contraction-relaxation procedure.

Results

Figure 3 depicts the effects of aging and nonenzymatic in vitro glycosylation on the contraction-relaxation characteristics. The effect of 1 mmol/l glucose changes the 12-month curves to a shape which be characteristic of approximately 30 months. A concentration of 2 mmol/l achieves a curve attributable to an age in the range of the maximum life span of the rat. Glucose concentrations of 4 and 100 mmol/l result in aging-like stabilizations far beyond those observed in vivo.

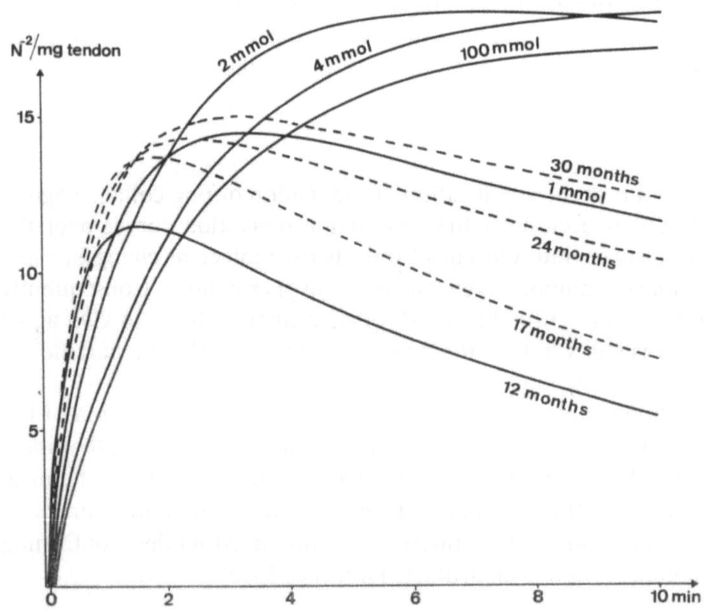

Fig. 3. Effects of age (12, 17, 24, and 30 months) and glucose (1, 2, 4, and 100 mmol/l) on the contraction-relaxation curves of rat tail tendons

All curves could be fitted exactly to the mathematical contraction-relaxation model. In the case of concentrations exceeding 2 mmol/l. k_1 became zero, thus giving the isolated contraction function predicted as the completion of posttranslational collagen aging.

The parameters of the model changed into the direction of a higher biological age. If we compare the effects of various glucose concentrations on the stability parameter k_1 (Fig. 4), concentrations of 1–2 mmol/l turn out to mimic in vivo

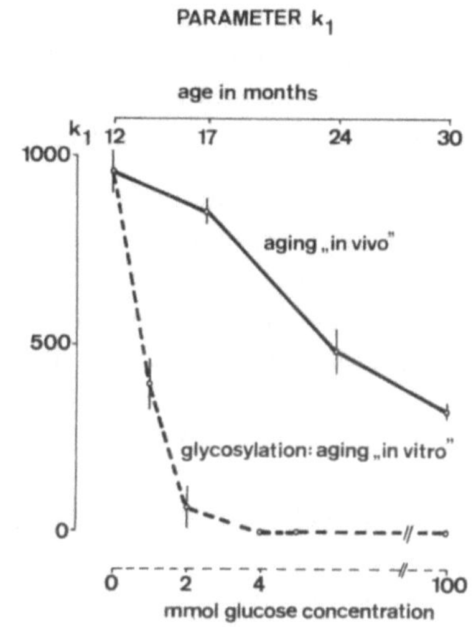

Fig. 4. Effects of age *(continuous line)* and glucose *(broken line)* on relaxation constant k_1

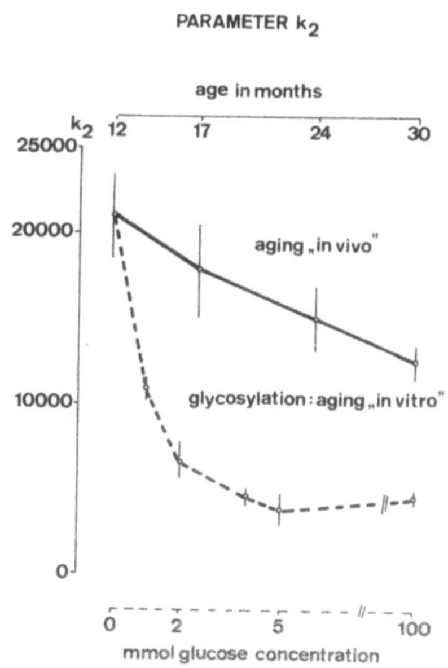

Fig. 5. Effects of age *(continuous line)* and glucose *(broken line)* on contraction constant k_2

aging between 12 and 30 months, and 4 mmol/l proves sufficient to achieve maximum stabilization. Parameter k_2, which is interpreted as a measure of the permeability of the fiber, displays a similar relation between in vivo and in vitro aging (Fig. 5). The crosslinking parameter y_o increases up to approximately 17 months, and shows a maximal in vitro aging at 2 mmol/l (Fig. 6).

In vitro nonenzymatic glycosylation clearly meets our criteria for being a model of in vivo aging and, therefore, allows us to hypothesize that this random process might be the basis of collagen aging. This result matches very well our earlier finding (Skalicky et al. 1987) that parameter k_1 decreases with age in a one-term exponential function that indicates a stochastic molecular change.

The concept put forward by Kohn and others that the formation of advanced glycosylation end products might be an important process not only in diabetes but also in normal aging is attractive for several reasons:

1. The transformation of reducible crosslinks into nonreducible ones is a developmental process and cannot account for the continuing structural change in senescence.
2. Some changes in connective tissue seen in diabetes, such as the thickening of the glomerular basement membrane, the stiffening of ligaments, and the increased susceptibility to atherosclerosis, are also features of advanced age.
3. Glucose tolerance decreases with normal aging (DeFronzo 1979). This is likely to increase the probability of stochastic glycosylation of long-lived proteins.
4. Severe caloric restriction retards collagen aging (Chvapil and Hruza 1959; Everitt et al. 1980). This effect could be due to lowered glucose levels or fewer and shorter postprandial glucose peaks.

Despite the attractiveness of this concept, it remains intriguing that glucose levels far below the normal blood glucose concentration of 4 mmol/l lead to

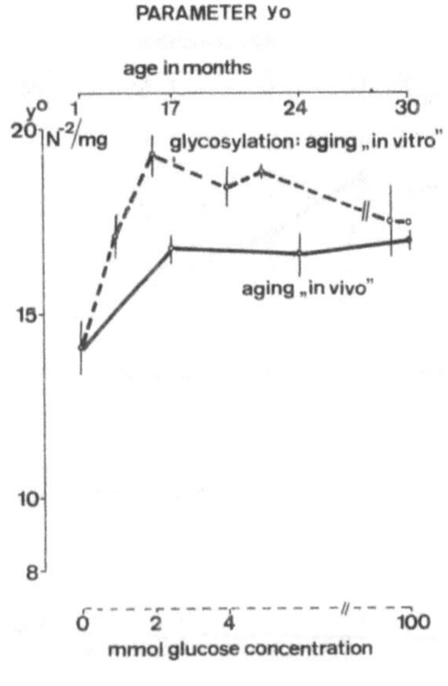

Fig. 6. Effects of age *(continuous line)* and glucose *(broken line)* on the crosslinking parameter y_o

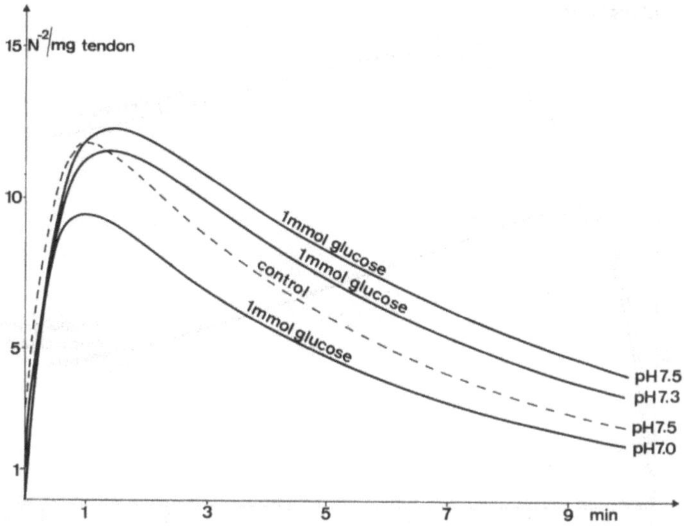

Fig. 7. Effects of pH on glucose-induced in vitro aging of tendons of a 12-month-old rat

accelerated collagen aging. This raises the question as to why aging proceeds less rapidly than we would expect from the actual glucose concentrations in the body.

One important factor might be the pH dependency of the nonenzymatic glycosylation. In order to test this effect, we incubated tendons of a 12-month-old rat in glucose solutions (1 mmol/l) buffered at different pH: 7.0, 7.3, and 7.5 (Fig. 7). At pH 7.5, contraction-relaxation curves changed toward a higher biological age. This effect was reduced at pH 7.3 and seemed to be reversed at 7.0. Though this factor seems to be important, a physiological pH of approximately 7.3 in the interstitial fluid obviously does not suffice to prevent proteins from being irreversibly crosslinked even by subphysiological glucose levels. It seems very probable that some unknown factor of the intercellular matrix protects the fibers, and probably cellular proteins, from accelerated aging. A drug providing this protection is aminoguanidine. As can be seen in Fig. 8, the effect of 2 mmol/l glucose was completely prevented by the addition of 2 mmol/l aminoguanidine.

Conclusions

We may conclude that nonenzymatic glycosylation performed in vitro mimics the normal aging changes of tendon fibers. Apparently, this process does not affect the lysyl-oxidase-induced crosslinks, but creates crosslinks of its own. Therefore, we feel that in the age-dependent changes of collagen fibers two posttranslational processes have to be kept apart: (a) The genetically programmed maturation, comprising the formation and stabilization of reducible crosslinks. (b) Nonenzy-

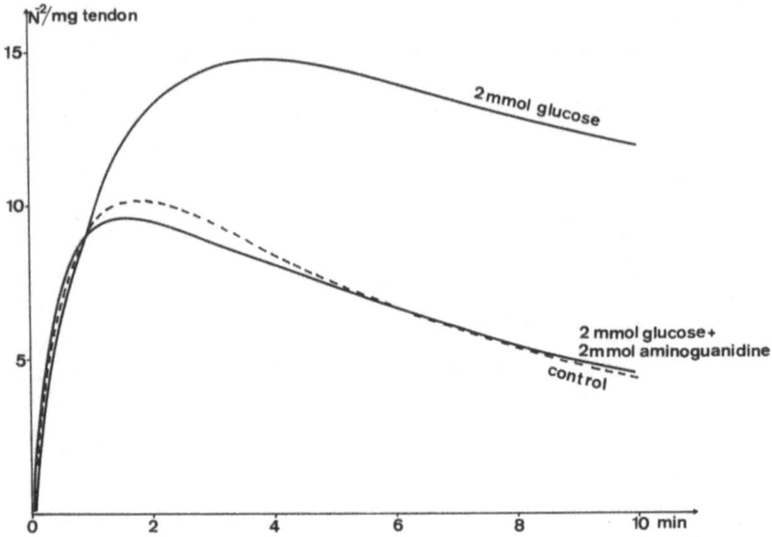

Fig. 8. Prevention of glucose-induced in vitro aging by aminoguanidine

matic stochastic events, such as glycosylation, normally producing crosslinks at a relatively low rate. The stabilization of the fiber connected with the slowing down of collagen turnover seems to enhance the change of stochastic events and the accumulation of their effects, thus setting the stage for collagen aging. The decreasing glucose tolerance at higher ages might contribute significantly to this process.

One fact that still remains to be explained is that glucose concentrations far below the normal blood glucose level accelerate in vitro tendon aging. We suspect that nonenzymatic glycosylation is counteracted in vivo by some unknown factor which retards the formation of advanced glycosylation end products in a similar way to aminoguanidine. A deeper insight into this kind of mechanism would probably contribute to our understanding of aging, diabetes, and atherosclerosis.

Summary

In diabetes, collagen is stabilized by nonenzymatic glycosylation. Decreasing glucose tolerance during senescence suggests that the age-related stabilization of collagen after the attainment of maturity could be brought about by nonenzymatic glycosylation. The present study investigates whether nonenzymatic in vitro glycosylation of collagen fibers mimics the in vivo stabilization during senescence. As an indicator of the biological age of the tendons we used the isometric contraction-relaxation during chemical denaturation (5 M sodium perchlorate, 40 °C). Contraction-relaxation curves of tendons of all ages could be fitted exactly to the model $y = y_o (e^{-k_1 t} - e^{-k_2 t})$. It is postulated that in vitro stabilization may be regarded as a model of in vivo aging only if the contraction-relaxation curves of treated tendons can be described by the same function. This is, for instance, not the case with tendons stabilized by $NaBH_4$.

Tendon fibers of rats aged 12 months were immersed for 10 days in 0.5 M phosphate buffer (pH 7.4) containing 1, 2, 4, and 100 mmol/l glucose. Tail tendons of rats aged 12, 17, 24, and 30 months served as controls and were incubated in phosphate buffer for the same period of time. All glucose concentrations mimicked extreme aging of the fibers: the relaxation constant k_1 approached zero, as predicted from the normal aging changes. Contraction-relaxation curves could be fitted exactly to the mathematical model. The normal range of tendon aging was obtained by concentrations of 1–2 mmol/l glucose, which are far beyond the normal glucose levels in vivo. It is concluded that nonenzymatic glycosylation may play an important role in collagen aging but seems to be counteracted by some unknown factor which retards the formation of glycosylation end products.

Discussion

Frenzel

Which type of collagen is affected by glycosylation?

Hofecker

Cerami and others of that group have postulated that nonenzymatic glycosylation can affect practically every protein, and so we must assume that all collagen types are susceptible to this process. However, it has been studied mainly in type I and type IV collagen, probably because of their involvement in protein trapping, as has been described, for instance, in the glomerular basement membranes of the kidney. Glycosylated type I collagen of artery walls seems to contribute to atherosclerosis by trapping plasma proteins like LDL. Another clue to the relation between nonenzymatic glycosylation and atherosclerosis was presented at the last FECTS meeting in Amsterdam, where Nemeth-Csoka showed that glycosylated type I collagen of arterial walls has an increased attractiveness for blood platelets. I have no information about type II and type III collagen.

Beischer

As a diabetologist I listened with great interest to your talk. Why is microangiopathy, in the pathogenesis of which glycosylation plays an important role, a diabetes-specific problem?

Hofecker

There is little information available on this problem. However, it seems sensible to assume that different proteins have a different susceptibility to this glycosylation process, depending on the type of sugar available, the number and positions of free amino groups, the microenvironment, and the pH. If the pH is lowered, for instance, in the environment of active cells, nonenzymatic glycosylation will be retarded. Also some unknown inhibitory factors may act differently in different tissues. So there should be a difference.

Rauterberg

Regarding the last question. A recent paper from a Finnish group reported that a part of the type IV collagen molecule is also due to glycosylation and that as a result of this further basement membrane formation is inhibited. This may be important in microangiopathy. And the other point which I want to make: The degree of glycosylation need not be different, but the consequences of glycosylation can be different, depending on the localization of additional crosslinks in the molecule.

Hofecker

Yes, I think that this is the case. In type IV collagen there is only a relatively small helical part and a big nonhelical part. Since nonenzymatic glycosylation is capable of forming interhelical crosslinks, which do not appear in crosslinking of the Schiff-base type, the structural difference between the collagen types may be responsible for different consequences of the same chemical process.

Hayflick

A number of years ago Dr. Holger von Hahn put forward the hypothesis that crosslinking of DNA may play an important role in aging. I was wondering whether you believe that this thesis is still tenable.

Hofecker

Bucala and his co-workers in Cerami's group have studied the effect of glucose on bacteriophage DNA, and found a reduced viral activity after in vitro glucose treatment. This suggests that amino groups of nucleic acids alone or togehter with amino groups of nuclear proteins may be a substrate for irreversible crosslinking. Thus the hypothesis of nonenzymatic glycosylation as an aging mechanism may well support von Hahn's ideas.

References

Andreassen TT, Seyrer-Hansen K, Bailey AJ (1981) Thermal stability, mechanical properties and reducible cross-links of rat tail tendon in experimental diabetes. Biochim Biophys Acta 677: 313–317

Bailey AJ, Light ND (1985) Intermolecular cross-linking in fibrotic collagen. In: Fibrosis (Ciba Foundation Symposium 114). Pitman, London, pp 80–96

Barnard K, Light ND, Sims TJ, Bailey AJ (1987) Chemistry of collagen cross-links. Origin and partial characterization of a putative mature cross-link of collagen. Biochemistry 1244: 303–309

Bjorksten J (1958) A common molecular basis for the ageing syndrome. J Am Geriatr Soc 6: 740–748

Brownlee M, Vlassara H, Kooney A, Ulrich P, Cerami A (1986) Aminoguanidine prevents diabetes-induced arterial wall protein cross-linking. Science 232: 1629–1632

Chvapil M, Hruza Z (1959) The influence of ageing and undernutrition on chemical contractility and relaxation of collagen fibres of rats. Gerontologia 3: 241–252

DeFronzo RA (1979) Glucose intolerance and aging: evidence for tissue insensitivity to insulin. Diabetes 28: 1095–1101

Everitt AV, Seedsman NJ, Jones F (1980) The effects of hypophysectomy and continuous food restriction begun at ages 70 and 400 days, on collagen aging, proteinuria, incidence of pathology and longevity in the male rat. Mech Ageing Dev 12: 161–172

Hofecker G (1975) Untersuchungen zur isometrischen Messung und mathematischen Analyse des Altersparameters. Chemische Kontraktion-Relaxation von Rattenschwanzsehnen. Habilitationsschrift, Veterinärmedizinische Universität Wien

Hofecker G, Moser P, Verzár F (1972) Chemische Spannungsänderungen von Kollagenfasern. Gerontologia 18: 28–35

Hofecker G, Niedermüller H, Skalicky M, Jahn J (1979) Die chemische Kontraktion-Relaxation von Schwanzsehnenfäden der Ratte als Altersparameter. Akt Gerontol 9: 469–476

Kohn RR, Cerami A, Monnier V (1984) Collagen aging in vitro by nonenzymatic glycosylation and b/Browning. Diabetes 33: 57–59

Skalicky M, Niedermüller H, Hofecker G (1987) Multivariate methods in the assessment of the biological age. In: Ruiz-Torres A (ed) Biological age and aging risk factors. Technipublicaciones, Madrid, pp 73–81

Verzár F (1957) The ageing of connective tissue. Gerontologia 1: 363–378

Vogel HG (1980) Influence of maturation and aging on mechanical and biochemical properties of connective tissue in rats. Mech Ageing Dev 14: 283–292

Age-Dependent Changes in Structure, Properties, and Biosynthesis of Collagen

J. RAUTERBERG[1]

Aging is closely linked to a number of connective tissue alterations, the aging skin being the predominant visual manifestation of an aging human being. Other age-related changes are of more clinical relevance, e.g., the osteoporetic aging bones or the aging vessel wall, "aging" being an additional important risk factor in arteriosclerosis. There is no doubt that collagen, the main structural protein of these tissues, must be involved in aging processes. Thus it is only natural that research has long been directed towards the disclosure of connections between age-related changes in collagen and the aging process. Indeed, the mere possibility of a connection between aging and collagen first brought this protein into the sights of medical research. Before that it had been more the domain of the leather and gelatine chemists.

Since the time of Professor Verzar, who first clearly showed an age-related change in collagen (Verzar 1964), knowledge about this remarkable protein family has grown tremendously. However, compared to that which we know today about the structure and biology of the different collagen types (for recent reviews see: Kühn and Timpl 1984; Mayne 1984; Miller and Gay 1987), the number of reports about age-specific alterations of collagens have remained relatively small. Nevertheless, a number of changes which can be correlated to age have been discovered. Some of these may be of importance for age-related impairments of tissue functions, and I will try to give a review of the most important recent findings in this field.

Under the headline "Aging of collagen" the following quite different aspects can be summarized.

1. Age-related Changes in Deposited Collagen. In most tissues collagen has a very slow turnover; its mere longevity favors the accumulation of changes induced by extraneous factors. Most of these changes represent alterations of amino acid side chains within the collagenous polypeptide chains, e.g., nonenzymatic glucosylation or crosslink formation. In addition, degradative processes due to the activity of tissue proteases or nonenzymatic cleavage mechanisms may alter collagen struture and function.

[1] Institut für Arteriosklerosefórschung an der Universität Münster, Domagkstr. 3, D-4400 Münster / FRG

Gerontology
Ed. by D. Platt
© Springer-Verlag Berlin Heidelberg 1989

2. Changes Arising from Altered Biosynthesis. Cellular aging leads to various changes in collagen biosynthesis which in turn result in altered collagens in the aging organism. The following alterations may occur:

a) Quantitative alteration of biosynthesis leading to changes in overall concentration of collagen and to changing ratios of the different collagen types
b) Modifications of primary structure due to age-related loss of accuracy in DNA replication, transcription to mRNA, and/or translation to polypeptide chains
c) Structural modification due to changes in posttranslational processing, e.g., in the enzymatically controlled hydroxylation of proline and lysine residues

3. Age-related Modifications in Collagen Functions Due to Alterations of Components Which Interact with Collagen. In this respect the following points may be important:

a) Interaction with other extracellular proteins changed due to age
b) Altered degradation due to changes in protease activities
c) Interaction with aging cells
d) Induction of immunological reactions, e.g., induction of autoantibody synthesis.

Especially with reference to aging of collagen, two different processes should be distinguished: the process of maturation and the process of senescence. Probably this distinction is a matter of course for all gerontology-related research, but it must be emphasized here, because in the collagen literature many of the reported age-related changes do refer more to maturation than to senescence. Indeed, for many age-related changes there is no basic difference between maturation and senescence; changes in very late years often arise from the fact that maturation-related processes do not stop after maturation is reached, but continue in the same direction, thus leading to a kind of overmaturation. This applies, for instance, to the main age-related structural change which occurs on already existing collagen fibrils: the propagation of crosslinking. Crosslinking is an important process in collagen maturation. It is essential for the mechanical stability of collagen fibers. But excessive increase in intermolecular crosslinking can lead to a decrease in elasticity and to the impediment of repair processes, for which fast degradation is essential.

If we look to the diversity of the family of collagens, as seen in Table 1, we become aware of the fact that practically all knowledge about age-related changes collected so far refers to only a few of the members of this family, namely to the so-called interstitial collagens. These are the fibril-forming collagens I, II, and III. No data concerning age-related differences are available on type V collagen, which contributes in an as yet unknown manner to fibril formation, or on the similar type XI collagen, which is cartilage specific. Recently some reports have appeared on quantitative and also qualitative changes in type IV collagen, the collagenous component of basement membrane (Karttunen et al. 1986). No data about aging are available about the other, so-called minor collagen types. On the other hand, some of these should be very interesting in this respect. Type VI collagen, for instance, is an extremely protease-resistant protein and may therefore accumulate under conditions in which proteolytic activity is present. An example of the involvement of type VI collagen in pathological processes which are favored by age is the glaucomatous eye (Lütjen-Drecoll et al. 1988). In glaucoma a thickening and morphological change of the trabecular network occurs, which regulates the pressure of the eye chamber. Type VI collagen, which forms typical 100-nm banded fribrils in places of occurrence in high concentration, is an essential component of this trabecular meshwork, as can be demonstrated by immunoelectron microscopy. In glaucomatous eyes there is considerable proliferation of type VI collagen-related matrix structures (Fig. 1).

Table 1. Types of collagen

Type	Chains	Chain composition	Main occurrence	Morphological equivalent	Functions(s)
I	α1 (I) α2 (I)	[α1 (I)]$_2$ α2 (I)	Bone, tendon, skin, most connective tissues	Collagen fiber	Tensile strength (preferably in one dimension); tissue mineralization
II	α1 (II)	[α1 (II)]$_3$	Cartilage	Thin fibrils	"Framework" of cartilage
III	α1 (III)	[α1(III)]$_3$	Together with type I; vessel wall, skin, interstitial connective tissue	"Reticular fibrils", composite fibrils with type I	Tensile strength (preferably in two dimensions) Induction of blood coagulation
IV	α1 (IV) α2 (IV)	[α1 (IV)]$_2$ α2 (IV)	Basement membranes	Basement membranes (lamina densa)	Support of endothelia and epithelia; filter
V	α1 (I) α2 (V) α3 (V)	[α1 (V)]$_2$ α2 (V), α1 (V) α2 (V) α3 (V)	Vessel wall, muscle, skin, bone	Together with type I in collagen fibrils? Cellular "exocytoskeleton"?	Support of cell movement(?) Participation in type I fibril formation(?)
VI	α1 (VI) α2 (VI) α3 (VI)	α1 (VI) α2 (VI) α3 (VI)	Vessel wall, placenta, interstitial connective tissues	"Microfibrils"? 100-nm banded fibrils	Linkage between connective tissue components?
VII	α1 (VII)	[α1 (VII)]$_3$	Placenta (fetal membranes)	Anchoring fibrils	Anchoring of basement membranes to extracellular matrix
VIII	?	?	Subendothelium in vessel walls (?) Descemet's membrane	Endothelial basement membranes (?)	?
IX	α1 (IX) α2 (IX) α3 (IX)	α1 (IX) α2 (IX) α3 (IX)	Cartilage	Linkage structures between type II fibrils	Stabilization of type II fibrillar network in cartilage
X	α1 (X)	[α1 (X)]$_3$	Cartilage (hypertrophic)	?	Cartilage-bone transition (?)
XI	1α.2α.3α	1α.2α.3α	Cartilage	?	?

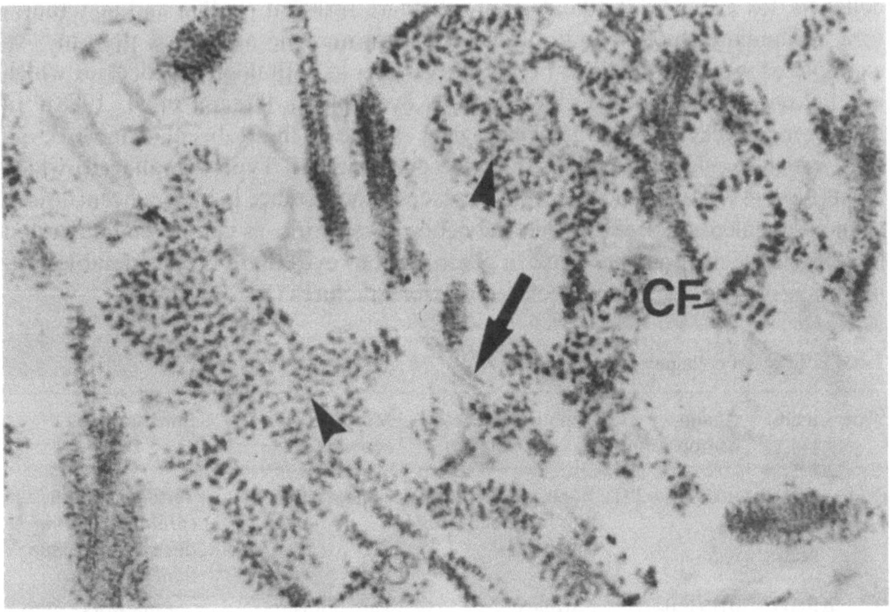

Fig. 1. Accumulation of type VI collagen-specific 100-nm banded fibrils within the trabecular meshwork of a human glaucomatous eye. Electron micrograph of a trabeculectomy, stained with anti type VI antibodies and peroxidase-linked second antibodies. Note positive staining of clumps of long spacing collagen (*arrowheads*), of small bandels, of periodic structures resembling connecting fibriles (*CF*) and of fine fibriles (*arrow*). (Lütjen-Drecoll et al. 1988)

The collagen types IX and XI seem to be essential for maintenance of cartilage structure. Possible contributions of these three collagens to aging phenomena in cartilage may be expected (Nemeth-Csoka and Meszaras 1983).

The age-related changes of collagen structures and synthesis described in the following refer to type I collagen, the major component of fibrillar collagen. As pointed out already, we have to distinguish between changes in collagen fibers which are deposited in the tissue and changes which occur due to alterations in biosynthesis.

Three main phenomena have been related to collagen aging:

1. Changes in mechanical properties. These were studied as long ago as the 1950s by F. Verzar (1964). Growth in tensile strength, which already occurs in the maturation period, is succeeded more and more by increasing stiffness and decreasing elasticity and flexibility (Rigby 1983).
2. Increasing thermal stabilitiy (Snowden et al. 1983; Flandin et al. 1984).
3. Increasing resistance against proteolysis (Rickert and Forbes 1972; Hamlin et al. 1978a, b; Holton et al. 1983; Miyahara et al. 1982).

All three changes are mainly due to an increase in intermolecular crosslinking within the collagen fibers. Morphological alterations of collagen fibrils have also been related to collagen aging: Parry et al. (1978) described remarkable changes in fibril diameters and shape in senescent human skin.

Collagen crosslinking represents the final stage in collagen biosynthesis. Induced by the enzymatically controlled oxidation of lysine-amino groups to aldehyde moieties, it proceeds without further enzymatic catalysis. The first reaction products between lysine-derived aldehydes among each other and with unchanged lysines are borohydride reducible and have been well characterized (for review see: Bentley 1979; Eyre et al. 1984). There was, however, a long period of uncertainty concerning the nature of the final stable forms of the crosslinks. Recently a major breaktrough has been achieved. Fujimoto was the first to isolate from tendon a fluorescent component derived from three residues of hydroxylysine and containing a 3-hydroxypyridinium ring which he named pyridinoline (Fujimoto et al. 1978). Pyridinoline and its analogue dehydroxypyridinoline (Henkel et al. 1987) represent the major collagen crosslinks in most tissues, especially in cartilage, tendon, ligaments, and bone (Fujimoto and Moriguchi 1978; Fujimoto et al. 1982; Eyre et al. 1984).

In skin only very low amounts of this crosslink could be detected. In 1987 Mechanic et al. described a trimeric crosslink which arises from one lysine, one hydroxylysine, and one histidine residue. It could be shown that this compound represents the major stable crosslink of mature skin collagen. W. Henkel (personal communication) in our group was recently able to demonstrate that two isoforms occur in isolated crosslinked peptides. It has become clear by now that this compound, histidino hydroxylysinonorleucine, represents the major stable crosslink in skin, whereas pyridinoline is the major crosslink in most other connective tissues.

An interesting age dependency in the amount of these crosslinks has been described: Pyridinoline (mainly the hydroxy form) increases during maturation at approximately the same rate as reducible crosslinks decrease (Barnard et al. 1987). After maturation is reached the increase in pyridinoline flattens and, especially in old human tissues, it declines considerably (Moriguchi and Fujimoto 1978). This decrease, however, does not occur in all tissues: in dentin a continuous increase can be demonstrated (Walters and Eyre 1983). The increase of histidino hydroxylysinonorleucine is similar. After maturation is reached, the increase flattens but proceeds further so that there remains a significant dependence on age (Yamauchi et al. 1988).

That the process of crosslink maturation is independent of the presence of enzymes or other connective tissue components is demostrated by the phenomenon of aging in vitro. In reconstituted collagen fibers reducible crosslinks are replaced in vitro by stable nonreducible forms (Barnard et al. 1987). But in this system the increase of stable crosslinks stops if the reducible crosslinks are used up. In vivo, however, lysyl oxidase is present in the extracellular space and can induce new formation of aldehydes, so that further generation and maturation of crosslinks remains possible.

In addition of these "physiological" crosslinks, other forms are induced which are common to all long-lived proteins. Crosslinking after nonenzymatic glucosylation or "glycation" represents the most frequent form (Monnier and Cerami 1981). The bulk of evidence indicates that glycation of collagen leads to enhanced crosslinking, as evidenced, for instance, by decreased solubility (Hamlin et al.

1975; Kohn 1983; Monnier et al. 1984). Glycation seems to be a normal process in aging; it is accelerated considerably in diabetes (Monnier et al. 1988). Another non-lysine-derived crosslink was described by Fujimoto to occur in collagen: histidino-alanine (Fujimoto et al. 1982). This kind of crosslinking was also described for other long-lived proteins and increases with age. Participation of tyrosine in additional crosslinking was described by Vancikova and Deyl (1974), but there have been no further reports on this phenomenon.

Age-related changes in collagen due to altered biosynthesis are probably as important as the aging phenomena of collagen fibrils, but research on these changes is by no means so far advanced.

In the first place, quantitative alterations have to be mentioned. Fibrotic conditions may result from overproduction of collagen. Loss of tissue strength may occur in the case of a decrease in the production of collagen fibrils. The balance between too much and too little is dependent on synthesis as well as on degradation and both may vary. In normal tissue, collagen synthesis is downregulated by keeping the messenger RNA level very low. By in situ hybridization, a method used to detect cytoplasmatic mRNA by hybridization with labeled transcripts from cDNA probes followed by radioautographic detection, no collagen I or III mRNA can be detected in normal human skin (Scharfetter et al., in press) or in normal human arterial wall (Jaeger et al., in preparation). In the case of tissue activation, e.g., in skin of scleroderma patients or in high pressure induced intimal thickening in the human aorta (Jaeger et al., in preparation), significant labeling can be seen. Contact with the surrounding matrix seems to be an important factor governing the inhibition of collagen synthesis in normal tissues because cells turn down the collagen synthesis if brought into a dense collagen lattice (Nusgens et al. 1984). It may well be that age-induced connective tissue changes impair this strict regulation. This may lead to enhanced biosynthesis which may result in the slow but continuous increase in collagen in many organs of the aging organism. The degree of collagen synthesis stimulation by external factors was found to be age dependent (Silbermann et al. 1987).

On the other hand, the ability to synthesize collagen in culture seems to decrease with the age of the cells. This applies for cell aging both in vitro (McCoy et al. 1982) and in vivo (Hildebran et al. 1983; Johnson et al. 1986). Total protein as well as collagen synthesis declines with increasing age of the donor; the decrease in collagen synthesis is steeper than that of total protein synthesis. Different results have been obtained by Klaus Bayreuther and co-workers: in their hands, fibroblasts at a late stage of differentiation in cultures after a high number of population doublings and also in cell preparations from aged donors show enhanced collagen synthesis as compared to fibroblasts in cultures at low population doubling ranges (Rodemann et al., in press).

An important aspect of overall collagen synthesis is the capacity of cells to degrade collagen. In this respect, a recent report by Sottile and co-workers is interesting. These authors describe considerably higher levels of collagenase production in late passage cultures. Furthermore, the ability to enhance collagenase production by stimulation with a certain factor is tremendously higher in the late passage cultures (Sottile et al. 1988). Of course, enhanced collagenase production does not mean a decrease in the amount of collagen in the tissue. Enhanced proteolysis in the tissues may even lead to enhanced biosynthesis of collagen due to disturbance of the regulation by cell matrix interactions. Alternatively, enhanced collagenase production must not necessarily lead to enhanced degradation, because it is often accompanied by enhanced inhibitor synthesis.

Changes in biosynthesis may not be equivalent for different collagen types and this may lead to a shift in their ratio. This phenomenon has been observed in some tissues (Lovell et al. 1987). In the case of the aorta there is a distinct shift in the ratio of type I and type III collagen during growth and maturation from relatively low to higher proportions of type III collagen (Fig. 2). With further aging, a further increase in type III can be observed in the human aorta as well as in a smaller vessel, the arteria poplitea (Fig. 3).

There are only a few reports on age-related changes of collagen in basement membranes. Typ IV collagen is a main component of this immensely important

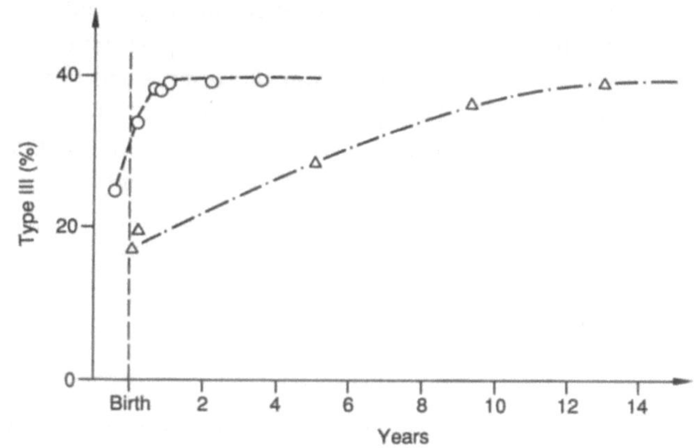

Fig. 2. Age dependency of the ratio of type III to type I collagen during maturation in bovine (– ○ – · ○ –) and human (–Δ–Δ–) aorta thoracalis

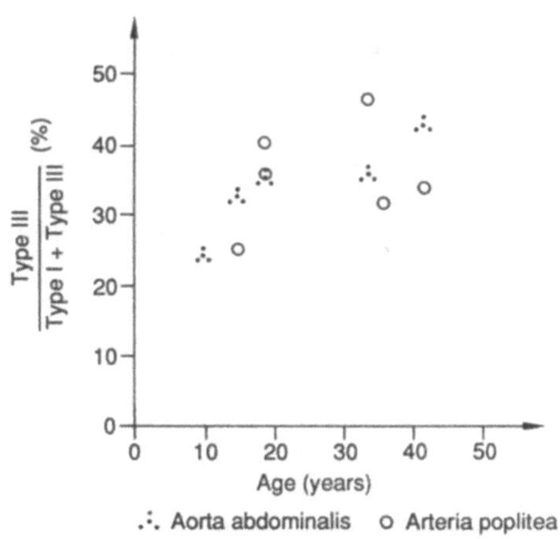

Fig. 3. Age dependency of the ratio of type III to type I collagen beyond maturation in human aorta abdominalis and arteria poplitea

extracellular structure, which, for instance, is responsible for filtration processes in the kidney and in blood capillaries.

During the process of aging a significant thickening of basement membranes has been observed (Ashworth et al. 1960; Kilo et al. 1972; Vracko 1978; Xi et al. 1982). Such basement membrane thickening may impair normal function (Harrison and Archer 1983). This demonstrates a further parallelism between aging and diabetes, in which basement membrane thickening is a major complication.

Quantitative determinations of basement membrane components have been performed on human and rat specimens of different ages (Kovanen et al. 1988). The authors found a common tendency in both species: type IV collagen increases relative to laminin, the major structural glycoprotein of basement membranes.

In the beginning I mentioned as a third possibility of age-related changes in collagen functions the alteration of matrix and cell components which interact with collagen. I will touch this point only very briefly. The possible role of cell activation due to matrix degradation has already been mentioned. No published data are available so far on the changes in matrix-cell interactions due to cellular aging. Thomas Krieg at the Dermatology Department of the University in Munich has observed that fibroblasts from old donors are less capable of contracting a collagen lattice (T. Krieg, personal communication). Since contraction and inhibition of collagen synthesis mostly go hand in hand, this phenomenon may be important for the regulation of matrix components in the aged organism.

Discussion

Linke

I would like to ask a general question. You used the terms maturation, overmaturation, and senescence. Could you comment on these terms with respect to their clear distinction; in particular, what do you think is normal and what is pathological?

Rauterberg

The term maturation covers all those processes which are part of the normal development of an organism in reaching a certain functional state; senescence means that there are changes after reaching this state which mostly are not functional, creating a status which is not appropriate for the organism.

Platt

I think that is very important because you said that men of 50 years are old. I'm 52; I don't feel old. That's a very important question, what is old and what is not old, and likewise what is maturity and what is not, and therefore the question of Dr. Linke must be clarified. Looking at animals is not the same as looking at men.

Rauterberg

The time of maturation is different in different species. The stage after maturity has been reached is a very characteristic age for each species.

Haug

Only one brief remark: Generally it is accepted that the basement membrane in the capillaries of the brain cortex thickens with age. In fact we have investigated people up to 92 years old and found basement membranes that were not thickened. We were astonished at these results, but I think there is a change in the distribution of laminin and collagen. However, at present we are unable to say more.

Klotz

Just following up the initial comments: Is there any biochemical marker for classifying the age of the subjects or an animal, for example a kind of enzyme activity or morphological feature, so that we can characterize aging more objectively than just by chronological age?

Rauterberg

That's a difficult question. In the paper about histidinolysinonorleucine it was emphasized that in reference to skin this component may be a kind of biological clock, because it increases continuously throughout life. But I believe that it is just too early to say that. And as you heard from Dr. Hofecker, some mechanical properties, for instance thermostability in relation to mechanical stress, may also serve as a reliable biological clock.

References

Ashworth CT, Erdman RR, Arnold NJ (1960) Age changes in the renal basement membrane in rats. Am J Pathol 36: 165–179

Barnard K, Light ND, Sims TJ, Bailey AJ (1987) Chemistry of the collagen cross-link, Origin and partial characterization of a putative mature cross-link of collagen. Biochem J 244: 303–309

Bentley JP (1979) Aging of collagen. J Invest Dermatol 73: 80–83

Eyre D, Paz AM, Gallop PM (1984a) Cross-linking in collagen and elastin. Ann Rev Biochem 53: 717–748

Eyre D, Koob TJ, Van Ness KP (1984b) Quantitation of hydroxypyridinium crosslinks in collagen by high-performance liquid chromatography. Anal Biochem 137: 380–388

Flandin F, Buffevant C, Herbage D (1984) A differential scanning calorimeter analysis of the age-related changes in the thermal stability of rat skin collagen. Biochim Biophys Acta 791: 205–211

Fujimoto D, Moriguchi T (1978) Pyridinoline, a non-reducible crosslink of collagen. Quantitative determination, distribution and isolation of a crosslinked peptide. J Biochem (Tokyo) 83: 863

Fujimoto D, Moriguchi T, Ishida T, Hayashi J (1978) The struture of pyridinoline, a collagen crosslink. Biochem Biophys Res Commun 84: 52–57

Fujimoto D, Hirama M, Iwashita T (1982) Histidinoalaline, a new crosslinking amino acid, in calcified tissue collagen. Biochem Biophys Res Commun 104: 1102–1106

Hamlin CR, Kohn RR, Lushin JH (1975) Apparent accelerated aging of human collagen in diabetes mellitus. Diabetes 24: 902–904

Hamlin CR, Luschin JH, Kohn RR (1978a) Partial characterization of the age-related stabilizing factor of post-mature human collagen – 1. By the use of bacterial collagenase. Exp Gerontol 13: 403–414

Hamlin CR, Luschin JH, Kohn RR (1978b) Partial characterization of the age-related stabilizing factor of post-mature human collagen – II. By the use of trypsin. Exp Gerontol 13: 415–423

Harrison DE, Archer JR (1983) Physiological assays for biological age in mice: relationship of collagen, renal function, and longevity. Exp Aging Res 9: 245–251

Henkel W, Glanville RW, Greifendorf D (1987) Characterization of a type-I collagen trimeric cross-linked peptide from calf aorta and its cross-linked structure: detection of pyridinoline by time-of-flight secondary ion-mass spectroscopy and evidence for a new cross-link. Eur J Biochem 165: 427–436

Hildebran JN, Absher M, Low BL (1983) Altered rate of collagen synthesis in in vitro aged human lung fibroblasts. In Vitro 19: 307–313

Holton JS, Litt MH, Kohn RR, Hamlin CR (1983) Human collagen digestion kinetics as a function of age and structure. Exp Gerontol 18: 477–483

Johnson BD, Page RC, Narayanan AS, Pieters HP (1986) Effects of donor age on protein and collagen synthesis in vitro by human diploid fibroblasts. Lab Invest 55: 490–496

Karttunen T, Risteli J, Autio-Harmainen H, Risteli L (1986) Effect of age and diabetes on type IV collagen and laminin in human kidney cortex. Kidney Int 30: 586–591

Kilo C, Vogler N, Williamson JR (1972) Muscle capillary basement membrane changes related to aging and to diabetes mellitus. Diabetes 21: 881–905

Kohn RR (1983) Effects of age and diabetes mellitus on cyanogen bromide digestion of human dura mater collagen. Connect Tiss Res 11: 169–173

Kovanen V, Suominen H, Risteli J, Risteli L (1988) Type IV collagen and laminin in slow and fast skeletal muscle in rats – effects of age and life-time endurance training. Coll Relat Res 8: 145–153

Kühn K, Timpl R (1984) Collagens: molecular and antigenic structure. In: Myelofibrosis and the biology of connective tissue. Alan R. Liss, New York, pp 45–59

Lovell CR, Smolenski KA, Duance VC, Light ND, Young S, Dyson M (1987) Type I and III collagen content and fibre distribution in normal human skin during ageing. Br J Dermatol 117: 419–428

Lütjen-Drecoll E, Rittig M, Rauterberg J, Jander R, Mollenhauer J (1988) Immunoelectron microscopical study of type-VI collagen in the trabecular meshwork of normal and glaucomatous eyes. Exp Eye Res 48: 138–147

Mayne R (1984) The different types of collagen and collagenous peptides. In: The role of extracellular matrix in development. Alan R. Liss, New York, pp 33–42

McCoy BJ, Galdun J, Cohen IK (1982) Effects of density and cellular aging on collagen synthesis and growth kinetics in keloid and normal skin fibroblasts. In Vitro 18: 79–86

Mechanic GL, Katz EP, Masayuki H, Noyes C, Yamauchi M (1987) Locus of a histidine-based, stable trifunctional, helix to helix collagen cross-link: stereospecific collagen structure of type I skin fibrils. Biochemistry 26: 3500–3509

Miller EJ, Gay S (1987) The collagens: an overview and update. Methods Enzymol 144: 3–41

Miyahara T, Murai A, Tanaka T, Shiozawa S, Kamayama M (1982) Age-related differences in human skin collagen: solubility in solvent, susceptibility to pepsin digestion, and the spectrum of the solubilized polymeric collagen molecules. J Gerontol 37: 651–655

Monnier VM, Cerami A (1981) Nonenzymatic browning in vivo: possible process for aging of long-lived proteins. Science 211: 491–493

Monnier VM, Kohn RR, Cerami A (1984) Accelerated age-related browning collagen in diabetes mellitus. Proc Natl Acad Sci USA 81: 583–587

Monnier, Sell DR, Abdul-Karim FW, Emancipator SN (1988) Collagen browning and cross-linking are increased in chronic experimental hyperglycemia: relevance to diabetes and aging. Diabetes 37: 867–872

Moriguchi T, Fujimoto D (1978) Age-related changes in the content of collagen crosslink, pyridinoline. J Biochem 84: 933–935

Nemeth-Csoka M, Meszaros T (1983) Minor collagens in arthrotic human cartilage. Change in content of 1 alpha, 2 alpha, 3 alpha and M-collagen with age and in osteoarthrosis. Acta Orthop Scand 54: 613–619

Nusgens B, Merrill C, Lapiere C, Bell E (1984) Collagen biosynthesis by cells in a tissue equivalent matrix in vitro. Coll Relat Res 4: 351–364

Parry DA, Barnes GR, Craig AS (1978) A comparison of the size distribution of collagen fibrils in connective tissues as a function of age and a possible relation between fibril size distribution and mechanical properties. Proc R Soc Lond (Biol) 203: 305–321

Reiser KM, Hennessy SM, Last JA (1987) Analysis of age-associated changes in collagen cross-linking in the skin and the lung in monkeys and rats. Biochim Biophys Acta 926: 339–348

Rickert WS, Forbes WF (1972) Changes in collagen with age — VI. The extraction of soluble collagen from human lung. Exp Gerontol 7: 387–396

Rigby BJ (1983) Aging pattern in collagen in vivo and in vitro. J Soc Cosmet Chem 34: 439–451

Rodemann HP, Bayreuther K, Francz PI, Dittmann K, Albiez M (in press) Selective enrichment and biological characterization of seven human skin fibroblast cell types in vitro. Exp Cell Res

Scharfetter K, Lankat-Butgereit B, Krieg T (1988) Localization of collagen mRNA in normal and sclerodermic skin by in-situ hybridization. Eur J Clin Invest 18: 9–17

Schnider SL, Kohn RR (1980) Glucosylation of human collagen in aging and diabetes mellitus. J Clin Invest 66: 1179–1181

Schnider SL, Kohn RR (1981) Effects of age and diabetes mellitus on the solubility and nonenzymatic glucosylation of human skin collagen. J Clin Invest 67: 1630–1635

Silbermann M, von der Mark K, van Menxel M, Reznik AZ (1987) Effect of short-term physical stress on DNA and collagen synthesis in the femur of young and old mice. Gerontology 33: 49–65

Snowden JM, Eyre DR, Swann DA (1982) Vitreous structure, VI: age-related changes in the thermal stability and crosslinks of vitreous, articular cartilage and tendon collagens. Biochim Biophys Acta 706: 153–157

Sottile J, Hoyle M, Millis AJT (1988) Differential response of early and late passage fibroblasts on collagenase stimulatory factor in conditioned media. Coll Relat Res 8: 361–374

Vancikova O, Deyl Z (1974) Disappearance of tyrosine residues in collagen with age. Suggestion of a possible reaction mechanism. Exp Gerontol 9: 123–130

Verzar F (1964) Aging of the collagen fibre. In: Hall ED (ed) International review of connective tissue research, vol 2. Academic, New York, pp 243–300

Vracko R (1978) Effects of aging and diabetes on basal lamina thickness of six cell types. In: Kefalides NA (ed) Biology and chemistry of basement membranes. Academic, New York, pp 483–493

Walters C, Eyre DR (1983) Collagen crosslinks in human dentin: increasing content of hydroxypyridinium residues with age. Calcif Tissue Int 35: 4–5

Xi Yu-Ping, Nette G, King DW, Rosen M (1982) Age-related changes in normal human basement membrane. Mech Ageing Dev 19: 315–324

Yamauchi M, Woodley DT, Mechanic GL (1988) Aging and crosslinking of skin collagen. Biochem Biophys Res Commun 152: 898–903

Cellular Aspects of Aging

Advances in Cytogerontology

L. HAYFLICK[1]

Introduction

The field of research in aging has only recently emerged as a legitimate area for scientific inquiry. Twenty-five years ago only a few dozen people in the United States conducted research in gerontology. At that time the stigma of working in a field recognized for centuries as a black art commanded little scientific respect. Those using cell cultures in gerontological research 25 years ago were doubly damned because cell culture itself was then just emerging from condemnation as a black art.

One excellent example of how far gerontology still has to go is to sample some of the hundreds of biology textbooks now in use in the United States (Krupka and Vener 1982). No mention is made of aging in 85% of all high school biology textbooks and from one to six pages are devoted to the subject in the remaining texts. Fifty-one percent of today's college biology textbooks do not mention aging. Of the 19 books that do, from one to four pages are devoted to the subject. This is despite the fact that aging is as universal a biological phenomenon as is development or reproduction. It is because of this enormous neglect that gerontology is still a subject rife with popular misconceptions held even by biologists themselves.

One good example can be found in the plant kingdom. On the California–Nevada border are to be found what are alleged to be the oldest living things – the bristlecone pines. These trees, along with the redwood trees in California, are believed by virtually everyone to be several thousand years old. Yet that is not true. Anyone older than 30 years is older than the oldest redwood tree or bristlecone pine.

The basis for my heresy is the fact that the cells that are alleged to be several thousand years old in those trees are dead. The living cells are found only in the peripheral cambium layer and in the needles. And they are no more than 30 years old. What is claimed to be thousands of years old is dead and that is a spurious argument when determining the age of *living* things. The living cells in these trees represent the leading edge of an ancient cell lineage, but that is not unique. You and I represent the leading edge of an ancient cell lineage also. The redwood trees

[1] University of California, San Francisco School of Medicine, Cell Biology and Aging Section (151E), 4150 Clement Street, San Francisco, California 94121, USA

Gerontology
Ed. by D. Platt
© Springer-Verlag Berlin Heidelberg 1989

and bristlecone pines do not even need the thousand-year-old dead cells to survive because many trees have had their dead tissue destroyed by fire yet they remain alive because the ring of living cambium tissue survives. These trees are truly only 30 years old because the thousand-year-old cells are not even present.
But there are other more important misconceptions.

The Biology of Aging

Aging is generally believed to be a universal property of all living things. Yet this is not true. There are animals in which aging is rare or has never been demonstrated. Only those animals that reach a fixed size after maturation age. Many fish, amphibians, and reptiles that have an indeterminate size also have an indeterminate life span. Animals like the shark, the sturgeon, or the Galapagos tortoise do not age but they are not immortal. Although normal age changes may not occur they will die eventually of disease, predation, or accidents at an annual rate similar to the half-life curve of radioactive decay. Such a curve is not a curve of true aging. In fact, extreme old age only occurs in humans and the domestic and zoo animals that we choose to protect. If aging occurs at all in feral animals its expression is brief because the physiological decrements of aging quickly make these animals vulnerable to disease and predation. Few feral animals live long enough after sexual maturation to experience old age. As soon as they incur even slight decrements in, say, running speed or jumping ability they are culled by predators. Similarly, as soon as their immune system becomes less capable, they may die of disease. Or, what is more likely, they will be culled by predators when disease has even slightly reduced their ability to elude capture. The likelihood is remote therefore that evolution could have selected for the aging process. There are simply too few feral old animals on which selective pressure could have been applied (Hayflick 1985, 1987). There is no selective advantage for a species to have its members live much beyond the age of sexual maturity and child rearing. From the standpoint of simple survival of the species, their is no advantage for humans to live much beyond the age of, say, 30. Life expectation at birth from the earliest hominid *Australopithecus* to *Homo sapiens* in the iron and bronze age never exceeded 18 years; therefore the human species has survived millions of years longer with an 18-year life expectation than it has with the current 75. Thus humans have survived for a much longer period of time with rare, or no, old members than we have with many old members.

Aging and Disease

It is most important to distinguish the aging process from disease. Age changes are not diseases, they are natural losses of function. Loss and graying of the hair, reduced exercise capacity and stamina, wrinkled skin, the menopause, presbyopia, loss of short-term memory, and hundreds of other similar decrements of old age are not diseases. They do not increase our vulnerability to die. Other "normal" decrements in vital organs do produce increased vulnerability to pathological change. For example, normal age-related decrements in immune system functions increase vulnerability to diseases that in youth would be easily resolved. Or, antigens recognized as self in youth might be recognized by an aging immune system as nonself, thus producing many of the chronic autoimmune diseases of old age.

Etiology of Aging

As in the study of development, aging must be studied using normal cells. It would be just as absurd to study abnormal or cancer cells in the pursuit of an understanding of developmental changes as it would be to study abnormal cells in the expectation that one would learn something about the aging process.

An essential element in considering the role of the cell as the origin of age changes is whether or not cells are capable of normal functions, including division, for an indefinite period of time. That is, are normal somatic cells intrinsically immortal? If they are immortal then age changes must result from causes that are extrinsic to the cell.

Centennial of the Controversy

The controversy that arose in efforts to answer this fundamental question actually began about 100 years ago. In 1881 the great German biologist August Weismann proposed that the somatic cells of higher animals will be found to have a limited doubling potential (Kirkwood and Cremer 1982). Although he provided no experimental evidence for his surmise, Weismann stated "... death takes place because a worn-out tissue cannot forever renew itself, and because a capacity for increase by means of cell division is not everlasting but finite" (Weismann 1891).

There are at least two ways in which the immortality of normal cells can be determined. First, vertebrate cells can be serially cultured in laboratory glassware, and second, similar cells, containing specific markers allowing them to be distinguished from host cells, can be serially transplanted in isogenic laboratory animals. The transplanted tissue is regrafted to a younger host when the present host becomes old. The goal of such studies has been to answer this fundamental question: Can normal vertebrate cells that function and replicate under ideal conditions escape from the inevitability of aging and death that is obligatory for the animals from which they were derived?

Immortal Heart Cells?

In respect to studies undertaken in cell culture, one investigation stood out as the classic response to this question before 1960. In the early part of this century, Alexis Carrel, a noted cell culturist, surgeon, and Nobel Laureate, described experiments purporting to show that fibroblasts derived from chick heart tissue could be cultured serially indefinitely. The culture was voluntarily terminated after 34 years (Ebeling 1942).

The importance of this experiment to gerontologists was this: If true, it strongly implied that cells released from in vivo control could divide and function normally for a period of time in excess of the life span of the species. So aging must result from cell interactions only when they are organized as tissues or organs or from changes in the intracellular matrix. In any case Carrel's results and their interpretation were of vital concern to biogerontologists because they strongly suggested that aging is not the result of events occurring within individual cells.

In the years that followed Carrel's observations, support for his experimental results seemed to be forthcoming from many laboratories in which it was observed that several cell populations appeared to have the striking ability to replicate apparently indefinitely. Immortal cell populations derived from a variety of human and animal tissues were reported to occur spontaneously in dozens of laboratories. They are best known by the prototype cell lines HeLa and L that, after about 40 years, continue to flourish to this day in cell culture laboratories throughout the world.

Nevertheless, what seemed to be incontrovertible evidence for the existence of immortal cells soon fell to new insights and a preponderance of opposing information.

Aging Under Glass

It has been almost 30 years since Paul Moorhead and I described the finite replicative capacity of normal human fibroblasts and interpreted the phenomenon as aging at the cell level (Hayflick and Moorhead 1961). We demonstrated that when normal human embryonic cells are grown under the most favorable conditions, aging and death are the inevitable consequences after about 50 population doublings. We called this the Phase III phenomenon. We also showed that the death of cultured normal human cells was not due to some trivial cause involving medium components or culture conditions but was an inherent property of the cells themselves. This observation has been confirmed in hundreds of laboratories (Hayflick 1977; Norwood and Smith 1985).

At the time that our observation was made the paramount dogma in cell biology was that the failure of cells to proliferate indefinitely in vitro must be attributable to errors in the "art" required to keep cells dividing forever. That dogma was so well entrenched that our original manuscript (Hayflick and Moorhead 1961) was rejected in 1960 by *The Journal of Experimental Medicine* with the statement that "The largest fact to have come out from tissue culture in the last fifty years is that cells inherently capable of multiplying will do so indefinitely if supplied with the right milieu in vitro." That belief was tantamount to the belief that, given the right milieu in vivo, human beings also will live forever. Ponce de Leon called the right milieu in vivo "The Fountain of Youth" and those who believe that cultured normal cells must be immortal if only the right medium can be found are, like Ponce de Leon, still searching for that fountain of youth.

Having demonstrated that normal cells are mortal, how can we explain the classic experiment of Carrel? Several years ago we proposed an explanation that has been supported by several people familiar with Carrel's work. The alleged immortal chick heart cell culture was fed at that time with freshly prepared chick embryo extract. The preparation of this crude material permitted the addition of fresh new cells to the so-called immortal culture at each feeding. Even if this explanation is invalid it is correct to say that no one has ever confirmed Carrel's work even to the extent of keeping continuously proliferating normal chick cells alive for as short a period of time as 2 or 3 years. Since confirmation is lacking and the scientific method demands this, Carrel's studies are invalid. Others have suggested more sinister reasons for Carrel's alleged success (Witkowski 1979, 1980, 1985).

In our description of the human diploid cell strains (Hayflick and Moorhead 1961; Hayflick 1965) we reported that these strains have several interesting properties:

First, if derived from human embryos, cell strains undergo about 50 population doublings. The potential cell yield from 50 population doublings is about 20 million metric tons.

Second, we found that human diploid cells undergo a number of population doublings inversely proportional to donor age. This suggested to us that the finite replicative capacity of cultured normal cells is an expression of aging at the cell level (Hayflick and Moorhead 1961; Hayflick 1965, 1977). This notion received considerable experimental support in subsequent years and is now the basis for the field of cell aging that we named cytogerontology.

We showed that, if derived from normal tissue, cell strains have the diploid karyotype and unlike immortal cell lines like HeLa, normal cell strains are incapable of replication in suspension culture. This property is now called anchorage dependence (Hayflick and Moorhead 1961; Hayflick 1965).

We also demonstrated that human cell strains will not produce tumors when inoculated into the hamster cheek pouch or even when directly inoculated into terminal human cancer patients (Hayflick and Moorhead 1961).

In addition we showed that human diploid cell strains can be cryogenically preserved. When, for example, our first widely distributed normal human diploid cell strain WI-38, which we developed in 1962, is preserved at a particular doubling level and then reconstituted, the number of doublings remaining is equivalent to 50 minus the number of doublings spent prior to preservation (Hayflick and Moorhead 1961; Hayflick 1965). The cells have an extraordinary memory and "remember" at what doubling level they were preserved even after 26 years of continuous storage in liquid nitrogen. WI-38 has been preserved longer than any other normal human or animal cell population.

As a result of this characterization we suggested (Hayflick and Moorhead 1961; Hayflick 1965) that all cultured animal and human cells be classified into three groups: (a) the primary cell culture, derived from intact tissue and undergoing no subcultivations; (b) the cell strain, which has a finite capacity to replicate, does not produce tumors when inoculated into experimental animals, has the karyology of the tissue of origin, and is anchorage dependent; and (c) the cell line, which is a population of immortal cells that may produce tumors when inoculated into laboratory animals, do not have the karyology of the tissue of origin, and are usually anchorage independent.

There Are No Immortal Cells

Prior to our finding that normal cells have a finite capacity to function and replicate it was believed that all cultured cells were immortal and therefore aging has nothing to do with events taking place at the cell level. Since we had conclusively shown that normal cells *are* mortal, the focus of attention in the field of aging began to be directed to the cell itself and the dogma of 60 years' duration began to die a slow death. But is it really true that cell immortality exists in vitro? Is HeLa, for example, immortal? In fact, it has never been proven.

There are two kinds of immortality that are frequently confused or misunderstood. These are immortality of individuals and immortality of populations. The immortality of a population depends upon a periodic exchange or rearrangement of genetic information. The immortality of individual organisms or cells, however, depends on providing evidence that exchange of genetic information has not occured. That seems self-evident but it is frequently ignored. For example, humans as individuals are mortal but humans as a population are immortal. That concept applies equally well to all animals and most plants. We frequently see it stated that bacteria and protozoa are immortal. That is not so. Like human populations, unicellular populations are immortal, but like individual humans, unicellular organisms are mortal.

No one has ever demonstrated that an allegedly immortal cell line, like HeLa, is actually immortal, i.e., that individual HeLa cells undergo continuous cell divisions *without* periodic exchange of genetic information. The importance of this point is that immortalization or transformation may be dependent upon a gene, virus, chemical, or radiation source that confers upon normal cells the ability to exchange genetic information which is the prerequisite for population immortality.

Cytogerontology

Several major observations have been made that support the concept of cell aging. In 1965 I reported that cultured fibrolasts derived from older humans replicated fewer times than those derived from embryos (Hayflick 1965). Martin and his colleagues derived cultures from human donors ranging from fetal to 90 years of age and observed that for each increase in year of life there was a loss of 0.2 of a population doubling (Martin et al. 1970). Since then at least ten studies have confirmed the finding that the number of population doublings of cultured human cells is inversely proportional to donor age using such diverse normal human cells and tissues as lung, skin, liver, arterial smooth muscle, vascular endothelium, biceps muscle myoblasts, keratinocytes, melanocytes, lens, and most recently T-lymphocytes (Hayflick 1984).

More than 200 changes in biological activity have been shown to occur in cultured normal human fibroblasts as they age in vitro (Hayflick 1980). Of great importance is that many of these changes are identical to changes recognized as characteristic of aging in intact humans.

Recent Developments

In the past few years several important observations have been made in efforts to understand why normal human cells have a finite capacity to function. Several laboratories have contributed to this work and I will present some of the more important findings.

Growth Factors

Cristofalo's group has analyzed the proliferative requirements of our human diploid cell strain in WI-38 and has identified three classes of mitogens used by these cells (Workshop on Control of Cell Proliferation in Senescent Cells 1988). Class 1 includes EGF, FGF, PDGF, and thrombin, which all act through separate receptor systems. Class 2 includes insulin-like growth factor-I (IGF-I), IGF-II, and insulin, all of which act through IGF-I receptors. Class 3 includes dexamethasone or hydrocortisone. Any class 1 mitogen in combination with any class 2 or 3 mitogen stimulates DNA synsthesis to levels found in 10% serum supplemented medium. Despite these findings using replicating cells, senescent cells will not enter S phase in response to any of the mitogens.

Seshradi and Campisi have found that there is no known growth factor that will cause normal human cells to escape from senescence despite the fact that senescent cells possess the normal numbers of growth factor receptors and binding characteristics (Workshop on Control of Cell Proliferation in Senescent Cells 1988). They have found that several growth factor-inducible mRNAs are expressed at three- to fivefold higher levels in senescent human cells than at earlier population doubling levels. These mRNAs include those encoding the c-myc proto-oncogene, fibronectin and ornithine decarboxylase. However, c-fos mRNA was induced to high levels in young cells but not in senescent cells.

In an effort to better understand the regulation of growth factor-inducible gene expression in senescent cells, Seshradi and Campisi monitored the synthesis of ornithine decarboxylase activity and fibronectin. Despite high levels of mRNA, senescent cells were deficient in ornithine decarboxylase activity and synthesized fibronectin at about one-half the rate found in young cells. These results lead to the speculation that a selective inhibition of the induction and translation of specific growth factor-inducible mRNAs in senescent cells could play a role in their failure to proliferate.

Hybridization Studies

Several years ago Pereira-Smith and Smith (1983) reported on cell hybridization studies in which they showed that in human cells mortality is a dominant trait over immortality. By hybrid analysis they have now assigned 24 different immortal human cell lines to at least four complementation groups for indefinite division (Pereira-Smith and Smith 1983; Workshop on Control of Cell Proliferation in Senescent Cells 1988). Thus four distinct genes must be involved in normal growth control. With one exception SV 40 immortalized cells are in one complementation group, suggesting that SV 40 immortalizes different human cells by the same process. They found that there was no increase in constitutive c-myc or c-H-ras expression in any of the complementation groups. Studies are now underway to determine whether the insertion of a single normal chromosome into immortal human cells is capable of reversing the immortal phenotype.

Inhibitors

The Smith laboratory has also found that senescent human cells produce a DNA synthesis inhibitor not expressed in young cells. The inhibitor appears to be localized on the outside surface of the cell membrane and may be a glycoprotein. They have also found that when poly A+ RNA is extracted from senescent cells and microinjected into young proliferation-competent cells, these cells are inhibited from synthesizing DNA. DNA and monoclonal antibody probes are now being used in an effort to isolate this inhibitor of DNA synthesis (Workshop on Control of Cell Proliferation in Senescent Cells 1988).

A few years ago Wang, now at the Lady Davis Institute in Montreal, Canada, reported the identification of a protein that apparently maintained the senescent state in normal human cells (Wang and Lin 1986). The protein was later identified by her as statin, a protein of 57 kD, found in most nonreplicating cells of animals including rat, mouse, dog, and human. Statin is present in the nuclei of senescent or quiescent normal cells arrested at the G_0/G_1 stage and is absent in young replicating cells (Wang and Lin 1986; Workshop on Control of Cell Proliferation in Senescent Cells 1988). Statin is a marker for cells that are no longer involved in division, like terminally differentiated keratinocytes, cardiac muscle cells, and mature chondrocytes.

Wang found statin to be a highly insoluble component of the nuclear envelope identifiable by staining with monoclonal antibody. Statin is synthesized as a monomer with an isoelectric point of 3.5. Statin has been isolated in relatively large amounts from rat liver. It has also been partially purified and the sequencing of a statin cDNA clone reveals high homology with the human elongation factor I-α. At the amino terminus, the two proteins are homologous; however, the COOH termini of the two sequences diverge significantly, resulting in drastic changes in hydrophobicity. In vitro synthesized statin from a cDNA clone shows similarity, by V-8 peptide mapping digestion, to the statin found in senescent fibroblasts. While the statin sequence is highly homologous to human elongation factor I-α, the two proteins are distinctly different by the unique nuclear location of statin and the hyrophobicity changes at the COOH end.

Giordano and Foster have isolated what appears to be a senescence-specific clone (pSEN) from a cDNA library constructed from senescent WI-38 cells that accounts for about 1% of the recombinants (Workshop on Control of Cell Proliferation in Senescent Cells 1988). Northern analysis of poly a(+) RNA from several intermediate population doubling levels shows that a 2.2-kb transcript hybridizes to pSEN but is expressed prior to PDL 40 at very low levels. The transcript begins to accumulate at PDL 40 and is induced approximately 50-fold just prior to senescence. Cell cycle northern blot analysis of total cellular RNA confirms the presence of the 2.2-kb species at high levels during G_0 of late PDL cells. Nucleotide sequence analysis of the 1300-bp pSEN insert shows 100% homology to 1050 bp of human elongation factor I-α. The pSEN cDNA lacks the 5′ end of the transcript and has an additional 246 bp at the 3′ end of the molecule. This 3′ extension appears to be unique to the pSEN transcript.

Methylation

One intriguing hypothesis put forward recently as the cause of senescence in human cells is the possibility of progressively increasing DNA methylation (Razin and Riggs 1980; Wilson and Jones 1983). The methylation of DNA affects gene expression and the patterns of methylation appear to be species specific (Wilson and Jones 1983). It has been speculated that alterations in the inherited DNA methylation patterns could cause changes in gene expression that might be related to aging (Wilson and Jones 1983).

When normal diploid fibroblast strains from mice, hamsters, and humans are grown in culture the 5-methylcytosine content of their DNAs markedly decreases as they approach the senescent state (Wilson and Jones 1983). On the other hand immortal cells maintain a constant level of 5-methylcytosine.

Fairweather et al. (1987) have reported that accelerating 5-methylcytosine loss by using 5-azacytidine induces demethylation and results in a marked reduction of the in vitro life span of normal human cells. The reduction is not the result of toxicity. A 22% lowering of 5-methylcytosine was associated with a striking 25% loss in life span. Hypomethylation itself therefore causes the reduction in life span.

Fairweather et al. describe three lines of evidence suggesting that DNA is related to in vitro aging:

1. 5-Methylcytosine levels fall as senescence approaches in all mortal cell strains studied from several animal species.
2. The rate of fall of 5-methylcytosine appears to be related to the in vitro life span of the cell strain.
3. Acceleration of hypomethylation shortens the life span of the cell strain.

Fairweather et al. propose that the 5-methylcytosine loss is a random phenomenon which would fit with the stochastic nature of in vitro aging. The acquisition of de novo methylase activity would confer immortality. Immortal SV 40-transformed human diploid cell strains have been found to have stable 5-methylcytosine levels for up to 700 population doublings (Fairweather et al. 1987).

At this time, however, there is no convincing evidence that DNA methylation of any specific gene locus changes with age.

We have now entered a period in the development of the field of cytogerontology where an understanding of cell longevity and aging at the molecular level is becoming possible. Many laboratories are now engaged in the quest to understand these phenomena at the most fundamental level. I expect that within the next decade we will know as much about longevity and aging at the cellular level as we know today about embryology and development.

Discussion

Platt

Is there any information on how the inhibitor outside the membrane acts by second messenger?

Hayflick

No, that's an area that's being studied now by Eugenia Wang and by James Smith and his wife.

Platt

And the second question: Can we find this inhibitor in all cells or in cells without nuclei, for instance in red cells, too?

Hayflick

The Smiths haven't looked for the inhibitor in many cell types. Wang calls the new protein "statin". It is found in every nondividing cell that she has looked at so far. It's a striking thing to see because the appearance of statin is brought out by using a monoclonal antibody and so you see the entire nuclear membrane glowing in all static cells, whereas in dividing cells there is no appearance of this material whatsoever. It has very obvious potential. If, in fact, this protein turns out to be either the cause of or somehow involved in a cascade of proteins associated with turning cell division off, then I think all of us here can readily speculate on the uses to which statin might be put.

Rauterberg

Are there any data available about age-related changes in growth factor receptors? That may be another point – that the cell membrane alters and the old cell cannot react with the growth factors in the same way that the young cell does.

Hayflick

Work in that area has been done by Vincent Cristofalo at the Wistar Institute and he finds that although there are growth factor receptors present in aging cells, there are quantitatively fewer than in younger cells.

Barrows

Is there any evidence that the cells get smaller and have a lower rate of protein synthesis in your Phase III?

Hayflick

A good question. In fact the reverse happens. The cells actually get larger. This has been found in many laboratories. The cells become much bigger as they age.

Barrows

Does protein synthesis go up then?

Hayflick

Well it depends on whether you're talking about, total protein synthesis or rate of synthesis. Individual cell's total synthesis does go up because cell mass increases, but the rate of protein synthesis may actually diminish when compared to young cells.

Hofecker

Would you say that as the cell size varies so too would the protein synthesis in the cell?

Hayflick

Apparently, but the cells definitely become larger. Some become at least twice as large in Phase III.

Hofecker

When mitotically active cells stop dividing, they age and die. When postmitotic cells have terminated their division, they can survive for a whole life, for 80 to 100 years. What accounts for such a difference, do you have any idea?

Hayflick

I wish I could answer that question with scientific accuracy but obviously I can't. I think it's important to point out that cell division is simply another functional capacity of cells. The loss of division capacity in dividing cells is, I think, equivalent to the loss of any functional property in postmitotic cells. It's simply an accident of circumstances that we first measured loss of cell division in the cell populations that we worked with initially. But over a period of time I think it's fair to say that any nondividing cell whose functional capacity can be measured (and these might even include neurons) declines over time. I think the same fundamental mechanism is operable when the decrement occurs, whether a cell's metabolism is directed toward replication or some other kind of function.

References

Ebeling AH (1942) Dr. Carrel's Immortal Chicken Heart, Sci. Am. 166: 22–24

Fairweather DS, Fox M, Margison GP (1987) The in vitro lifespan of MRC-5 cells is shortened by 5-azacytidine-induced demethylation. Exp Cell Res 168: 153–159

Hayflick L (1965) The limited in vitro lifetime of human diploid cell strains. Exp Cell Res 37: 614–636

Hayflick L (1977) The cellular basis for biological aging. In: Finch C, Hayflick L (eds) Handbook of the biology of aging. Van Nostrand Reinhold, New York, pp 159–186
Hayflick L (1980) Cell aging. In: Eisdorfer C (ed) Annual review of gerontology and geriatrics. Springer, New York.
Hayflick L (1984) The coming of age of WI-38. Adv Cell Culture
Hayflick L (1985) Theories of biological aging. Exp Gerontol 20: 145–159
Hayflick L (1987) Developmentally programmed aging, In: Warner HR, Butler RN, Sprott RL, Schneider E (eds) Modern biological theories of aging vol 31. Raven, New York, pp 21–34
Hayflick L, Moorhead PS (1961) The serial cultivation of human diploid cell strains. Exp Cell Res 25: 585–621
Kirkwood TBL, Cremer T (1982) Cytogerontology since 1881: a reappraisal of August Weismann and a review of modern progress. Hum Genet 60: 101–121
Krupka IR and Vener AM (1982) Aging in American Textbooks. The American Biology Teacher 41: 264–269
Martin GM, Sprague CA, Epstein CJ (1970) Replicative lifespan of cultivated human cells. Effect of donor's age, tissue, and genotype. Lab Invest 23: 86–92
Norwood TH, Smith R (1985) The cultured fibroblast-like cell as a model for the study of aging. In: Finch CE, Schneider EL (eds) Handbook of the biology of aging. Van Nostrand Reinhold, New York, pp 291–321
Pereira-Smith OM, Smith J (1983) Evidence for the recessive nature of cellular immortality. Science 221: 964–966
Razin A, Riggs AD (1980) DNA Methylation. Science 210: 1350
Wang E, Lin SL (1986) Disappearance of statin, a protein marker for non-proliferating and senescent cells, following serum-stimulated cell cycle entry. Exp Cell Res 167: 135–143
Weismann A (1891) Essays upon heredity and kindred biological problems, 2nd edn. Clarendon, Oxford
Wilson VL, Jones PA (1983) DNA methylation decreases in aging but not in immortal cells. Science 220: 1055–1057
Witkowski JA (1979) Alexis Carrel and the mysticism of tissue culture. Med Hist 23: 279–296
Witkowski JA (1980) Dr. Carrel's immortal cells. Med Hist 24: 129–142
Witkowski JA (1985) The myth of cell immortality. Trends Biochem Sci 10: 258–260
Workshop on Control of Cell Proliferation in Senescent Cells (1988) Abstracts, National Institute on Aging, NIH and The Bloomfield Center for Research in Aging, Lady Davis Institute and McGill University, Montreal, Canada, 12–13 August 1988

Red Blood Cell Membrane – Composition and Aging

T. BROSCHE[1]

Introduction

One mechanism which could contribute to the aging process is the alteration in cell membrane composition associated with aging. As a consequence of such alteration, a variety of functions of membranes are also altered, including regulation of enzyme activities, transport processes, and signal recognition and transduction (Packer et al. 1967; Strehler 1969; Masoro 1975; Zs-Nagy 1979; Kay 1985). Considerable interest has been focused on erythrocytes as a simple model for gaining insight into mechanisms of aging at the cellular as well as the organism level. Erythrocytes present the same sort of membrane structure as typically nucleated cells, consisting of an asymmetrical lipid bilayer, various categories of membrane proteins, glycoproteins, and a complex cytoskeleton. In mammals the potential life span of red blood cells ranges from 51 days in the mouse to 175 days in cattle and 240 days in the guanaco; in man it reaches 120 days (Vácha 1979). The aging of individual red cells is characterized by certain biochemical and biophysical changes, such as decreased flexibility and osmotic resistance, increased density, and structural modifications of the membrane (see also chapter by T. Vömel, this volume). Different pathways for the elimination of old or damaged red blood cells from the circulation are discussed. Beside the nonspecific mechanism of aggravated passage through capillaries of the liver and spleen, specific mechanisms have also been suggested, such as a physiological desialylation of the old cells and their recognition in liver and spleen (Gattegno et al. 1975) and the senescent cell antigen mechanism. By modification of a preexisting protein the antigen appears on the surface of the senescent red blood cell, is recognized by a specific IgG auto-antibody in serum, and induces the removal by macrophages (Kay 1985).

[1] Institute of Gerontology, University of Erlangen-Nürnberg, Heimerichstr. 58, D-8500 Nürnberg 90 / FRG

Gerontology
Ed. by D. Platt
© Springer-Verlag Berlin Heidelberg 1989

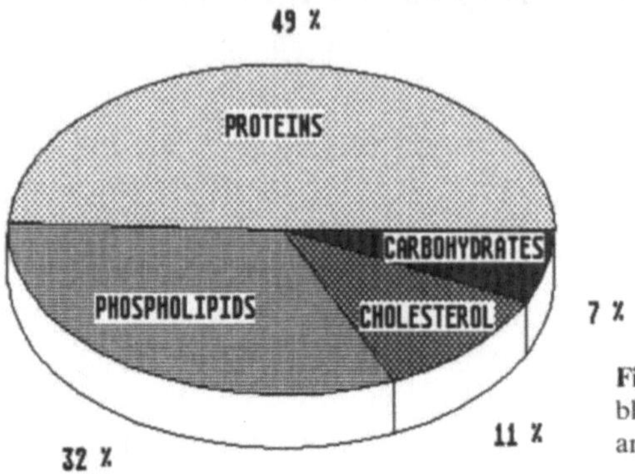

Fig. 1. Composition of pooled human red blood cell ghosts. (Adapted from Rosenberg and Guidotti 1968)

Table 1. Lipid composition of human erythrocyte membranes (according to Hanahan 1969)

Lipid class	% of total lipid	% plasmalogen form of phospholipid class
Cholesterol	25	
Phosphatidyl-ethanolamine	22	35
Phosphatidyl-serine	6	
Phosphatidyl-inositol	6	
Phosphatidyl-choline	19	2
Sphingomyelin	20	
Gangliosides	<5	
Glycolipids	<5	

Composition of Human Red Cell Membranes

The human erythrocyte membrane is composed of approximately 50% protein, 7% carbohydrate, and 43% lipid (Fig. 1). The lipids provide a dynamic network which may affect the mobility, orientation, and function of receptors, enzymes, and antigens on the membrane surface. The lipid composition of human erythrocyte membranes is given in Table 1. The arrangement of red cell membrane components is highly heterogeneous with respect to lateral distribution and asymmetry between the two leaflets. Carbohydrates are exposed to the outer cell surface exclusively. The four main phospholipid classes are distributed asymmetrically between the two membrane leaflets: phosphatidylcholine and sphingomyelin are exposed predominantly to the outer side, whereas phosphatidylethanolamine and phosphatidylserine are confined to the cytoplasmic side (Bretscher

1973; Zwaal et al. 1975). Cholesterol has been suggested to be concentrated preferentially both in the inner leaflet (Brasaemle et al. 1988) and in the outer leaflet (Flamm and Schachter 1982). These contradictory findings may be due to experimental problems caused by a translocation rate of cholesterol of $t_{1/2} < 60$ min (Heckers and Platt 1988).

Dynamic Exchange of Red Cell Lipids and Aging

Plasma lipoproteins transport lipid for delivery to cells and help maintain a normal cell membrane lipid composition. The free cholesterol and phospholipid (mainly lecithin and sphingomyelin) molecules on the surface of lipoproteins exchange with their counterparts in the plasma membrane of the cells. Similar exchanges occur between the plasma membrane and intracellular organelles (Shinitzky 1987). Mature mammalian erythrocytes have a very limited ability to synthesize phospholipids de novo from simple precursors (Strunecka and Folk 1988) and no biosynthetic capacities for cholesterol production. Therefore, alterations of the plasma lipoproteins are reflected in the composition of erythrocyte membranes,

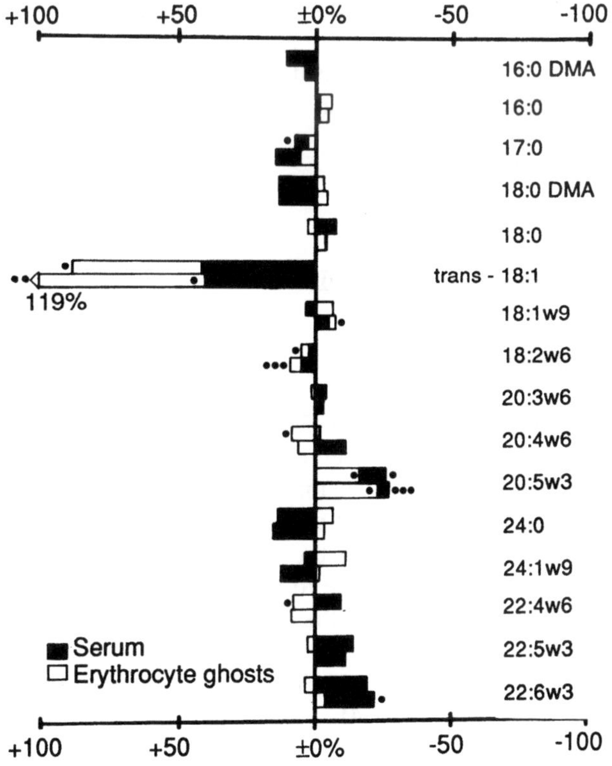

Fig. 2. Effect of delivery of a diet, supplemented with a margarine based on a partially hydrogenated sunflower oil, on relative changes of fatty acid concentrations in phospholipids of erythrocyte membranes *(open bars)* and plasma *(filled bars)* of geriatric subjects. Data are given as delta percent to 2-week *(upper bars)* and to 3-week *(lower bars)* diet period values. n=5; •, $P<0.025$; ••, $P<0.005$; •••, $P<0.0005$; t-test for paired data. (Adapted from Brosche et al. 1986)

which in turn affects the function of red cells as well as that of other tissues. An important determinant of membrane function is the fluidity, which can be influenced by the cholesterol to phospholipid ratio, the lecithin to sphingomyelin ratio, and the fatty acid composition of the phospholipids. Both compositional and positional changes of fatty acids in acylglycerols have been noted upon aging. In man these alterations are difficult to evaluate because of the contribution of diseases, drug therapy, and dietary lipids: In a study on the effect of different fat-supplemented diets on the erythrocyte ghost composition of geriatric subjects we found statistically significant changes in the erythrocyte and plasma phospholipid fatty acid patterns (Brosche et al. 1986). As an example Fig. 2 shows the observed variation of fatty acid concentrations of blood phospholipids, induced by a 3-week dietary period with administration of a margarine based on partially hydrogenated sunflower oil. The high concentration of linoleic acid (18:2w6, Fig. 2) and trans-configurated octadecenoic acids (trans-18:1, Fig. 2) in the margarine is reflected in the erythrocyte membranes. In comparison to our results, studies in the yeast *Lipomyces lipoferus,* which can be grown on chemically defined medium, have shown that each position of the glycerophospholipids has a unique distribution of fatty acids which changes to a varying degree with age (Phornpiboonya and Jack 1980). The net decrease in phospholipid–fatty acid double bonds of aging cells of *Lipomyces lipoferus* suggests that aging in this yeast is accompanied by reduced membrane fluidity. There is ample evidence that age-dependent changes in membrane lipids of many tissues are associated with a relative increase in rigidifying lipids, e. g., free cholesterol, sphingomyelin, and saturated fatty acids (Hegner 1980; Shinitzky 1987).

Conflicting data in the literature concerning the changes in human erythrocyte membrane lipid levels that occur in association with donor age led us to reconsider this problem.

Materials and Methods

Experimental Design

Blood was obtained from 95 volunteers (70 female and 25 male), aged 70–90 years and living in seven different homes for the aged in the Nuremberg region. No patients were included in this study. Participants who suffered from hematological or liver disease and those who were under a lipid-lowering therapy were excluded, as were diabetics. Over the course of 5 years experimental groups of no more than ten volunteers were formed and analyzed successively. Some of the blood donors were included in the study a second time at a different point in time. Blood samples were taken in the fasting state, the heparinized plasma was separated by centrifugation, and hemoglobin-free red cell ghosts were prepared according to Platt and Schoch (1974).

Erythrocyte Lipid Analyses

Lyophilized erythrocyte ghosts were extracted, and the crude lipid extracts were separated on Silica Sep-Pak cartridges (Waters Assoc., Milford, CT, USA) into fractions of free cholesterol, glycolipids, and phospholipids as described previously (Brosche et al. 1986). Aliquots of the phospholipid eluates were analyzed in duplicate, using a phosphorus test kit (Boehringer Mannheim, FRG), and the results were converted into the corresponding phospholipid values by multiplication.

The free cholesterol in the eluates was determined by capillary gas chromatography after derivatization to trimethylsilylethers with dihydrocholesterol as internal standard.

Analyses were recorded and integrated on a Hewlett Packard HP-5880A instrument, equipped with a flame ionization detector. A DB210 15 m × 0.25 mm i.d. fused silica column (J.+W. Scientific Inc., Rancho Cordova, CA) was used with helium as the carrier gas (0.70 bar). The injector and detector were kept at 280 °C; the oven temperature was 220 °C. All samples were analyzed in triplicate and the results are given as means.

Results

Table 2 shows the results of analyses of human erythrocyte ghost lipids derived from blood samples of the volunteers aged 70–90 years. The subjects were divided into four age groups, each covering 5 years. When the Kruskal-Wallis test was employed as a nonparametric one-way analysis of variance, no statistically significant differences were revealed in red cell membrane phospholipid concentrations

Table 2. Erythrocyte membrane lipid composition of donors aged 70–90 years

Age group (years)	I (70 to <75)	II (75 to <80)	III (80 to <85)	IV (85 to <90)
Donors:				
Total	24	31	28	12
Male	4	6	6	4
Female	20	25	22	8
No. of samples	46	46	47	26
Erythrocyte membrane components:				
Cholesterol (CH; nmol/mg ghost)[a, b]	326 ± 37	315 ± 29	310 ± 27	296 ± 36
Phospholipids (PL; nmol/mg ghost)[c]	338 ± 33	336 ± 30	336 ± 28	349 ± 41
PL/CH ratio[d]	1.035 ± 0.097	1.068 ± 0.120	1.089 ± 0.084	1.186 ± 0.0155

[a] Values are means ± SD of all samples; [b] $P < 0.01$, Kruskal-Wallis test; [c] NS; [d] $P < 0.001$.

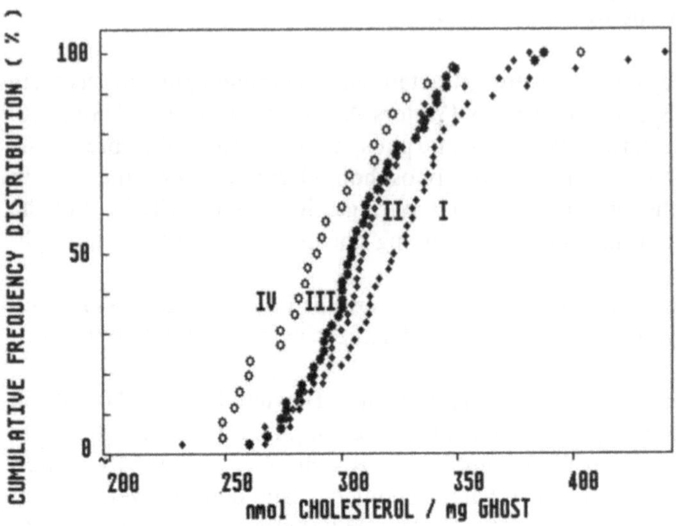

Fig. 3. Cumulative frequency distribution of cholesterol concentrations in lyophilized erythrocyte ghosts of 95 elderly subjects. Samples and age groups as in Table 2: 70 to below 75 years (*I*, *n*=46), 75 to below 80 (*II*, *n*=46), 80 to below 85 (*III*, *n*=47), and 85 to below 90 years of age (*IV*, *n*=26)

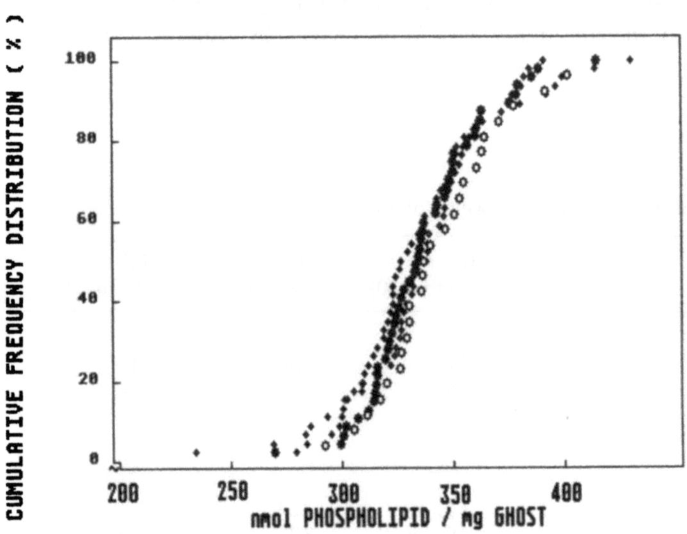

Fig. 4. Cumulative frequency distribution of phospholipid concentrations in red cell membranes. Donors and age groups as in Fig. 3

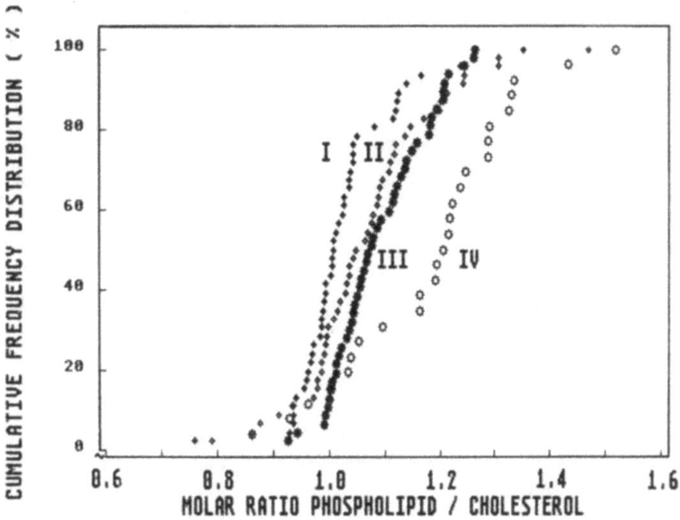

Fig. 5. Cumulative frequency distribution of the molar phospholipid to cholesterol ratio in human erythrocyte ghosts. Donors and age groups as in Fig. 3

between the four age groups. But the test yielded values of $P < 0.01$ for membrane cholesterol and of $P < 0.001$ for the molar phospholipid to cholesterol ratio (Table 2).

The cumulative frequency distributions of the individual values of the membrane cholesterol and phospholipid concentrations and the molar phospholipid to cholesterol ratio are depicted in Figs. 3–5 for each age group.

Discussion of Results

The dynamic exchange processes involving the red blood cell (RBC) membrane cholesterol and the different body pools, as well as the pool sizes, have been reported to be associated with age (Malhotra and Kritchevsky 1975; Miller 1987; Van Meer 1987). Therefore, RBC membranes have been suggested as a tool for monitoring the other cells (Rifkind et al. 1985; Shinitzky 1987). But the alterations of erythrocyte lipids with donor age are still subject to controversy (Table 3), as is the RBC membrane fluidity (Hegner et al. 1979; Butterfield et al. 1982). In a comparative study Hegner et al. (1979) disclosed age-dependent physiochemical and biochemical alterations of human red cell membranes. They compared young (< 30 years) and old (> 70 years) persons. The phospholipid content in red cell membranes of old donors was significantly lower than in the young ones. Cholesterol and fatty acid composition revealed no difference between the two donor groups. However, there was no differentiation of the old donors with respect to age. In general, attention has to be paid to some basic features when comparing reports of age-associated alterations of red cell lipids (Table 4).

Table 3. Changes of lipid composition in red cell membranes with donor age

Donor age (years)	No.	Tissue	Cholesterol	Phospholipids	Reference
18 – 95	68	Red cells	+	0	Araki and Rifkind (1980)
<30, >70	10, 35	Ghosts	0	–	Heger et al. (1979)
70 – 95	9	Red cells	NR	–	Gold and Altschuler (1972)[a]
20 – 40	10				Dodge and Phillips (1967) Jaffé and Gottfried (1968)
70 – 95	9	Plasma	NR	–	Gold and Altschuler (1972)[b]
20 – 40					Boon et al. (1969) Phillips and Dodge (1967)

+, increase; –, decrease; 0, constant.
[a] As compared to Dodge and Phillips (1967) and Jaffé and Gottfried (1968).
[b] As compared to Boon et al. (1969) and Phillips and Dodge (1967).
NR = not reported.

Table 4. Basic features for donor age-specific comparisons of red cell lipids

1. Participants' age	Age limit settings Size of age intervals
2. Participants' health status	Relatively fit elderly Geriatric patients
3. Reference base for expressing analytical results	Volume of packed cells Cell number Protein content Weight of lyophilized ghosts

Many studies in developed countries around the world have demonstrated in both sexes a uniform pattern of mean plasma total cholesterol and low density lipoprotein (LDL) cholesterol concentrations with age (Fig. 6): the lowest levels in early adulthood rise gradually to a maximum in the sixth decade of life, and decline thereafter (Keys et al. 1950; Masoro 1976; Gillibrand et al. 1980; Jacobs et al. 1980; Connor et al. 1982; Miller and Miller 1983; Heckers and Platt 1985; Mattila et al. 1986; Hayashi et al. 1987; Kasim and Kreisberg 1988; Vallés et al. 1988). There are some variations as to the age at which peak levels occur and the extent to which the concentrations fall in the last period of life. These trends, observed in cross-sectional studies, have been confirmed by longitudinal surveillance (Miller 1984). It was postulated that the age-related rise in serum cholesterol level is due to an acquired decline in LDL receptor activity (Miller 1984), but a contribution of both fractional clearance rates of LDL and production rates of apo-LDL has been reported (Grundy et al. 1988). The progressive increase in plasma total and LDL cholesterol levels with age does not occur in all societies, suggesting that dietary, environmental, and ethnic factors could, among others, account for the plasma cholesterol rise in developed countries (Masoro 1976;

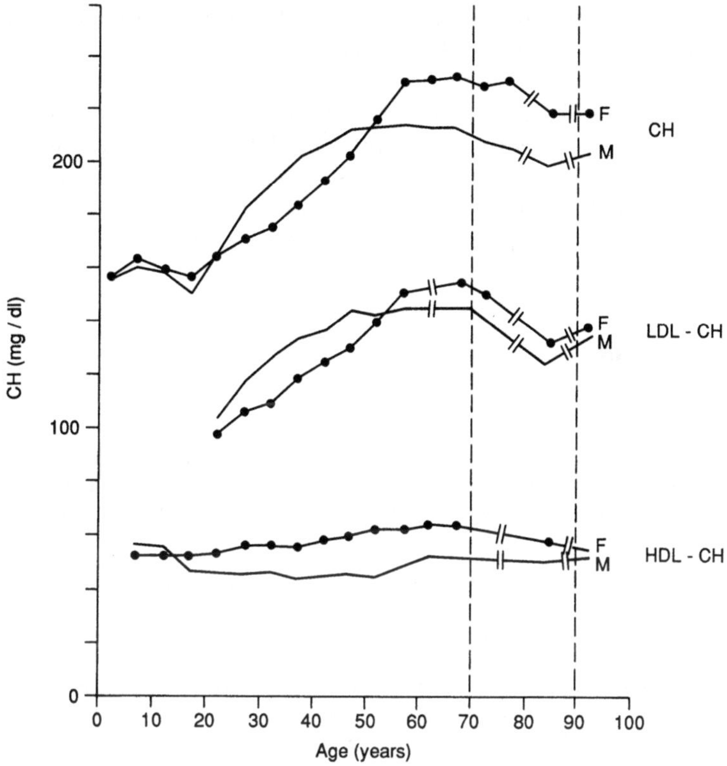

Fig. 6. Mean values of plasma total cholesterol *(CH)*, low density lipoprotein cholesterol *(LDL-CH)*, and high density lipoprotein cholesterol *(HDL-CH)* in males *(M)* and females *(F)* of different age groups (according to Heckers and Platt 1985). The age range of participants of the present study is indicated by *dashed lines*

Kasim and Kreisberg 1988). These factors also may be responsible for the decline in the serum cholesterol concentration in late adulthood, but the possibility that this decline is a survival artifact due to atherosclerotic accidents cannot be excluded.

Figure 3 demonstrates that at the age of 70 years and over one can observe a gradual decrease in cholesterol concentrations in RBC membranes, in parallel to the known plasma pattern with further advancing donor age. As a consequence, the molar phospholipid to cholesterol ratio increases with age (Fig. 5). These alterations do not necessarily indicate any increase in membrane fluidity, since (a) no measurements of fluidity have been performed with our material and (b) membrane microviscosity is regulated by different processes, which not only have been observed to vary with age but also are reported to compensate the effects of each other to guarantee homeostasis (Popp-Snijders et al. 1986). A reduced activity of lecithin-cholesterol-acyltransferase (LCAT) may provide a mechanism for the regulation of the exchangeable cholesterol pool in the plasma in old age. A decline in LCAT activity with age has been noted (Takeuchi et al. 1983). In old age the red cells' age distribution in man is normal (Woodford et al. 1962; Hurdle and Rosin 1962), but recently Glass et al. (1985) reported evidence of increased, well-compensated red cell turnover in elderly humans, with almost twice as many reticulocytes in the circulation and an increased percentage of low density young erythrocytes. Whether such an increase with donor age is responsible for our observations has not yet been proven. However, these results indicate why one might get different results in studies of age-dependent membrane lipid alterations if only rough age group divisions are made (e. g., subjects under age 60 vs those over age 60, or subjects younger than 30 years vs those older than 70 years).

Discussion

Linke

I've a question concerning the membrane composition. Do you know whether it changes with the diet? Do you control for it, or what is the variation of the membrane composition due to diet? Perhaps young people eat a different diet, a more modern one, than older individuals.

Brosche

The last point of your question seems to me very important. But you can't change the phospholipid content of erythrocyte lipids simply by eating another diet. If you have a diet enriched with lecithin it may be possible, but normally you don't see any significant change. With dietary cholesterol and healthy test persons it's all the same: you see no difference in the medium range of time in the membranes. We have controlled the diets by the way we designed the study: the study was done within 5 years and we had low numbers of participants in groups at different places, which were analyzed successively. We suppose that changes in diet are compensated in this way, if any have occurred.

Frenzel

Aging in respect to erythrocytes may have two meanings: aging of the individual erythrocyte and aging of the patient. What is known about the aging effect on the membrane of erythrocytes?

Brosche

There are numerous changes in cell aging of erythrocytes. Density is higher in older cells and there is some loss of membrane material by vesiculation, but there is no preferential loss of distinct subclasses of lipids; a loss is observed over the entire classes.

Platt

Perhaps I can add to this. It is not the same if you have a red cell of a young person or of an old person. We looked – I think 15 years ago – at the activities of ATPases depending on the age of the proband and depending on the age of the red cell and there were quite substantial differences. There was a decrease in the activities depending on the proband's age but not depending on the age of the isolated cell. So we must distinguish between red cell aging per age of the cell and of the patient or proband. This is very important.

Brosche

It has been believed that the age distribution of the red cells is constant within donor age, but Gershon's group has shown in recent years that there is a well compensated increase in turnover of red cells in old age. Perhaps this fact is responsible for some age-associated changes, but there are probably other reasons.

Frenzel

I want to come back to the individual erythrocyte. Why is an old erythrocyte filtered out of the bloodstream by the spleen or by the Kupffer cells in the liver? Are membrane alterations responsible for this selection process?

Brosche

The next presentation (Vömel) will deal with this topic.

Greiling

Have you evidence that there are age-dependent changes in the biosynthesis of the lipoproteins, or is there an age-dependent process in the degradation processes? My second question: Do plasma lipoproteins influence the biosynthesis or degradation processes of the lipoproteins in the cell membrane? This would be an age-dependent regulatory effect on the biosynthesis or degradation of the lipoproteins.

Brosche

One can speculate that the enzyme LCAT (lecithin-cholesterol acyltransferase) is involved in these processes. LCAT has been reported by a Japanese group [N. Takeuchi et al. (1983) Arch Gerontol Geriatr 2: 41–48] to show a donor age-dependent decline in activity. It is believed to be involved indirectly in the exchange processes between the plasma membrane and the lipoproteins, and in this way to remove free cholesterol from the cell membrane. This would be one possibility of regulation. The work on lipoprotein biosynthesis and degradation in old age is in progress; I have no clear answer to this point.

Hager

Did you compare your data with data from a control group of young people? I ask because we did some studies on the lipid compositon of platelet membranes and we also found an increase in the phospholipid to cholesterol ratio with donor age. But we compared a group of young people aged about 22 years and an older age group with a mean age of, I think, 72 years.

Brosche

We did compare four age groups, from 70 to 90 years, each covering 5 years.

Hager

I have another point. I think that your results are somewhat in contrast to those of Professor Hegner. Hegner showed an increase in the cholesterol-phospholipid ratio in red blood cells.

Brosche

No. Hegner and co-workers compared the age groups below 30 and over 70 years as a whole. If there is a decline in cholestrol values in very old age, then the values, which at first are quite different from those of younger people, become progressively more similar to them again.

Platt

The point is that one must distinguish between whether one is studying the 70- to 90-year age group as a whole or different subgroups within this range. I was one of the co-authors of Hegner and Heckers, and we only looked at a total group compared with 20- to 30-year-olds. This new work by Brosche and myself was to distinguish between 5-year age groups at the higher age.

Hofecker

I think there is one more interesting aspect: if we study populations at a high age and compare, for instance, ages of 70 to 90, we find an "age selection effect," so that the values may change to what we could say is a lower biological age. I think that this is the case with the curves you have shown for LDL cholesterol, which increases up to 70 years and then goes down. Here, statistics can cause the impression that the individuals become biologically younger but I think that this is rather a question of "age selection," which means that only those survive who possess a better functionality of their body systems.

Brosche

I totally agree with you and would add a second point of criticism: the question is whether this increase in plasma cholesterol values is a physiological one. There are populations in which it doesn't occur.

Medvedev

Does the life span of red blood cells decline in these very old individuals or is it the same as in the young?

Brosche

The Ghershon group says there is a decline, but other groups say there is none. I didn't make measurements.

References

Araki K, Rifkind JM (1980) Erythrocyte membrane cholesterol: an explanation of the aging effect on the rate of hemolysis. Life Sci 26: 2223–2230

Boon J, Broekhuyse RM, van Münster P, Schretlen E (1969) Abnormal patterns of the phospholipids of plasma and erythrocytes in four children with obstructive jaundice with abnormal spontaneous hemolysis. Clin Chim Acta 23: 453–456

Brasaemle DL, Robertson AD, Attie AD (1988) Transbilayer movement of cholesterol in the human erythrocyte membrane. J Lipid Res 29: 481–489

Bretscher MS (1973) Membrane structure: some general principles. Science 181: 622–629

Brosche T, Heckers H, Platt D, Summa JD (1986) The effect of different fat supplemented diets on the erythrocyte ghosts and plasma lipid composition of geriatric subjects. Arch Gerontol Geriatr 5: 83–95

Butterfield DA, Ordaz FE, Markesbery WR (1982) Spin label studies of human erythrocyte membranes in aging. J Gerontol 37: 535–539

Connor SL, Connor WE, Sexton G, Calvin L, Bacon S (1982) The effects of age, body weight and family relationships on plasma lipoproteins and lipids in men, women and children of randomly selected families. Circulation 65: 1290–1298

Dodge JT, Phillips GB (1967) Composition of phospholipids and of phospholipid fatty acids and aldehydes in human red cells. J Lipid Res 8: 667–675

Flamm M, Schachter D (1982) Acanthocytosis and cholesterol enrichment decrease lipid fluidity of only the outer human erythrocyte membrane leaflet. Nature 298: 290–292

Gattegno L, Bladier D, Cornillot P (1975) Ageing in vivo and neuraminidase treatment of rabbit erythrocytes: influence on half-life as assessed by ^{51}Cr labelling. Hoppe-Seyler's Z Physiol Chem 356: 391–397

Gillibrand D, Grewal D, Blattler DP (1980) Chemistry reference values as a function of age and sex, including pediatric and geriatric subjects. In: Dietz AA (ed) Aging – its chemistry. The American Association for Clinical Chemistry, Washington DC, pp 366–389

Glass GA, Gershon D, Gershon H (1985) Some characteristics of the human erythrocyte as a function of donor and cell age. Exp Hematol 13: 1122–1126

Gold M, Altschuler H (1972) Red blood cell and plasma phospholipids in aged humans. J Gerontol 27: 444–450

Grundy SM, Vega GL, Bilheimer DW (1988) Kinetic mechanisms determining variability in low density lipoprotein levels and rise with age. Arteriosclerosis 5: 623–630

Hanahan DJ (1969) Characterization of the erythrocyte membrane. In: Jamieson GA, Greenwalt TJ (eds) Red cell membrane, structure and function. JB Lippincott Company, Philadelphia & Torontp, pp. 83–92

Hayashi R, Kogure S, Sakaibori K, Kurihara S, Kasagi J, Murata K (1987) Serum cholesterol level in normal people-association of serum cholesterol level with age and relative body weight. Jpn J Med 26: 153–157

Heckers H, Platt D (1985) Lipide und Lipoproteine im Alter und hohen Alter. Einflußfaktoren, Prävalenzen von Abnormitäten und prognostische Bedeutung. Akt Endokrinol Stoffw 6: 11–24

Heckers H, Platt D (1988) Red cell membrane lipids and aging. In: Platt D (ed) Blood cells, rheology and aging. Springer, Berlin Heidelberg New York, pp 18–28
Hegner D (1980) Age-dependence of molecular and functional changes in biological membrane properties. Mech Ageing Dev 14: 101–118
Hegner D, Platt D, Heckers H, Schloeder U, Breuninger V (1979) Age-dependent physiochemical and biochemical studies of human red cell membranes. Mech Ageing Dev 10: 117–130
Hurdle ADF, Rosin AJ (1962) Red cell volume and red cell survival in normal aged people. J Clin Pathol 15: 343–345
Jacobs DR, Hunninghake DB, Dempsey ME et al. (1980) Blood lipids and lipoproteins in a Minnesota urban population. J Chron Dis 33: 395–406
Jaffé ER, Gottfried EL (1968) Hereditary nonspherocytic hemolytic disease associated with an altered phospholipid composition of the erythrocytes. J Clin Invest 47: 1375–1388
Kasim S, Kreisberg RA (1988) Lipoprotein metabolism and aging. In: Sowers JR, Felicetta JV (eds) The endocrinology of aging. Raven, New York, pp 175–194
Kay MMB (1985) Aging of cell membrane molecules leads to appearance of an aging antigen and removal of senescent cells. Gerontology 31: 215–235
Keys A, Mickelsen O, Miller EO, Hayes ER, Tood RL (1950) Concentration of cholesterol in blood serum of normal man and its relation to age. J Clin Invest 29: 1347–1353
Malhotra S, Kritchevsky D (1975) Cholesterol exchange between the red blood cells and plasma of young and old rats. Mech Ageing Dev 4: 137–145
Masoro EJ (1975) General considerations of membranes. In: Cristofalo VJ, Roberts J, Adelman RC (eds) Explorations in aging. Plenum, New York, pp 81–84
Masoro EJ (1976) Lipids and lipid metabolism as a function of aging. In: Elias MF, Eleftherion BE, Elias PK (eds) Special review of experimental aging research. EAR, Bar Harbor, Maine, pp 199–215
Mattila KS, Marniemi J, Mäki J, Juva K (1986) Lipids, lipoproteins and apoproteins in the elderly. Scand J Lab Invest 46: 131–136
Miller NE (1984) Why do plasma low density lipoprotein concentration in adults increase with age? Lancet I: 263–267
Miller NE (1987) On the associations of body cholesterol pool size with age, HDL cholesterol and plasma total cholesterol concentration in humans. Atherosclerosis 67: 163–172
Miller NE, Miller GJ (1983) Lipids and lipoproteins throughout the human lifespan in relation to ageing and atherosclerosis. In: Stout RE (ed) Medicine in old age – arterial disease. Churchill Livingstone, London, pp 32–56
Packer L, Deamer DW, Heath RL (1967) Regulation and deterioration of structure in membranes. Adv Geront Res 2: 77–120
Phornpiboonya Y, Jack RC (1980) Changes in stereospecific distribution of yeast fatty acids with age. Chem Phys Lipids 26: 57–66
Phillips GB, Dodge JT (1967) Composition of phospholipids and phospholipid fatty acids of human plasma. J Lipid Res 8: 676–681
Platt D, Schoch P (1974) Effect of age and cardiac glycosides on the activity of ATPase (EC 3.6.1.3) of red cell ghost membranes. Mech Ageing Dev 3: 245–252
Popp Snijders C, Schouten JA, Van Blitterswijk WJ, Van der Veen EA (1986) Changes in membrane lipid composition of human erythrocytes after dietary supplementation of (n-3) polyunsaturated fatty acids. Maintenance of membrane fluidity. Biochim Biophys Acta 854: 31–37
Rifkind JM, Araki K, Mohanty JG, Suda T (1985) Age dependent changes in erythrocyte membrane function. In: Eaton JW, Konzen DK, White JG (eds) Cellular and molecular aspects of aging: the red cell as a model. Alan R Liss, New York, pp 159–170
Rosenberg SA, Guidotti G (1968) The protein of human erythrocyte membranes. J Biol Chem 243: 1985–1992
Shinitzky M (1987) Patterns of lipid changes in membranes of the aged brain. Gerontology 33: 149–154
Strehler BL (1969) Molecular biology of aging. Naturwissenschaften 56: 57–61
Strunecka A, Folk P (1988) Phospholipid biosynthesis in mature human erythrocytes. Gen Physiol Biosphys 7: 205–216

Takeuchi N, Matsumoto A, Katayama Y, Arao M, Koga M, Nakao H, Uchida K (1983) Changes with aging in serum lipoproteins and apolipoprotein C subclasses. Arch Gerontol Geriatr 2: 41–48

Vácha J (1979) Critical comparative review of the life span of red blood cells in mammals. Acta Sc Nat Brno 13 (5): 1–47

Vallés J, Aznar J, Santos MT (1988) Composition of platelet fatty acids and their modulation by plasma fatty acids in humans: effect of age and sex. Atherosclerosis 71: 215–225

Van Meer G (1987) Plasma membrane cholesterol pools. TIBS 12: 375–376

Woodford WE, Webster D, Dixon MP, Mackenzie W (1962) Red cell longevity in old age. Gerontol Clin 4: 183–193

Zs-Nagy I (1979) The role of membrane structure and function in cellular aging: a review. Mech Ageing Dev 9: 237–246

Zwaal RFA, Roelofsen B, Comfurius P, Van Deenen LLM (1975) Organization of phospholipids in human red cell membranes as detected by the action of various purified phospholipases. Biochim Biophys Acta 406: 83–96

Age-Dependent Phagocytosis by Short-Term Cultured Kupffer Cells

T. VÖMEL [1]

Introduction

The reticulohistiocytic system (RHS), first described by Aschoff (1924), is distributed among all organs and tissue structures of the body. This leads to extraordinary difficulties in conducting investigations under standardized conditions, especially as the different cells of the RHS possess their own age kinetics (Wisse and Knook 1979). The liver constitutes a practical test organ, as it contain 80% – 90% of the cellular and functional capacity of the RHS (Munniksma et al. 1980).

Investigations of the phagocytic capacity can take place in the whole organism, in one organ (isolated liver perfusion), or in the cell culture. The exact standardization of complete organisms creates great problems. However, several questions could be answered by the isolated liver perfusion method, leaving other questions still open. For example, different ways of recognizing erythrocytes of various ages were found. Surprisingly, young erythrocytes were eliminated from the perfusion medium faster than old ones (Vömel and Platt 1982). But it is impossible to differentiate between the activity of old and young Kupffer cells in the isolated perfused liver.

After a reliable method for separating and isolating liver macrophages had been developed by Knook and Sleyster (1976), the short-term cultivation of Kupffer cells became a working model for studying the influence of macrophage age on the phagocytic reactions.

Material and Methods

Sprague-Dawley rats of our own extraction were used in these experiments (Vömel 1987). The liver preparation resembled the procedure for the perfusion of the whole organ (Vömel et al. 1981). The liver vein catheter was omitted, since there was no need to control perfusion flow.

Cell preparation was in accordance with the method of Knook and Sleyster (1976): First the prepared liver was perfused for 5 min in the open system with

[1] Hüttenhospital Dortmund-Hörde, Am Marksbach 28, D-4600 Dortmund / FRG

Gerontology
Ed. by D. Platt
© Springer-Verlag Berlin Heidelberg 1989

2% pronase buffer. Then followed 30 min cyclic perfusion with 0.05% pronase buffer and 0.5% collagenase at 37 °C. After this perfusion the Glisson capsule was removed and the liver was suspended in 0.02% pronase and 0.05% collagenase for 30 min at 37 °C. After two gauze filtrations the cells were centrifuged for 10 min at 500 × *g*. The liquid upper layer was sucked off and the remaining bottom layer containing the cells was mixed with 5 ml Hanks buffer and 7 ml 30% metrizamide solution. The resulting 17% metrizamide solution was overlaid with 2 ml Hanks buffer and centrifuged for 15 min at 2000 × *g*. This cleared the liver cells from cell detritus and erythrocytes and assembled them between the metrizamide solution and the buffer. The liver cells were collected from there into 10 ml buffer, centrifuged again for 10 min at 2000 × *g*, resuspended in a small volume, and checked for the intactness and number of the cells.

The cells were introduced into the rotor with a flow rate of 13.5 ml/min. The following flow rates for the extraction of different liver cell fractions were applied in accordance with Knook and Sleyster (1976). The lymphocytes left the rotor first at the initial 13.5 ml/min. The endothelial cells were elutriated at a flow rate of 22.5 ml/minute, and the intermediary cells at a flow rate of 33 ml/min. The Kupffer cells appeared at a flow rate of 43–45 ml/min. The elutriation volume amounted to 150 ml each time. After elutriation the cells were washed three times in Hanks buffer. The homogeneity of each fraction was controlled by the peroxidase reaction in accordance with Wisse (1974).

Homologous and heterologous erythrocytes of different ages were won by ultracentrifugation as described by Platt et al. (1979). The ink particles had a mean diameter of 5 μm. The mean diameters of the polyvinylpyrrolidone (PVP) particles were 0.51 and 1.1 μm, respectively.

The Kupffer and the endothelial cells resulting from the elutriation were cultured as liver cells, while the lymphocyte and the intermediary cell fractions were cast away. Pure fractions were defined as containing at least 95% endothelial cells or 80% Kupffer cells.

The endothelial cells were placed on a slide for cell cultures (Schirmer Labtec 4008) and cultured for 24 h at 37 °C in a medium evolved by Dulbecco and Vogt (1954). Each culture chamber contained 5×10^5 to 2×10^6 endothelial cells in 400 μl. Either 10 μg of ink or 10 μg of PVP particles or 10×10^6 erythrocytes was added to a chamber.

After 24 h cultivation the medium was decanted, the chamber tops were removed, and the cells were left to dry by air. Then the cell cultures were dyed according to May and Grünwald (1899) and put under the microscope for counting the number of colloidal particles adhering to or incorporated into macrophages.

Homologous erythrocytes of all age groups were offered for phagocytosis to the liver cells from ten animals aged 8–12, 22–26, and 30–36 months, forming nine groups. Heterologous human red blood cells (blood group 0 Rh negative) of all age groups were presented to liver cells from 8–12 and 30–36 month old rats. Ink and PVP particles of both diameters were used in all three age groups.

This led to 24 combinations with ten animals each, two slides and eight culture chambers per animal.

Results

The combinations described above showed significant differences between the phagocytosis of red blood cells and inert particles. Figures 1–3 demonstrate different slides. Previously the livers were perfused with colloidal carbon (Fig. 2), homologous red blood cells (Fig. 1), and PVP particles (Fig. 3). While ink and PVP were incorporated completely (Figs. 1, 3), erythrocytes only adhered to the macrophages (Fig. 2). Controls using fresh plasma for a culture fluid instead of

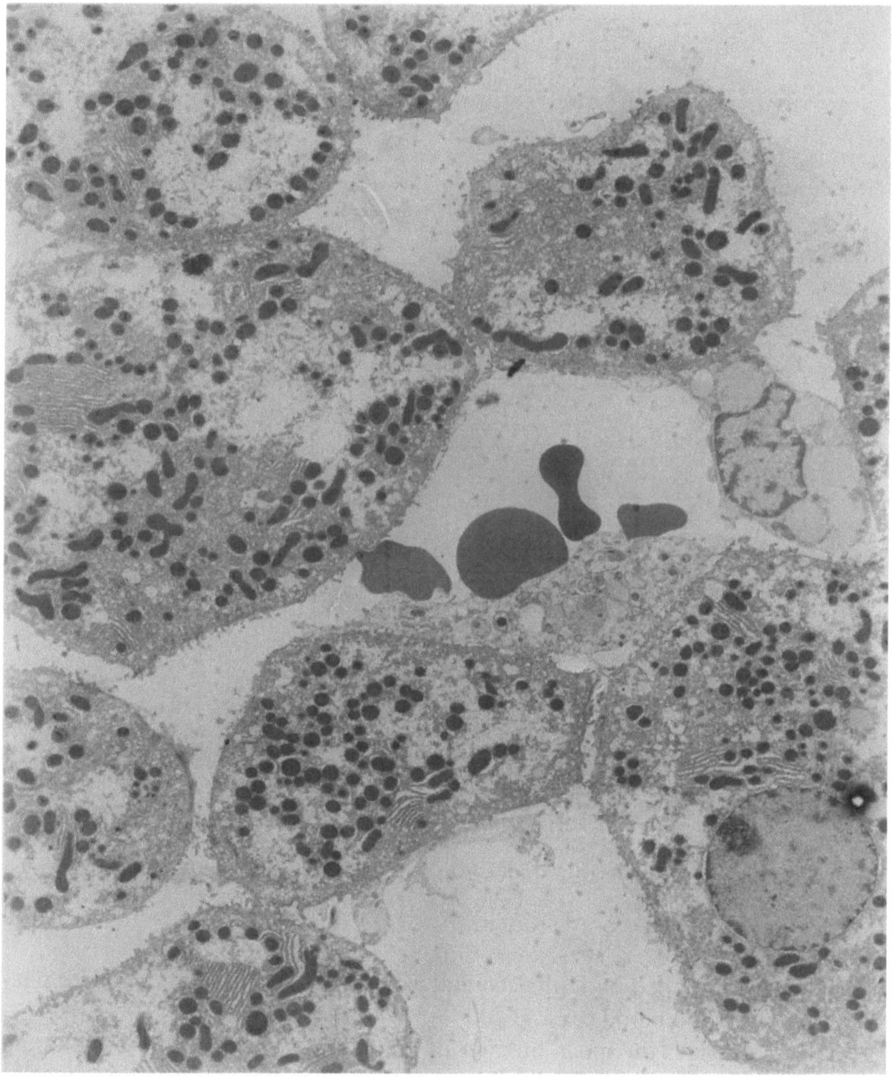

Fig. 1. Electron micrograph (× 8500) of a liver slide which shows a Kupffer cell with adhered red blood cells.

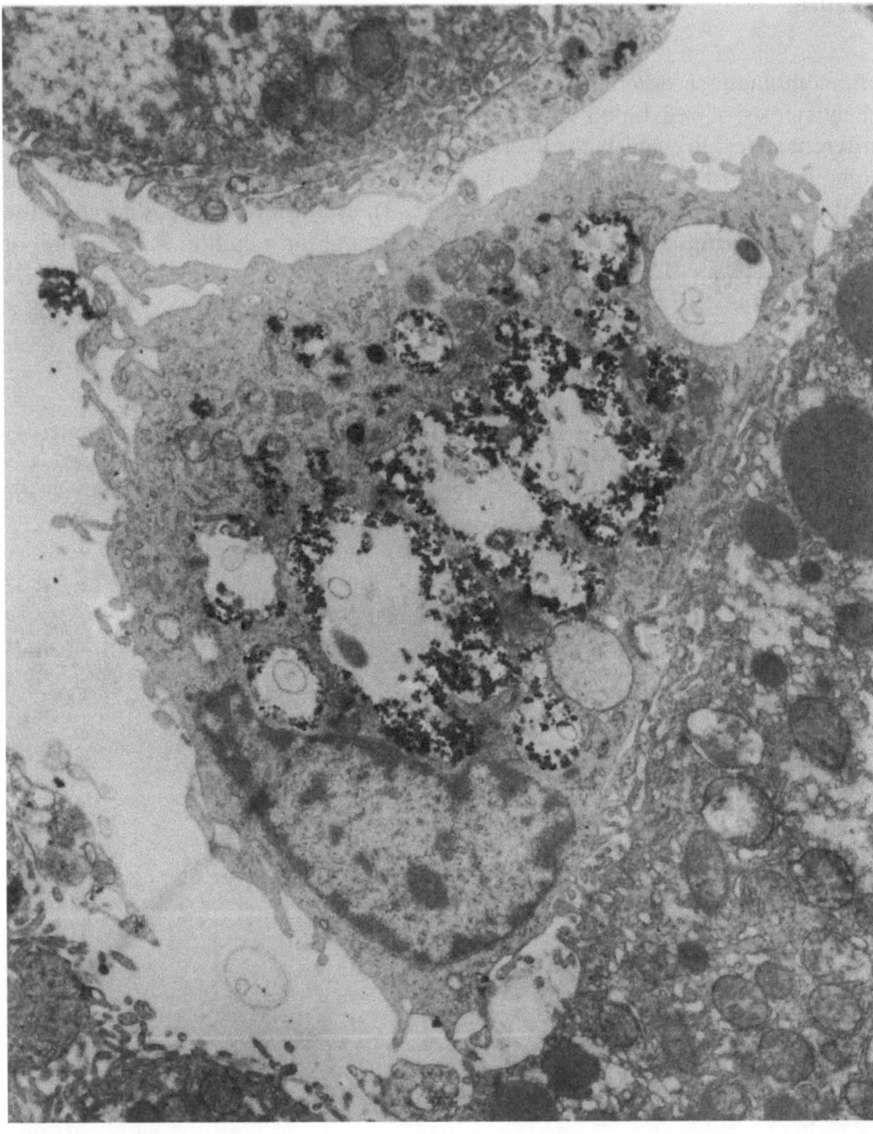

Fig. 2. Electron micrograph (× 10500) of a liver slide which shows a Kupffer cell with ingested colloidal carbon

the medium developed by Dulbecco and Vogt (1954) resulted in complete phagocytosis of the red blood cells, also.

Table 1a-d gives the mean number of particles phagocytosed by of adhering to the Kupffer cells. Table 2a-d demonstrates the significance of these values as won by the variance analysis with the comparison of multiple mean values (Sachs 1978).

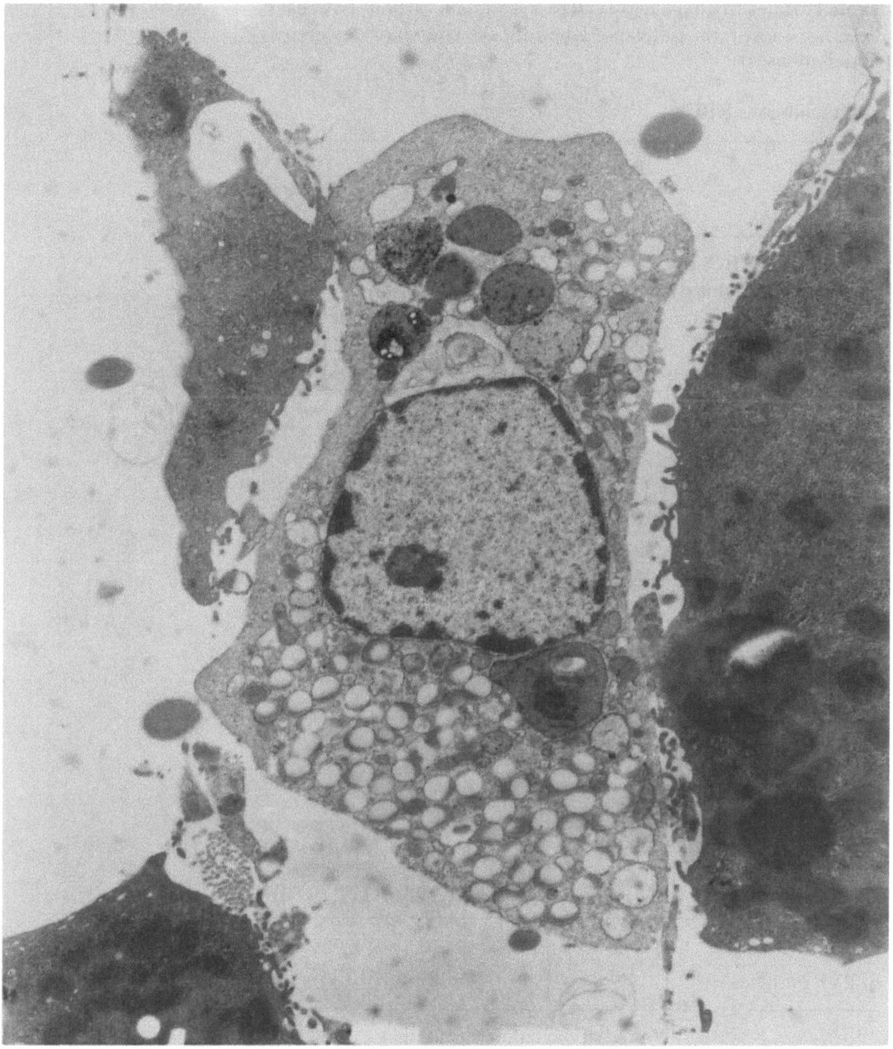

Fig. 3. Electron micrograph (× 12500) of a liver slide which shows a Kupffer cell with ingested PVP particles

Discussion

Approximately 56% of the monocytes change into Kupffer cells and continue to live in the liver for about 21 days (Crofton et al. 1978). The liver contains 80%–90% of the cellular and functional phagocytic capacity of the rat organism (Vömel and Platt 1981). This makes the liver an excellent model organ for studying phagocytosis. But investigations in the whole animal as well as in the isolated

Table 1. Rates of phagocytosis (RBCs, colloidal carbon, PVP particles) of short-term cultivated Kupffer cells (standard deviations in parentheses)

a. Homologous RBCs

	Age of the animals (months)		
	8–12	22–26	30–36
Homologous RBCs from animals aged (months)			
8–12	3.45 (0.21)	3.44 (0.23)	0.56 (0.23)
22–26	3.23 (0.31)	3.20 (0.33)	0.66 (0.26)
30–36	3.88 (0.32)	3.82 (0.34)	0.92 (0.55)

b. Human RBCs

	Age of the animals (months)		
	8–12	22–26	30–36
Young	1.31 (0.34)	∅	0.63 (0.19)
Middle aged	1.02 (0.36)	∅	0.66 (0.20)
Old	1.89 (0.39)	∅	1.12 (0.28)

c. Colloidal carbon

	Age of the animals (months)		
	8–12	22–26	30–36
Colloidal carbon	3.11 (0.88)	3.30 (0.79)	1.62 (0.82)

d. PVP particles

	Age of the animals (months)		
	8–12	22–26	30–36
∅ 0.51 μm	4.22 (0.69)	4.10 (0.76)	1.03 (0.62)
∅ 1.10 μm	3.36 (0.88)	3.34 (0.62)	1.30 (0.56)

perfused rat liver leave several questions open. In particular, it is impossible to differentiate clearly between the role of the hepatocytes and the Kupffer cells in phagocytosis. These questions can be further studied by cultivating isolated Kupffer cells and offering various phagocytic stimulants to them. Different phagocytic kinetics with regard to adherence as well as ingestion exist for the many colloidal particles (Vömel 1987), which makes it interesting to study them singly. Contrary

Table 2. Statistical evaluation of phagocytic activity of short-term cultivared Kupffer cells, depending on age of the animal and age of the RBCs. Age of the animals; y = 8–12 months; ma = 22–26 months; o = 30–36 months. * $P = 0.05$; ** $P = 0.01$; NS, not significant

a. Homologous RBCs

Animals/RBC	y/y	y/ma	y/O	ma/y	ma/ma	ma/O	O/y	O/ma	O/O
y/y	NS	*	*	NS	*	*	**	**	**
y/ma		NS	*	*	NS	*	**	**	**
y/a			NS	*	*	NS	**	**	**
ma/y				NS	*	*	**	**	**
ma/ma					NS	*	**	**	**
ma/O						NS	**	**	**

b. Human RBCs

RBC/animals	Young/y	Middle-aged/y	Old/y	Young/O	Middle-aged/O	Old/O
Young/y	NS	*	*	**	**	NS
Middle-aged/y		NS	*	*	*	NS
Old/y			NS	**	**	**

c. Colloidal carbon

Animals (age)	y	ma	O
y	NS	NS	*
ma		NS	*

d. PVP particles

Animals/PVP	y/0.51	y/1.10	ma/0.51	ma/1.10	O/0.51	O/1.10
y/0.51	NS	*	NS	*	**	**
y/1.10		NS	NS	**	**	*
ma/0.51			NS	NS	**	**
ma/1.10				NS	**	*
O/0.51					NS	NS
O/1.10						NS

findings on the activity of the phagocytic system have been reported in the literature. With advancing age Eder and Gedick (1974) found a reduced activity, while Vömel and Platt (1981) found an increase in the phagocytic activity. Everybody has agreed on a marked reduction in the phagocytic activity in very old organisms. This concurs with the findings in isolated Kupffer cells in this paper. But it was not possible to differentiate between the activity of old and young

Kupffer cells by referring to their liver life span. A reliable method for distinguishing these age groups still has to be developed.

The growth rate of the RHS cells is lower in old age, just like the reduplication rate of all other cell systems (Ueno 1971). But in the model of the isolated perfused liver as well as in the whole organism an age-dependent increase in the elimination of ink and cells was found by several authors (Perkins 1971; Hjelm 1974; Vömel and Platt 1981). However, the investigation of one substance cannot lead to valid overall statements on the RHS and its changes with age.

The elimination of erythrocytes presents a special case of phagocytosis. The whole organism as well as the phagocytosed and phagocytosing cells are subject to different, individual aging kinetics taking place at the same time. A host of models for the aging of red blood cells have been evolved from biochemical, biophysical, and morphological data. The age-dependent phagocytosis of erythrocytes acts mainly via two mechanisms: One trigger is formed by an increased rigidity due to a changed surface tension and a changed composition of the phospholipids in the membrane (Thomas and Vaez-Zadeh 1974; Bartosz 1981). The other mechanism starts with the removal of neuraminic acid from the end of the glycophorin molecules (Gattegno et al. 1975; Baxter and Beeley 1975). This reveals antigenetic structures, which are covered by immunoglobulins inducing phagocytosis (Kay 1985; Hunt et al. 1980). Until now, investigations of the whole organism and of the isolated perfused liver have shown the young and middle-aged fraction of erythrocytes to be phagocytosed faster than the fraction of old cells (Platt et al. 1979; Vömel and Platt 1981, 1982).

The results presented here demonstrate that the Kupffer cells are able to recognize erythrocytes of different ages without any extra help from other cells, the liver, or the whole organism. They prove the existence of an age-recognizing mechanism consisting of two components, the Kupffer cell and the red blood cell. The different rates of phagocytosis in various models is probably due to interactions between cells and organs in the whole organism. These interactions invite further investigations.

Summary

The age-dependent phagocytic activity of Kupffer cells from rat livers was investigated in the model of short-time cell culture. Homologous erythrocytes and human heterologous erythrocytes of different age groups, ink, and polyvinylpyrrolidone particles were offered for phagocytosis. The Kupffer cells from old animals showed a significantly lower rate of phagocytosis in all variations than the cells from young and middle-aged rats, which showed no significant difference. In the group of homologous erythrocytes the cells from old animals were eliminated significantly more than erythrocytes from young animals. In contrast to earlier findings in the isolated perfused liver and in the whole organism, old heterologous human erythrocytes were removed quicker than young and middle-aged ones. The results are discussed and related to other findings in literature.

References

Aschoff L (1924) Das Reticuloendothelialsystem. Ergeb Inn Med Kinderheilkd 25: 1–118
Barthosz G (1981) Aging of erythrocytes. Acta Biol Med Germ 40: 985–989
Baxter A, Beeley JG (1975) Changes in surface carbohydrate of human erythrocytes aged in vivo. Biochem Soc Trans 553: 132–136
Crofton RW, Diesselhoff-Den Dulk MC, van Furth R (1978) The origin, kinetics and characteristics of the Kupffer cells in the normal steady state. J Exp Med 148: 1–17
Dulbecco R, Vogt M (1954) Modified minimal essential medium for tissue culture. Cap Med 99: 167–182
Eder M, Gedick P (1974) Lehrbuch der allgemeinen Pathologie und der pathologischen Anatomie. Springer, Berlin Heidelberg New York
Gattegno L, Bladier D, Cornillot P (1975) Aging in vivo and neuraminidase-treatment of rabbit erythrocytes. Influence on half life. Hoppe Seyler's Z Physiol Chem 356: 3391–3397
Hjelm M (1974) Methodological aspects of current procedures to separate erythrocytes into age groups. In: Yoshikawa H, Rapoport S (eds) Cellular and molecular biology of erythrocytes. Urban & Schwarzenberg, Berlin, pp 427–444
Hunt JS, Beck ML, Hardmann JT, Tegtmeier GE, Bayer WL (1980) Characterization of human erythrocyte alloantibodies by IgG subclass and monocyte interaction. Am J Clin Pathol 74: 735–738
Kay MMB (1985) Aging of cell membrane molecules leads to appearance of an aging antigen and removal of senescent cells. Gerontology 91: 215–235
Knook DL, Sleyster EC (1976) Separation of Kupffer and endothelial cells of the rat liver by centrifugal elutriation. Exp Cell Res 99: 444–449
May R, Grünwald L (1899) Über Blutfärbungen. Centralbl Inn Med 23: 265–270
Munniksma JM, Noteborn M, Kooistra T et al. Fluid endocytosis by rat liver and spleen. Biochem J 192: 613–621
Perkins EH (1971) Phagocytic activity of aged mice. J Reticuloendothel Soc 9: 642–643
Platt D, Hofmann K-H, Vömel T (1979) Untersuchungen mit ^{59}Fe zur Frage der Lebensdauer von Kaninchen-Erythrozyten. Z Gerontol 12: 60–72
Sachs L (1978) Angewandte Statistik – statistische Methoden und ihre Anwendungen, Springer, Berlin Heidelberg New York
Thoms HL, Vaez-Zadeh V (1974) A homeostatic mechanism for the removal of antigen from the portal circulation. Immunology 26: 375–382
Ueno Y (1971) Radiosensitivities of the haematopoietic system in young and old mice. Exp Gerontol 8: 469–475
Vömel T (1987) Alter und Phagozytose – am Modell der isoliert perfundierten Rattenleber. Habilitationsschrift, Erlangen
Vömel T, Platt D (1981) Lifespan of rabbit erythrocytes and activity of the reticulohistiocytic system. Mech Ageing 17: 261–266
Vömel T, Platt D (1982) Age-dependent red cell phagocytosis and activity of the rabbit reticulohistiocytic system. Gerontology 28: 149–155
Vömel T, Platt D, Schnorr B (1981) Untersuchungen zur Phagozytoseaktivität der isoliert perfundierten Leber unterschiedlich alter Ratten. Fortschr Med 99: 261–266
Wisse E (1974) Observations on the fine structure and peroxidase cytochemistry of normal rat liver Kupffer cells. J. Ultrastruct Res 46: 393–426
Wisse E, Knook DL (1979) The investigation of sinusoidal cells: a new approach to the study of liver function. Prog Liver Dis 4: 153–171

Aging at the Organ Level

Changes of Myocardial Structure with Aging

H. Frenzel[1,2], R. Zweihoff[1], B. Schwartzkopff[1], and K.-F. Bürrig[1]

Introduction

The functional capacity of the heart declines with advancing age (Gerstenblith et al. 1976; Lakatta 1979; Lakatta und Yin 1982). The diminished cardiac adaptability to stress in senescence could provide an explanation why heart insufficiency and cardiac death occur in older people even upon only a minor increase in demand (Wei and Gersh 1987). Most of the morphological studies of the hearts of old people therefore have the aim of finding a structural correlate for the reduced functional capacity in old age. A whole range of findings on the hearts of elderly humans have been compiled (Pomerance 1968; Linzbach 1972): In autopsy studies, an increasing degree of coronary atherosclerosis was found with advancing age (Linzbach 1972) as well as increased fibrosis of the small intramural cardiac vessels (Rahlf 1980). Typical age-related changes of the cardiac valves are calcification of the mitral valve ring and the aortic valves (Pomerance 1967, 1970; Pomerance et al. 1978; Waller and Roberts 1983). Mitral valve prolapse and mucoid degeneration are further alterations which are observed more frequently in senescent people (Pomerance 1969).

It could be shown that the heart in senescence does not undergo atrophy; rather the heart weight increases as a consequence of an elevation of the blood pressure with advancing age (Linzbach and Akuamoa-Boateng 1973). The ability of the myocytes to develop hypertrophic growth which is characterized by an increase in DNA and protein synthesis is maintained even in old age (Rosenberg and Pfitzer 1983; Adler and Friedberg 1986). However, a decreased rate of RNA and protein synthesis in the aged myocardium has been reported by others (Johnson et al. 1975; Meerson et al. 1978).

Light and electron microscopic examination of the myocardium reveals additional findings which are common in old age (Frenzel 1985): amyloid deposits in the heart (Hodkinson and Pomerance 1977; Westermark et al. 1979; Cornwell et al. 1983; Linke 1983; Olson et al. 1987), a deposition of fine-fibrillar glycogen-like material in some of the myocytes, which is known as basophilic degeneration (Kosek and Angell 1970; Rosai and Lascona 1970), and an increase in lipofuscin pigment (Strehler et al. 1959; Ikeda et al. 1985). Lipofuscin particles are residual

---

[1] Pathologisches Institut der Universität Düsseldorf, Moorenstr. 5, D-4000 Düsseldorf 1 / FRG
[2] Present address: Institut für Pathologie des Städtischen Klinikums Karlsruhe, Postfach 6280, D-7500 Karlsruhe 1 / FRG

Gerontology
Ed. by D. Platt
© Springer-Verlag Berlin Heidelberg 1989

bodies of intracellular degradation of cell organelles, especially mitochondria, which change their structural composition with advancing age (Frenzel 1985; Ikeda et al. 1985). With the exception of Koobs et al. (1978) authors have supposed the increase in lipofuscin to be of minor or nonfunctional importance.

In a fine-structural study of myocardial biopsies from 15 tumor patients, aged between 28 and 75 years, who underwent biopsy before the commencement of adriamycin therapy, Unverferth et al. (1986) found larger nuclei and a more severe folding of the intercalated discs, which is said to indicate increased protein synthesis. In addition, as already reported in older animals (Travis and Travis 1972; Tomanek and Karlsson 1973), a greater number of fat droplets and dilated T tubuli were seen, while an increased collagen content of the interstitial space was not obvious.

Experimental Studies

None of the above-mentioned qualitative changes reported in the hearts of aged people can be regarded as the definitive age-specific change restricting the range of cardiac functional capacity. The explanation could be that growth and aging of the myocardium is more a quantitative than a qualitative phenomenon. So far, there are no comprehensive quantitative studies of the myocardium in old age.

The myocardium consists mainly of myocytes, interstitium, and the vascular system. From a morphological point of view these structural elements represent a functional-structural unit. Primary changes to any one of these structural elements can result in secondary changes to the remaining constituent parts of the myocardium. Even minor changes become important because not infrequently they affect the entire cardiac muscle. A change in the composition of the myocardium can substantially impair the pumping function of the heart.

As a rule hearts from autopsies are unsuitable for fine-structural studies of the myocardium because of advanced autolysis. Endomyocardial biopsies are indicated only with particular diseases of the heart and are therefore unavailable from people of various ages with healthy hearts. Using morphometric methods we compared the left ventricular myocardium from rats of various ages (Zweihoff et al. in preparation). The results are summarized in Tables 1 and 2.

The investigated male Wistar rats were 3, 8, and 30 months old. The spontaneous mortality for 30-month-old animals of this breed is about 38%. While the body weight continuously rose with advancing age, the heart weight significantly increased only during the growth period and merely showed a trend towards further increase with aging. Like heart weight, the thickness of the myocytes increased significantly during the growth period while the difference between adult and aged rats was not significant. During the physiological growth of the heart a disproportional increase in the myocyte mass and the interstitium occured: the volumetric proportion of the interstitium had increased in the adult rats whereas the volume density of myocytes had decreased as compared to the young animals. In the aged rats the proportion of the interstitium had further increased

Table 1. Quantitative analysis of left ventricular myocardium from rats of various ages

Parameter	Young rats (3 months)	Adult rats (8 months)	Old rats (30 months)
Body weight (g)	289 ± 10	391 ± 7[a]	535 ± 51[b]
Heart weight (g)	0.84 ± 0.09	1.16 ± 0.09[a]	1.24 ± 0.12
Body weight/ heart weight (mg/g)	2.89 ± 0.22	3.28 ± 0.5	2.34 ± 0.19[b]
Thickness of myocytes (μm)	17.37 ± 0.86	19.31 ± 0.81[a]	20.20 ± 1.02
Vv myocytes (%)	85.66 ± 1.18	83.62 ± 1.22[a]	81.00 ± 0.70[b]
Vv interstitium (%)	14.34 ± 1.18	16.38 ± 1.22[a]	19.00 ± 0.70[b]
Vv collagenous fibers (%)	1.85 ± 0.25	2.49 ± 0.29[a]	4.22 ± 0.75[b]
Calculated number of myocytes (× 10^6)	43.51 ± 3.45	43.09 ± 2.88	38.14 ± 2.92[b]
Capillary density (transversel sections) (1/mm^2)	3898 ± 499	3034 ± 169[a]	3121 ± 263
Capillary density (longitudinal sections) (1/mm^2)	332 ± 70	336 ± 101	298 ± 81
Sv capillaries (mm^2/mm^3)	63.22 ± 5.62	52.41 ± 2.65[a]	46.26 ± 3.53[b]
Vv capillaries (%)	10.49 ± 1.43	9.63 ± 1.12	7.68 ± 1.16[b]
Diameter of capillaries (μm)	5.28 ± 0.3	5.66 ± 0.27	4.93 ± 0.12[b]
Thickness of capillary basement membrane (nm)	42.10 ± 2.99	46.30 ± 2.88[a]	58.52 ± 4.14[b]
Thickness of capillary endothelial cells (nm)	141 ± 14.8	145 ± 15.6	157 ± 16.2
Intercapillary distance (μm)	12.02 ± 1.08	13.87 ± 0.46[a]	14.35 ± 0.71
Vv mitochondria, total (%)	28.94 ± 4.01	32.55 ± 2.92	33.31 ± 1.96
Vv mitochondria, subsarcolemmal compartment (%)	32.56 ± 5.11	37.75 ± 4.23	39.47 ± 2.58
Vv mitochondria, inner compartment (%)	27.20 ± 4.01	28.86 ± 3.05	30.13 ± 1.85

Vv, volume density; Sv, surface density.
[a] Difference between young and adult rats statistically significant ($P < 0.05$).
[b] Difference between adult and old rats statistically significant ($P < 0.05$).

while the volume density of the myocytes was correspondingly reduced. In preceding studies we had been able to show that the increase in the interstitium of the right ventricular wall surpasses that of the left ventricular wall significantly (Frenzel and Feimann 1984), which could be explained by a rising pressure load of the right ventricle due to pulmonary alterations with aging.

The interstitium consists of mesenchymal cells, collagenous fibers, and capillaries. These structures are embedded in a ground substance containing proteoglycans, the composition of which is subject to age-related changes (Lindner 1983).

Table 2. Changes of myocardial structure of rats with growth and aging[a]

Parameter	Growth period	Aging
Body weight	35% ↑	37% ↑
Heart weight	38% ↑	NS
Thickness of myocytes	11% ↑	NS
Vv myocytes	2% ↓	3% ↓
Vv interstitium	14% ↑	16% ↑
Vv collagenous fibers	35% ↑	70% ↑
Calculated number of myocytes ($\times 10^6$)	NS	13% ↓
Capillary density (transversel sections)	22% ↓	NS
Capillary density (longitudinal sections)	NS	NS
Sv capillaries	17% ↓	12% ↓
Vv capillaries	NS	20% ↓
Diameter of capillaries	NS	13% ↓
Thickness of capillary basement membrane	10% ↑	26% ↑
Thickness of capillary endothelial cells	NS	NS
Intercapillary distance	15% ↑	NS
Vv mitochondria, total	NS	NS
Vv mitochondria, subsarcolemmal compartment	NS	NS
Vv mitochondria, inner compartment	NS	NS

[a] Percent values represent significant differences ($P < 0.05$) between young and adult rats (growth period) and adult and old rats (aging).
↑, increase; ↓, decrease; Vv, volume density; Sv, surface density.

The collagenous fiber content of the interstitium rises continuously with advancing age of the rats (Coleman et al. 1987). From the heart weight and morphometrically obtained data, a decrease of about 13% in the number of myocytes in the myocardium of old rats could be calculated. By counting the number of nuclei in the myocardium, Anversa et al. (1986b) determined a loss of myocytes at 18% in the subendocardial region of the left ventricle of 24-month-old-rats as compared to young rats. This cell loss led to compensatory hypertrophy of the remaining myocytes. In our study, however, the calculated loss of myocytes was in a lower range; correspondingly, there was only a tendency for the heart weight and the muscle fiber thickness to increase in the old animals. A patchy fibrosis was the only qualitative finding by which myocardium of adult and aged rats could be discriminated (Fig. 1). This replacement fibrosis is probably the consequence of a loss of myocytes in the aged myocardium. In hearts of old humans, however, a reduction of myocytes could not found to be an age-specific process (Adler and Friedburg 1986).

Sufficient vascularization of the myocardium is of great importance for unimpaired heart function. Enlargement of the heart during physiological and pathological growth is accompanied by a widening of the major epicardial coronary arteries, unless they have undergone pathological changes. It could be demonstrated that the diameter of the coronary arteries corresponds well with the volume of the heart and the heart weight (Hort et al. 1982; Thüroff et al. 1984). Using corrosion casts of human hearts of various weights it was calculated that the absolute number of small and very small intramural coronary arteries remains constant during heart growth (Reinecke and Hort 1988). However, little is known about the number of the minor coronary arteries in the aged myocardium. Capillaries serve as the final pathway for oxygen and substrate exchange. Substrate exchange between blood and tissue is mainly determined by the degree of capillarization. The knowledge of changes of capillarization during physiological growth and aging was expanded by our studies on rats of various ages.

Capillarization of the myocardium may be estimated from various morphometric parameters. Volume density of capillaries corresponds to flow capacity, surface density to oxygen delivery capacity. Capillary density is defined as the number of capillaries per area. It must be considered that the capillaries in the myocardium do not run exactly parallel to the myocytes, as is assumed for Krogh's model, and not randomly; rather they show a partially anisotropic arrangement. Therefore, evaluation of the number of capillaries on transversely and longitudinally cut myocardium is required. Evaluation of the myocardial capillaries on semithin sections has shown that the capillary density, i.e., the number of capillaries cut open in cross-sections of the myocardium, is lower in adult and elderly rats than in young animals, the difference between adult and elderly animals being nonsignificant. This finding is in accordance with those of Engelmann et al. (1987). On the other hand, Rakusan and Poupa (1964) and Tomanek (1970) found a further decrease in capillary density with aging and a reduced capillary/fiber ratio, which suggests that an obliteration of capillaries occurs. In longitudinal sections of the myocardium the number of circular transversely incised capillaries is largely constant in all three groups of animals. One can conclude from this that during physiological growth the numerical density of capillaries running longitudinally decreases on account of the thickening of the muscle fibers, whereas an increase occurs in the number of vascular branches as well as capillaries running transversely. The decrease in those capillaries running parallel to the myocytes results in an increased intercapillary distance in the myocardium of adult and old rats as compared to young animals. It is apparent that capillary density and intercapillary distance are influenced by growth but not by aging. The surface density of capillaries, however, continuously decreases with advancing age, and the volume density of capillaries has also diminished in old age, mainly as a result of a narrowing of the capillary lumina.

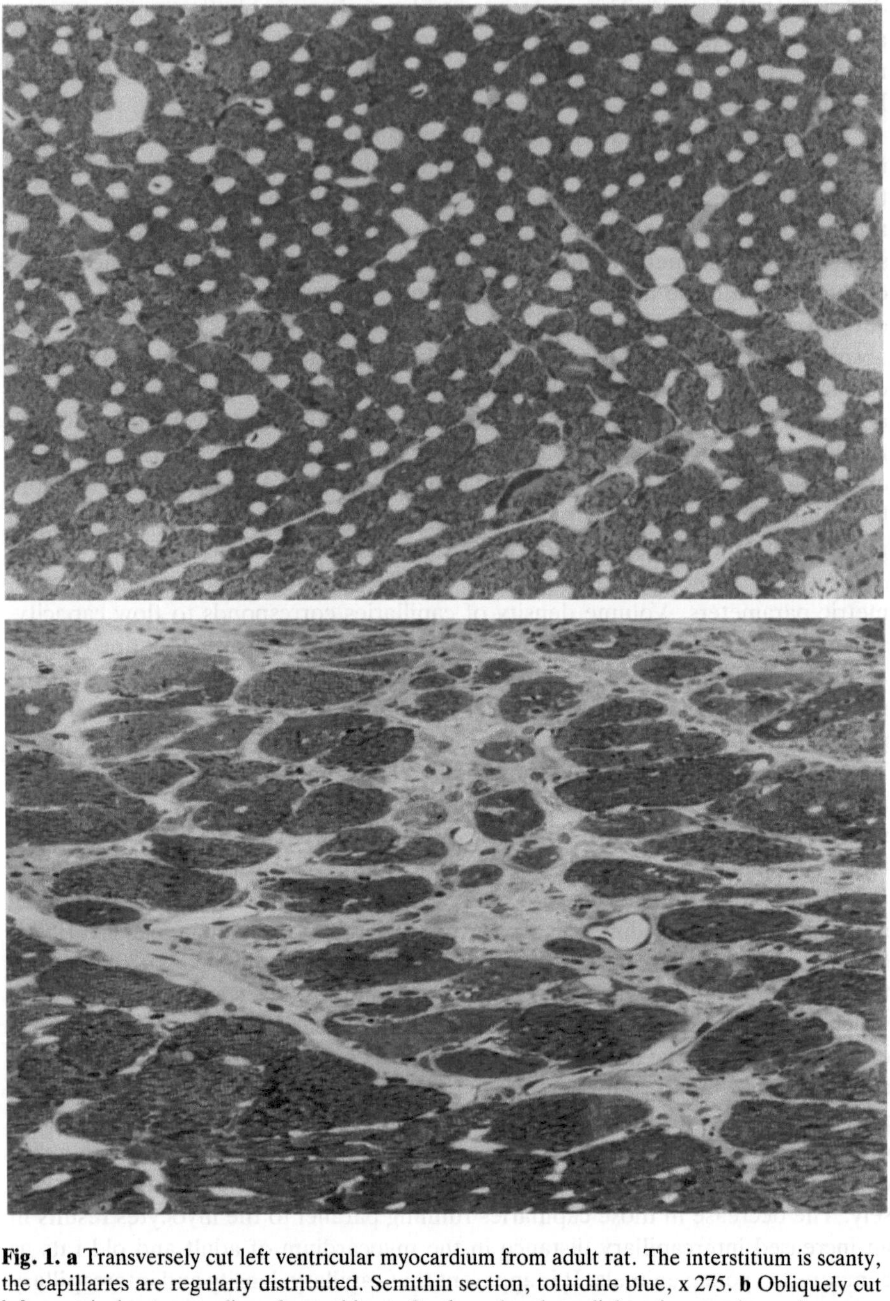

a

b

Fig. 1. a Transversely cut left ventricular myocardium from adult rat. The interstitium is scanty, the capillaries are regularly distributed. Semithin section, toluidine blue, x 275. **b** Obliquely cut left ventricular myocardium from old rat. In the subendocardial region patchy replacement fibrosis indicates a focal loss of myocytes. Semithin section, toluidine blue, x 200

Measurements on the capillary walls according to the method of Siperstein et al. (1973) have shown that the thickness of the basement membrane increases in old age. In the capillaries the basement membrane has a static function but probably also influences the permeability of the vessels. Age-related changes at the capillary wall could have an adverse effect on the exchange of oxygen and substrates between capillaries and myocytes. In this context, an interesting comparison can be made with diabetes mellitus, where a broadening of the capillary basement membrane also occurs in various organs. A nonenzymatic linking of glucose to free aminogroups is under discussion as the common priciple of these changes. The formation of glycosylation products appears to be a specific characteristic of diabetes but also of aging (Schnider and Kohn 1981).

The capillaries are the final route of the vascular system in which the exchange of oxygen and substrates between blood and parenchymal cells takes place. From morphometric studies on skeletal muscles it became evident that a relation exists between capillarization of a tissue unit and its oxidative capacity (Hoppeler and Kayar 1988). The oxidative capacity can be estimated by the mitochondrial volume per cell volume. The volume density of mitochondria corresponds well with the activity of mitochondrial enzymes and a positive linear relation has been demonstrated between the maximal oxygen consumption of the individual muscle and the volume density of mitochondria (Reichmann et al. 1985; Hoppeler et al. 1987). Quantitative studies on animals conditioned by strenuous endurance training have shown that in the event of training-induced hypertrophic growth of the heart a new formation of capillaries and an increase in the volume density of mitochondria are typical, which points to an adaptation to an increased demand (Anversa et al. 1986a; Mattfeldt et al. 1986; Frenzel et al. 1988). The volume density of mitochondria, however, is indicative of the oxidative capacity only under the precondition that no functional disorder of the mitochondria is present. With so-called mitochondriopathy, a functional inferiority results in compensatory hyperplasia of the mitochondria, i.e., mitochondriosis, although this is not an indication of an enhanced oxidative capacity (Egger et al. 1981).

Different results have been reported concerning age-dependent changes of mitochondria in myocytes. Sachs et al. (1977) found an increased volume density of mitochondria in aged Syrian hamsters, while Herbener (1976) was able to demonstrate an age-dependent decrease in mitochondrial volume density in myocytes of mice. No change of mitochondrial volume density in hearts of old rats was reported by Kment et al. (1966) and Schmucker and Sachs (1985). In our study, the volume density of mitochondria showed a trend towards an augmentation with advancing age, which was not significant. Previously it was established that there are differences in the mitochondrial size between young and old rats: in the elderly animals there was an increased number of mitochondria, with each individual mitochondrion being reduced in size (Kment et al. 1966; Frenzel and Feimann 1984). Tate and Herbener (1976), on the other hand, found a decreased number of mitochondria per volume unit of cytoplasm in aged mice, while mitochondrial average volume remained constant. The diminished mitochondrial cristae surface per volume unit of cytoplasm in old mice was only due to a decreased volume density of mitochondria (Tate and Herbener 1976). Sachs et al.

(1977), however, found a decreased area of mitochondrial inner membrane plus cristae per mitochondrial volume. These varying results may be explained by differences in the strain of the investigated animals, by their age and sex, and by different methodological procedures.

In this context, the arrangement of the mitochondria within the myocytes is of interest. Mitochondria are found in myocytes at three regions: perinuclear, intermyofibrillar, and under the sarcolemma. It has been demonstrated that subsarcolemmal and intermyofibrillar mitochondria isolated from cardiac muscle differ in their biochemical properties (Palmer et al. 1977). If one looks at a cross-section of the myocardium then it is apparent that there are differences in the topography of the mitochondria within the myocytes between young rats on the one hand and adult and elderly rats on the other. Whereas the mitochondria are relatively evenly distributed in the myocytes of the young animals (Fig. 2a), in adult and old animals mitochondrial clusters are frequently found under the sarcolemma and in the pericapillary region (Fig. 2b). We have determined the volume density of the mitochondria in an outer subsarcolemmal region, in a pericapillary area, and in the center of the myocytes. It could be shown that with growth and aging there is a greater increase in the volume density of the mitochondria in the subsarcolemmal region than in the mitochondrial volume density of the inner part of the myocytes. The trend towards an increase in total mitochondrial mass, the redistribution of the mitochondria with aging, and its significant increase in the outer cell compartment in the old rats is possibly to be regarded as an adaptive reaction of the myocyte in order to compensate for the diminished capillarization or a decreasing oxidative capacity of the individual mitochondrion. A decline in mitochondrial function has been demonstrated biochemically in old animals (Chen et al. 1972; Abu-Erreish and Sanadi 1978). Probably these compensatory structural alterations are mainly determined by the thickness of the myocytes but are not correlated to aging. However, Rakusan and Tomanek (1986) showed a decrease in the volume density of mitochondria in the subsarcolemmal region in rat hearts with hypertrophy due to renal hypertension.

Conclusion

After birth the heart is subjected to two physiological processes, growth and aging (Fig. 3, Table 2). In the growth period the thickness of the myocytes increases, myocytes and interstitium show a disproportional enlargement, and the collagenous fibers are augmented. The capillarization is reduced: capillary density is diminished, but the branching of capillaries is increased. In senescence, heart weight and thickness of myocytes show only a tendency for further increase. The

Fig. 2. Left ventricular myocardium with transversely sectioned myocytes and capillaries. **a** In young rats the mitochondria (*dark*) are evenly distributed in the myocytes. Electron micrograph, × 2100. **b** In adult (as well as in old) rats mitochondria (*dark*) are clustered in the subsarcolemmal region of the myocytes. Electron micrograph, × 2100

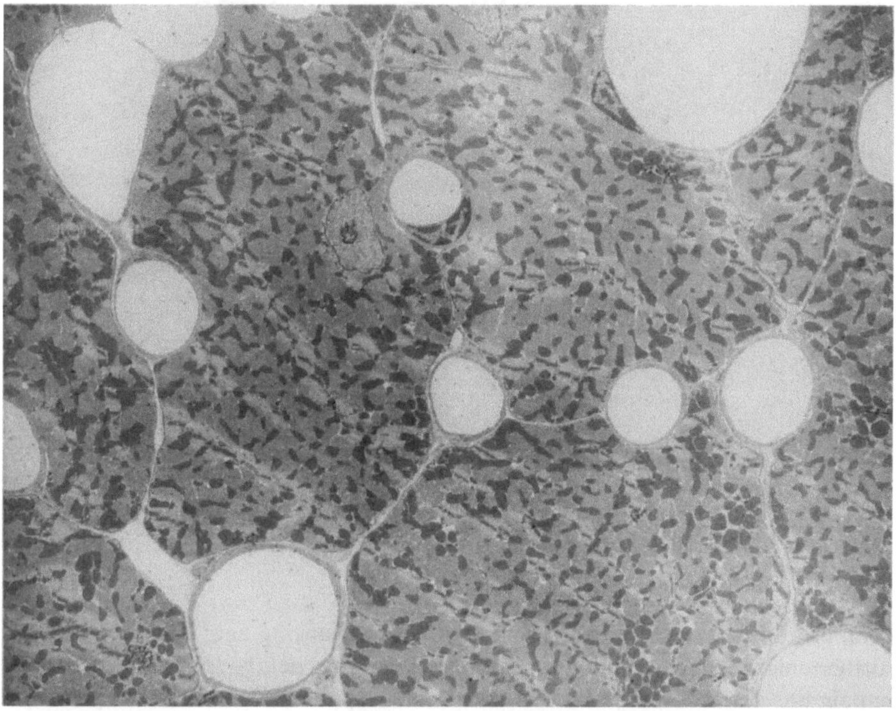

a

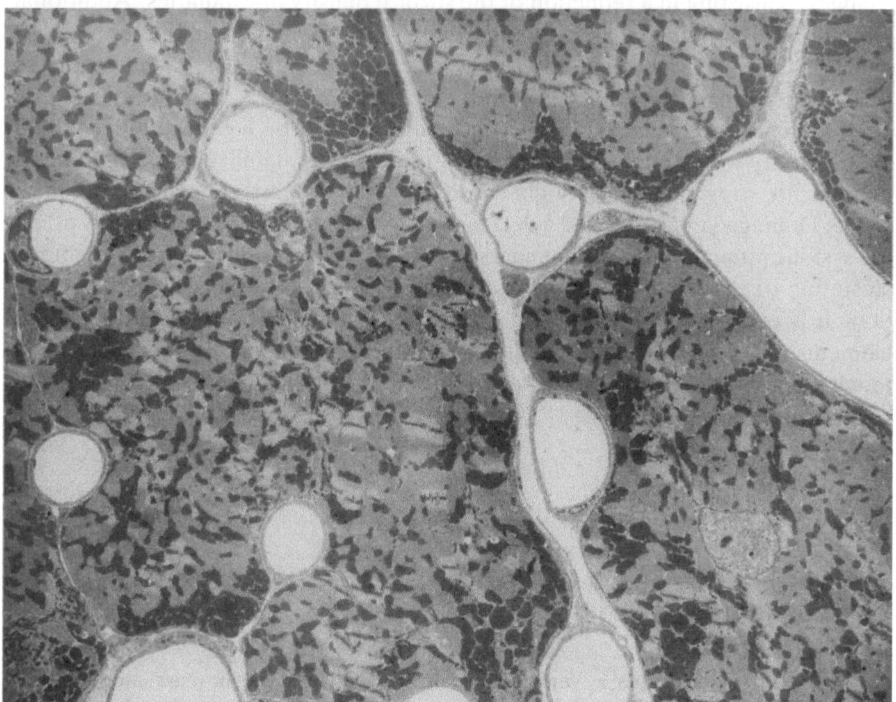

b

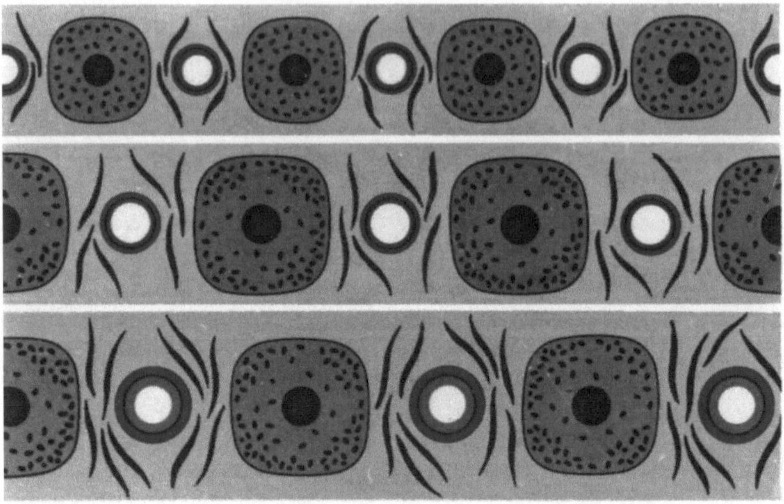

Fig. 3. Schematic drawing of the myocardium of young (*top panel*), adult (*midde panel*), and old rats (*botton panel*) according to the quantitative analysis (see conclusion)

composition of the myocardium changes with advancing age: The interstitium further enlarges and the amount of collagenous fibers nearly doubles, which may impair the diastolic properties of the heart. Capillarization shows only minor changes, consisting in a reduction of the surface density of capillaries. Additional alterations are related to the individual capillary. Basement membrane thickens, which may be of importance to the vascular permeability. The diameter of the individual capillary lumina is decreased, corresponding to a diminished capillary volume density in older age. The consequence could be a reduced myocardial flow capacity which might contribute to a reduced adaptability of the aged heart under acute stress and which might cause a progressive loss of myocytes in senescence. Damaged myocytes and a decreased myocytic mass may unfavorably affect the systolic pump function. An enlarged mitochondrial mass with subsarcolemmal clustering of mitochondria possibly compensates for the diminished capillarization. It is evident that even minor quantitative changes of any of the structural elements of the myocardium may induce a detrimental circle. It has to be shown to what extent these results are transferable to the human heart.

Discussion

Barrows

If I read your slides correctly, the mitochondria are only half as large in the senescent heart as in the young growing one. Is that correct?

Frenzel

The size of the mitochondria in younger animals is bigger than that in older animals. With advancing age the size becomes smaller but the number of mitochondria increases.

Barrows

Are they only half as large?

Frenzel

The size decreases by 36%.

Barrows

Do you know of any other tissue that shows such a change in mitochondrial size?

Frenzel

I'm not aware of changes of the mitochondrial size of that extent in other tissues, but under other conditions in the heart you can find similar changes in the size of mitochondria. During the hibernation of animals the mitochondria become smaller to a large extent.

Barrows

Have you done any biochemical studies of isolated mitochondria in senescent and young animals?

Frenzel

No, we have not done biochemical investigations on the mitochondria. But other authors have shown that the functional capacity of mitochondria is reduced in old age.

Barrows

That depends upon what biochemical system you are measuring.

Haug

Do the number and density of cristae in the mitochondria change with age?

Frenzel

We have not studied this question but the question has been answered by other authors. They found a diminished density of mitochondrial cristae per unit of cytoplasm but the surface density of mitochondrial cristae per unit of mitochondria was not altered in 36-month-old as compared with 9-month-old animals.

Beischer

Do the rats die from cardiac problems or do they die from something else?

Frenzel

We have not examined functional parameters in old animals but it is well known from investigations by Lakatta and by Weisfeldt that the functional capacity of old rats is diminished. They die, I suppose, from pulmonary complications and from cardiac insufficiency.

Rauterberg

One question regarding basement membranes: Are there any investigations about isolated endothelial cells from myocardium and what kind of basement membrane protein do they make?

Frenzel

I'm not aware of investigations of isolated endothelium in very old age and we have not carried out biochemical studies on the basement membrane. We have shown by electron microscopy that the structure of the basement membrane in old age is not changed; we can differentiate lamina densa and lamina rara. Thickening of basement membrane can be caused by two processes, diffuse thickening and lamination. The process in old age seems to be diffuse thickening, not lamination.

Rauterberg

I'm interested for one reason. There seems to be a considerable variation in the biosynthesis of proteins by cultured endothelial cells even within one species, e.g., between cells from aorta, from brain capillaries, from muscle capillaries, and so on. So I just wonder whether there are any data about endothelial cells from heart muscle.

Platt

This could be one point for future research. The title is "Present State and Future Perspective" and this would be a future perspective, I think.

Greiling

I would suppose that in this case your age-dependent changes in myocardium are also dependent on the oxygen supply. Do you know the oxygen lack theory of John Scott and Stockwell? They have proposed that under oxygen diminution there is a change in the proteoglycan pattern; therefore I don't believe that only the glycosylation process is important. I think the changes in keratan sulfate composition, which depends on the oxygen supply, are also most important, and I think that the swelling of the capillaries is dependent on the proteoglycan or glycosaminoglycan patterns. This is a hypothesis at the moment but I think that, as suggested by Professor Platt, there is a future research project here, namely: What is changed in the capillaries with age? Another example is the composition of glycosaminoglycans in CO poisoning (H. Ohishi et al. 1986). There are published results showing important changes in proteoglycans, especially keratan sulfate-chondroitin sulfate and heparan sulfate, after CO poisoning, and there was an increase in keratan sulfate, a substance not found in myocardium beforehand. So I think these biochemical processes are regulated and stimulated by the oxygen supply.

References

Abu-Erreish GM, Sanadi DR (1978) Age-related changes in cytochrome concentration of myocardial mitochondria. Mech Ageing Dev 7: 425–432

Adler CP, Friedburg H (1986) Myocardial DNA content, ploidy level and cell number in geriatric hearts: post-mortem examination of human myocardium in old age. J Mol Cell Cardiol 18: 39–53

Anversa P, Ricci R, Olivetti G (1986a) Quantitative structural analysis of the myocardium during physiologic growth and induced cardiac hypbertrophy: a review. J Am Coll Cardiol 7: 1140–1149

Anversa P, Hiler B, Ricci R, Guideri G, Olivetti G (1986b) Myocyte cell loss and myocyte hypertrophy in the aging rat heart. J Am Coll Cardiol 8: 1441–1448

Chen JC, Warshaw JB, Sandadi DR (1972) Regulation of mitochondrial respiration in senescence. J Cell Physiol 80: 141–148

Coleman R, Silbermann M, Gershon D, Reznick AZ (1987) Effects of long-term running stress on the ultrastructure of the aging mouse heart. Gerontology 33: 19–33

Cornwell GG, Murdoch WL, Kyle RA, Westermark P, Pitkänen P (1983) Frequency and distribution of senile cardiovascular amyloid. A clinico-pathologic correlation. Am J Med 75: 618–621

Egger J, Lake BD, Wilson J (1981) Mitochondrial cytopathy. A multisystem disorder with ragged red fibres on muscle biopsy. Arch Dis Child 56: 741–748

Engelmann GL, Vitullo JC, Gerrity RG (1987) Morphometric analysis of cardiac hypertrophy during development, maturation, and senescence in spontaneously hypertensive rats. Circ Res 60: 487–494

Frenzel H (1985) Das Herz im Alter. Licht- und elektronenmikroskopische Befunde. Z Kardiol 74 [Suppl 7]: 17–25

Frenzel H, Feimann J (1984) Age-dependent structural changes in the myocardium of rats. A quantitative light- and electron-microscopic study on the right and left chamber wall. Mech Ageing Develop 27: 29–41

Frenzel H, Schwartzkopff B, Höltermann W, Schnürch HG, Novi A, Hort W (1988) Regression of cardiac hypertrophy: morphometric and biochemical studies in rat heart after swimming training. J Mol Cell Cardiol 20: 737–751

Gerstenblith G, Lakatta EG, Weisfeldt ML (1976) Age changes in myocardial function and exercise response. Prog Cardiovasc Dis 19: 1–21

Herbener GH (1976) A morphometric study of age-dependent changes in the mitochondrial populations of mouse liver and heart. J Gerontol 31: 8–12

Hodkinson HM, Pomerance A (1977) The clinical significance of senile cardiac amyloidosis: a prospective clinico-pathologic study. Q J Med 46: 381–387

Hoppeler H, Kayar SR (1988) Capillarity and oxidative capacity of muscles. NIPS 3: 113–116

Hoppeler H, Hudlická O, Uhlmann E (1987) Relationship between mitochondria and oxygen consumption in cat muscles. J Phyiol (Lond) 385: 661–675

Hort W, Lichti H, Kalbfleisch H, Köhler F, Frenzel H, Milzner-Schwarz U (1982) The size of human coronary arteries depending on the physiological and pathological arteries of the heart, the age, the size of the supplying areas and the degree of coronary sclerosis. Virchows Arch [A] 397: 37–59

Ikeda H, Tauchi H, Sato T (1985) Fine structural analysis of lipofuscin in various tissues of rats of different ages. Mech Ageing Dev 33: 77–93

Johnson LK, Johnson RW, Strehler BL (1975) Cardiac hypertrophy, aging and changes in cardiac ribosomal RNA gene dosage in man. J Mol Cell Cardiol 7: 125–133

Kment A, Leibetseder J, Burger H (1966) Gerontologische Untersuchungen an Rattenherzmitochondrien. Gerontologia 12: 193–199

Koobs HD, Schultz RL, Jutzy RV (1978) The origin of lipofuscin and possible consequences to the myocardium. Arch Pathol Lab Med 102: 66–68

Kosek JC, Angell W (1970) Fine structure of basophilic myocardial degeneration. Arch Pathol 89: 491–499

Lakatta EG (1979) Alterations in the cardiovascular system that occur in advanced age. Fed Proc 38: 163–167

Lakatta EG, Yin FCP (1982) Myocardial aging: functional alterations and related cellular mechnisms. Am J Physiol 242: H927–H941

Lindner AJ (1983) Age dependent biochemical changes of connective tissue. In: Platt D (ed) Cardiology and ageing. Schattauer, Stuttgart, pp 37–55

Linke RP (1983) Senile cardiac amyloid: biochemical and immunohistochemical results. In: Platt D (ed) Cardiology and ageing. Schattauer, Stuttgart, pp 81–97

Linzbach AJ (1972) Das Altern des menschlichen Herzens. In: Altmann HW, Büchner F, Cottier H et al. (eds) Handbuch allgemeiner Pathologie, vol VI, 4. Springer, Berlin Heidelberg New York, pp 369–428

Linzbach AJ, Akuamoa-Boateng E (1973) Die Altersveränderungen des menschlichen Herzens. I. Das Herzgewicht im Alter. Klin Wochenschr 51: 156–163

Mattfeldt T, Krämer K-L, Zeitz R, Mall G (1986) Stereology of myocardial hypertrophy induced by physical exercise. Virchows Arch [A] 409: 473–848

Meerson FZ, Javich MP, Lerman MI (1978) Decrease in the rate of RNA and protein synthesis and degradation in the myocardium under long term compensatory hyperfunction and on aging. J Mol Cell Cardiol 10: 145–159

Olson LJ, Gertz MA, Edwards WD et al. (1987) Senile cardiac amyloidosis with myocardial dysfunction. Diagnosis by endomyocardial biopsy and immunohistochemistry. N Engl J Med 317: 738–742

Palmer JW, Tandler B, Hoppel CL (1977) Biochemical properties of subsarcolemmal and interfibrillar mitochondria isolated from cardiac muscle. J Biol Chem 252: 8731–8739

Pomerance A (1967) Ageing changes in human heart valves. Br Heart J 29: 222–231

Pomerance A (1968) Cardiac pathology in the aged. Geriatrics 23: 101–114

Pomerance A (1969) Ballooning deformity (mucoid degeneration) of atrioventricular valves. Br Heart J 31: 343–351

Pomerance A (1970) Pathological and clinical study of calcification of the mitral valve ring. J Clin Pathol 23: 354–361

Pomerance A, Darby AJ, Hodkinson HM (1978) Valvular calcification in the elderly: possible pathogenetic factors. J Gerontol 33: 672–675

Rahlf G (1980) Intramyocardial microarteriopathy. Virchows Arch [A] 388: 289–311

Rakusan K, Poupa O (1964) Capillaries and muscle fibres in the heart of old rats. Gerontologia 9: 107–112

Rakusan K, Tomanek RJ (1986) Distibution of mitochondria in normal and hypertrophic myocytes from rat heart. J Mol Cell Cardiol 18: 299–305

Reichmann H, Hoppeler H, Mathieu-Costello, von Bergen F, Pette D (1985) Biochemical and ultrastructural changes of skeletal muscle mitochondria after chronic electrical stimulation in rabbits. Pflugers Arch 404: 1–9

Reinecke P, Hort W (1988) Untersuchungen über das Wachstum der Koronararterienäste – Morphometrische Untersuchungen an Korrosionspräparaten des R. interventricularis der A. coronaria sinistra beim Schwein und Ferkel. Z Kardiol 77: 229–304

Rosai J, Lascona EF (1970) Basophilic (mucoid) degeneration of myocardium. A disorder of glycogen metabolism. Am J Pathol 61: 99–116

Rosenberg B, Pfitzer P (1983) Ploidy in the hearts of elderly patients. Virchows Arch [Cell Pathol] 42: 19–24

Sachs HG, Colgan JA, Lazarus ML (1977) Ultrastructure of the aging myocardium: a morphometric approach. Am J Anat 150: 63–72

Schmucker DL, Sachs HG (1985) Age-dependent alterations in rat ventricular myocardium: a quantitative analysis. Mech Ageing Dev 31: 89–101

Schnider SL, Kohn RP (1981) Effects of age and diabetes mellitus on the solubility and nonenzymatic glycosylation of human skin collagen. J Clin Invest 67: 1630–1635

Siperstein MD, Raskin P, Burns H (1973) Electron microscopic quantification of diabetic microangiopathy. Diabetes 22: 514–527

Strehler BL, Mark DD, Mildvan AS, Gee MV (1959) Rate and magnitude of age pigment accumulation in human myocardium. J Gerontol 14: 430–439

Tate EL, Herbener GH (1976) A morphometric study of the density of mitochondrial cristae in heart and liver of aging mice. J Gerontol 31: 129–134

Thüroff JW, Hort W, Lichti H (1984) Diameter of coronary arteries in 36 species of mammalian from mouse to giraffe. Basic Res Cardiol 79: 199–206

Tomanek RJ (1970) Effects of age and exercise on the extent of the myocardial capillary bed. Anat Rec 167: 55–62

Tomanek RJ, Karlsson UL (1973) Myocardial ultrastructure in young and senescent rats. J Ultrastruct Res 42: 201–220

Travis DF, Travis A (1972) Ultrastructural changes in the left ventricular rat myocardial cells with age. J Ultrastruct Res 39: 124–148

Unverferth DV, Baker PB, Arn AR, Magorien RD, Fetters J, Leier CV (1986) Aging of the human myocardium: a histologic study based upon endomyocardial biopsy. Gerontology 31: 241–251

Waller BF, Roberts WC (1983) Cardiovascular disease in the very elderly. Analysis of 40 necropsy patients aged 90 years or over. Am J Cardiol 51: 403–421

Wei JY, Gersh BJ (1987) Heart disease in the elderly. Curr Probl Cardiol 12: 1–65

Westermark P, Johansson B, Natvig JB (1979) Senile cardiac amyloidosis: evidence of two different amyloid substances in the ageing heart. Scand J Immunol 10: 303–308

Zweihoff R, Bürrig KF, Schwartzkopff B, Frenzel H (in preparation) Age-dependent changes in left ventricular myocardium of rats. A morphometric study

Regulation of Force of Contraction in the Aged and Diseased Myocardium

M. Böhm and E. Erdmann[1]

Introduction

Myocardial failure is characterized by an inadequate cardiac output, which leads to a compensatory activation of the sympathetic nervous system (Packer 1988). As a consequence, increased norepinephrine levels can be detected in the serum of patients with congestive heart failure (Chidsey et al. 1962). Moreover, the increase of norepinephrine in the blood is closely related to the severity of heart failure and the prognosis of these patients (Cohn et al. 1984). The increased activity of the sympathetic nervous system imposes a permanent β-adrenergic stimulus on the heart which is suggested to initiate a downregulation of cardiac β-adrenoceptors in the failing myocardium (Bristow et al. 1982; Bristow 1984; Ginsburg et al. 1983; Böhm et al. 1988a, b). The consequence is a reduced capability of β-adrenoceptor agonists to increase force of contraction in isolated cardiac preparations from failing hearts (Bristow et al. 1982; Bristow 1984; Feldman et al. 1987; Böhm et al. 1988a, b). In the treatment of patients with heart failure, the effectiveness of β-adrenoceptor agonists such as dobutamine is also reduced (Colucci et al. 1987). Similar alterations occur in the aged myocardium. Several reports indicate that in the aged rat heart there is a reduced effect of β-adrenoceptor agonists such as dobutamine on force of contraction (Lakatta et al. 1975). The response to Ca^{2+} was not reduced in the aged heart (cf. Lakatta and Yin 1982). Impaired adenylate cyclase-mediated positive inotropic effects, but unchanged effects of cAMP-independent mechanisms such as Ca^{2+} or cardiac glycosides, have also been observed in the failing human myocardium (Feldman et al. 1987; Böhm et al. 1988a–c). The latter findings indicate that in both failing and aging myocardium similar alterations occur, which affect the β-adrenoceptor–adenylate cyclase system, leaving the contractile apparatus itself more or less unchanged. For these reasons, it appears mandatory to investigate whether age-related changes contribute to the reduction of the density of β-adrenoceptors and the effectiveness of β-adrenoceptor agonists in the diseased human heart.

The present experiments were designed to study biochemical alterations in the failing human heart and to elucidate whether age-related changes contribute to these defects. Therefore, we studied the number of β-adrenoceptors and the

[1] Medizinische Klinik I der Universität München, Klinikum Großhadern, Marchioninistr. 15, D-8000 München 70 / FRG

Gerontology
Ed. by D. Platt
© Springer-Verlag Berlin Heidelberg 1989

positive inotropic effects of the β-adrenoceptor agonist dobutamine and the phosphodiesterase inhibitor isobutylmethylxanthine in isolated human myocardium with different stages of heart failure. Nonfailing hearts which could not be transplanted for technical reasons served as controls.

The density of α-adrenoceptors, which also mediate positive inotropic effects (Brückner et al. 1984; Aass et al. 1986; Böhm et al. 1988c) in the human heart, was studied as well. Experiments on cardiac α- and β-adrenoceptors were also performed in myocardium from spontaneously hypertensive rats (SHRs) which have increased norepinephrine levels in the myocardium (Head et al. 1985), resulting in β-adrenoceptor downregulation (Yamada et al. 1984; Böhm et al. 1988d). Moreover, SHRs develop cardiac failure in later stages of the syndrome (Pfeffer et al. 1976). Hence, this model for hypertensive cardiomyopathy exhibits pathophysiological alterations which have been suggested to be similar to those observed in the failing human heart.

Materials and Methods

Patients and Laboratory Animals

Myocardial tissue was obtained from patients undergoing cardiac transplantation because of terminal heart failure (NYHA IV) due to dilated or ischemic cardiomyopathy. Tissue from papillary muscles of patients with mitral valve disease was taken during mitral valve replacement. These patients were clinically in functional class NYHA II–III of heart failure. Myocardium from nonfailing hearts which could not be transplanted for technical reasons served as controls. Young and aged SHRs and normotensive Wistar-Kyoto rats (WKs) were purchased from Savo-Ivanovas Kiesslegg, FRG.

Contraction Experiments

Force of contraction was measured isometrically in isolated, electrically driven human papillary muscle strips or dissected rat left ventricular papillary muscles using field stimulation at 1 Hz. Further details of the method are published elsewhere (Böhm et al. 1988a–d).

Radioligand Binding Experiments

Cardiac α- and β-adrenoceptors were determined in cardiac membrane preparations from human left ventricular myocardium and left ventricles from SHRs and WKs. Alpha- and ß-adrenoceptors were determined with ^{3}H-prazosin and ^{3}H-CGP 12 177, respectively. For further details see Böhm et al. (1988 a,c,d).

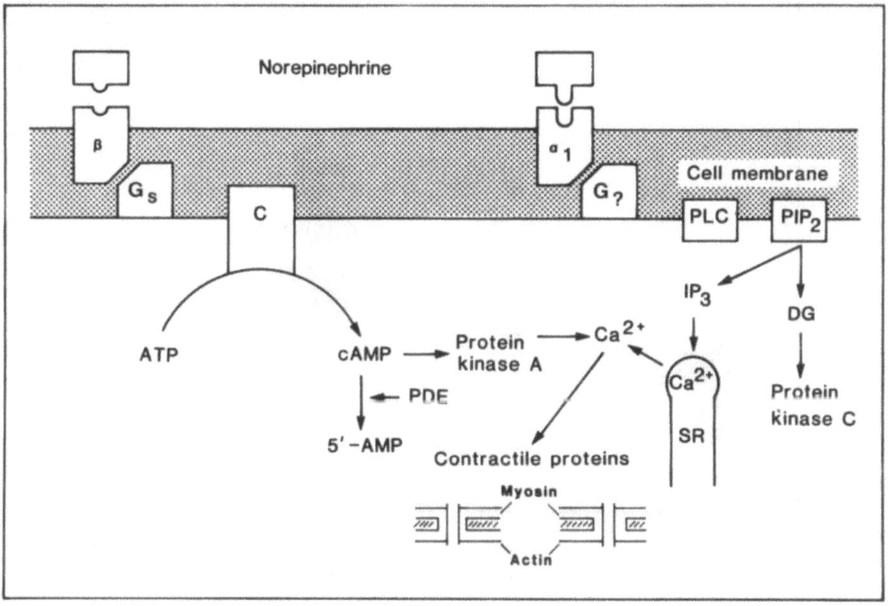

Fig. 1. Model of the mechanisms of action by which norepinephrine increases force of contraction by stimulation of α- and β-adrenoceptors. Occupation of the β-adrenoceptor (β) activates the catalytic subunit of the adenylate cyclase *(C)* by mediation of a stimulatory guanine nucleotide binding protein (G_s), thereby increasing cAMP formation from ATP. Cyclic AMP activates cAMP-dependent protein kinases (protein kinase A), which increase the slow Ca^{2+}-inward current. The action of cAMP is reversed by breakdown of cAMP to 5'-AMP by the cAMP-phosphodiesterase *(PDE)*. The action of norepinephrine on α_1-adrenoceptors (α) activates the activity of the phospholipase C, which hydrolyzes phosphoinositol triphosphate *(PIP_2)* to inositol triphosphate *(IP_3)* and diacylglycerol *(DG)*. IP_3 releases Ca^{2+} presumably from the sarcoplasmic reticulum *(SR)* and DG activates protein kinase C. Coupling of cardiac α_1-adrenoceptors involves a guanine-nucleotide binding protein ($G_?$) which is as yet not classified. Ca^{2+} finally acts on the contractile proteins to increase force of contraction

Results

Regulation of Myocardial Force of Contraction by Adrenoceptors

Myocardial force of contraction is adjusted to peripheral requirements by the activation of the sympathetic nervous system. At the level of the myocardial cell the effect is mediated by an activation of α- and β-adrenoceptors with sympathetic neurotransmitters such as norephinephrine. Figure 1 summarizes the events which follow the binding of the neurotransmitter to the adrenoceptors. After activation of cardiac β-adrenoceptors, the receptors couple to a stimulatory guanine nucleotide binding protein (G_s; Gilman 1984) which activates the catalytic subunit of the adenylate cyclase. Consequently, increased cAMP formation from ATP is initia-

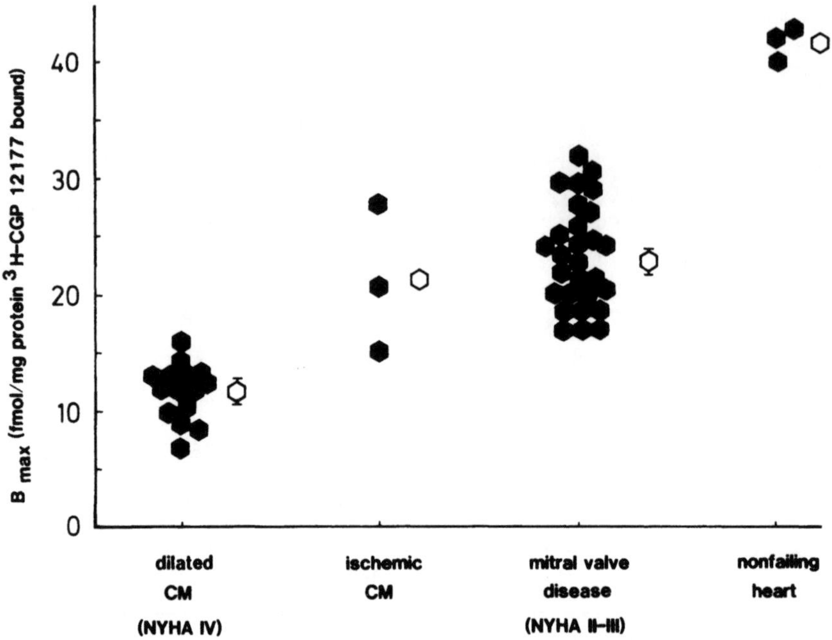

Fig. 2. β-Adrenoceptors in the human heart. The number of myocardial β-adrenoceptors in cardiac membranes from patients with dilated cardiomyopathy *(CM)*, ischemic heart disease with left ventricular dysfunction *(ischemic CM)*, mitral valve disease *(NYHA II–III)*, and non-failing hearts. (Modified from Böhm et al. 1988b)

ted. Cyclic AMP activates cAMP-dependent protein kinases which produce phosphorylation of functional membrane proteins, leading to an activation of the slow Ca^{2+} inward current (Reuter 1983). The enhanced free cytosolic concentration of Ca^{2+} finally produces a positive inotropic effect. In contrast, cardiac α-adrenoceptors produce positive inotropism independently of cAMP. Activation of the receptor is followed by a stimulation of phospholipase C, which increases the formation of inositol triphosphate and diacylglycerol from membrane-bound phospholipids (Scholz et al. 1988). Inositol triphosphate most likely acts as a second messenger to produce positive inotropism (Schmitz et al. 1987), probably by delivering Ca^{2+} from intracellular stores. In summary, in the myocardium force of contraction can be increased by two different types of adrenoceptor, with entirely different biochemical mechanisms of action.

β-Adrenoceptor in Human Myocardium

In vivo the regulation of force of contraction is mediated by norepinephrine (Packer 1988), which stimulates both cardiac α- and β-adrenoceptors. Since norepinephrine levels are elevated in the blood of patients with heart failure (Chidsey et al. 1962; Cohn et al. 1984), the heart might be exposed to a permanent stimulation of both receptor types. Therefore, both receptors could be subject to desensitization in the failing heart.

Figure 2 summarizes the numbers of β-adrenoceptors which were measured with radioligand binding experiments in cardiac membranes from patients with severe heart failure (NYHA IV) due to dilated cardiomyopathy, ischemic cardiomyopathy, or moderate heart failure (NYHA II–III) due to mitral valve disease. Three nonfailing donor hearts served as controls. There is a decline in the number of cardiac β-adrenoceptors which is dependent on the degree of heart failure. The number of receptors in severely failing myocardium was only about 25% of the number in nonfailing hearts. In ischemic cardiomyopathy or moderately failing myocardium, the decline was about 50%. These data show that not only in severe but also in moderate heart failure a reduction occurs in the number of β-adrenoceptors. Similar evidence was provided by determination of β-adrenoceptors in myocardial biopsy samples from patients undergoing cardiac catheterization (Fowler et al. 1986). In the latter and in the present study, there was no detectable difference in receptor composition between hearts with similar degrees of heart failure but different types of heart disease, such as mitral valve incompetence or mitral valve stenosis. Therefore, the severity of heart failure has the most important impact on β-adrenoceptor downregulation.

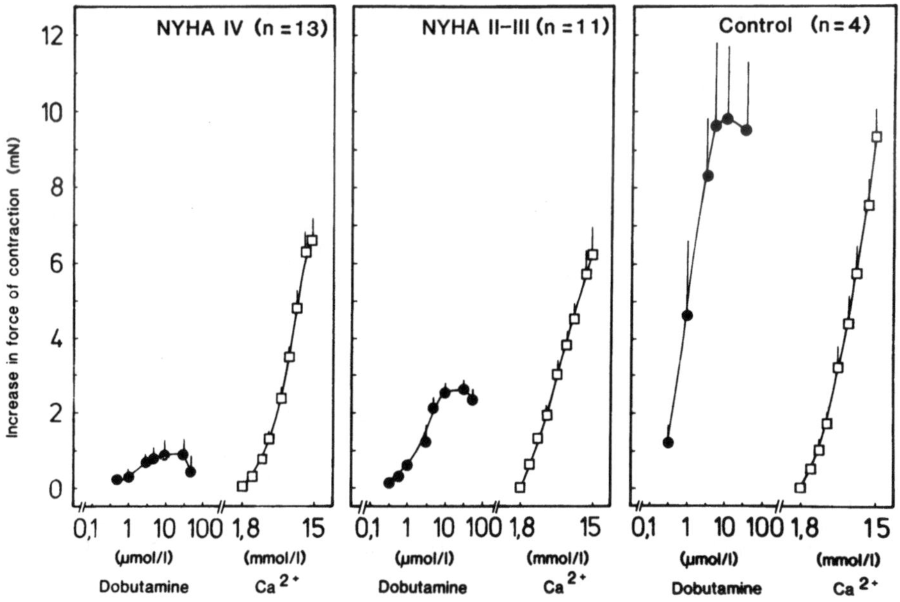

Fig. 3. Concentration–response curves for the positive inotropic effects of dobutamine (0.3–30 μmol/l) and Ca^{2+} (1.8–15 μmol/l) in 13 papillary muscle strips from five patients with severe heart failure *(NYHA IV)*, in 11 strips from four patients with moderate *(NYHA II–III)* heart failure, and in four strips from two nonfailing donor hearts *(Control)*. Concentration–response curves for Ca^{2+} are shown for comparison. Basal force of contraction was 2.9 ± 0.3 mN (n = 13; NYHA IV), 3.3 ± 0.1 mN (n = 11; NYHA II–III), and 2.4 ± 0.7 mN (n = 4; Control). (Modified from Böhm et al. 1988a)

The question arises of whether the decline in the number of β-adrenoceptors is functionally important in the failing heart. Therefore, the positive inotropic effect of dobutamine was studied in an isolated cardiac preparation. Figure 3 summarizes the data. As with the number of β-adrenoceptors, there is a decline in the positive inotropic effect of dobutamine depending on the severity of heart failure. The degree of β-adrenoceptor down-regulation and the decline of the effectiveness of dobutamine correlates closely.

If a decline in the number of β-adrenoceptors were to be the only alteration, one would expect that agents acting beyond the β-adrenoceptor–adenylate cyclase system to produce more pronounced effects in failing myocardium. Therefore, the effect of the phosphodiesterase inhibitor isobutylmethylxanthine (IBMX) was studied in preparations from severely failing, moderately failing, and nonfailing hearts. These results are shown in Fig. 4. A decline in effectiveness was observed not only with the β-adrenoceptor agonist dobutamine but also with the phosphodiesterase inhibitor IBMX. These findings indicate that in heart failure β-adrenoceptor downregulation might not be the only alteration of receptor-mediated regulation of force of contraction. Other defects in the adenylate cyclase system, such as a reduced basal activity of the adenylate cyclase system, might also play a role.

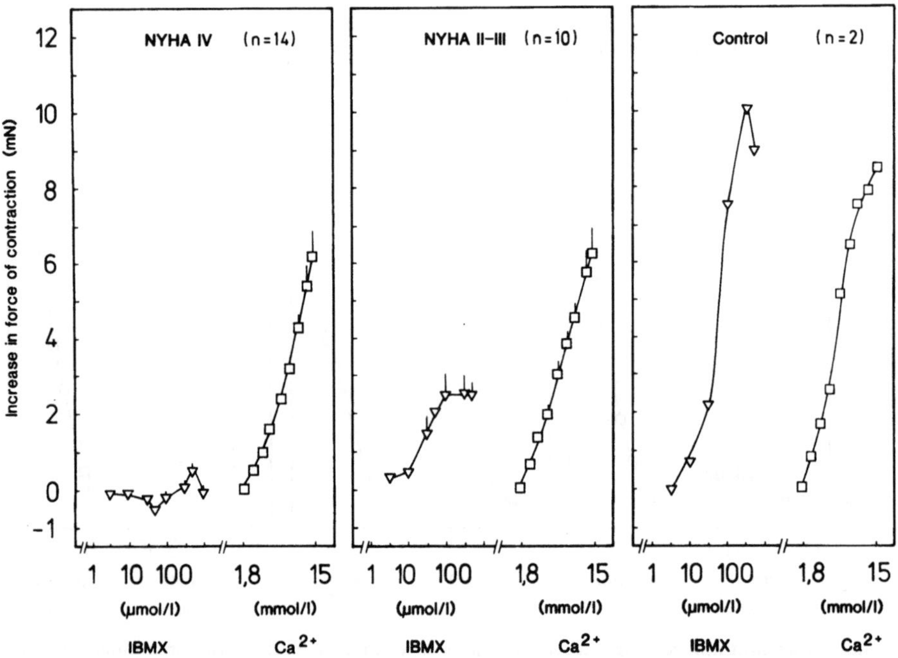

Fig. 4. Concentration–response curves for the positive inotropic effect of isobutylmethylxanthine (*IBMX*; 3–300 μmol/l) in papillary muscle strips from patients with severe *(NYHA IV)* or moderate *(NYHA II–III)* heart failure or a nonfailing donor heart *(Control)*. Concentration–response curves for calcium are shown for comparison. Basal force of contraction was 2.7 ± 0.2 mN ($n = 14$; NYHA IV) 1.6 ± 0.4 mN ($n = 10$; NYHA II–III), and 3.5 mN ($n = 2$; Control). (Modified from Böhm et al. 1988a)

α-Adrenoceptors in Human Myocardium

Cardiac α-adrenoceptors mediate positive inotropic effects in a variety of species (Schümann et al. 1974, 1975; Brodde et al. 1978), including humans (Brückner et al. 1984; Aass et al. 1986; Böhm et al. 1988c). However, the physiological role of α-adrenoceptors is not clear. In pathological situations in which β-adrenergic effects are compromised, such as hypothyroidism (Kunos et al. 1974; Kunos 1977) or treatment with β-adrenoceptor antagonists (Mügge et al. 1985), cardiac α-adrenoceptors are increased. Since an inverse regulation of α- and β-adrenoceptors occurs in a number of tissues (Kunos and Ishac 1987), it has been hypothesized that cardiac α-adrenoceptors serve as a reserve mechanism when β-adrenoceptor-mediated effects are diminished. However, the situation in the human heart is not clear. Figure 5 A shows that the number of α-adrenoceptors is not different in severely failing and moderately failing myocardium. In the same hearts, there is still a decline in the number of β-adrenoceptors (Fig. 5 B). The number of α-adrenoceptors is extremely low. Consistently, the α-adrenoceptor-mediated positive inotropic effect of phenylephrine in the presence of propranolol was found not to be different in severely and moderately failing myocardium (Fig. 6), whereas in the same hearts there was a decline in the positive inotropic effect of isoproterenol. Moreover, the potency and efficacy of the α-adrenoceptor-mediated

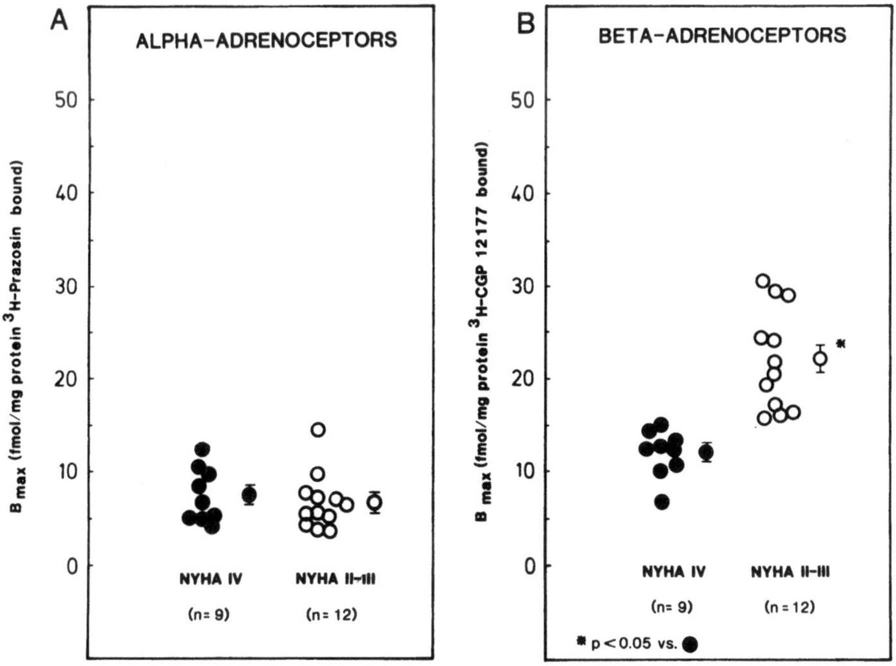

Fig. 5. A Cardiac α-adrenoceptors and **B** cardiac β-adrenoceptors in myocardial membranes from severely *(NYHA IV)* and moderately *(NYHA II–III)* failing myocardium. Alpha- and β-adrenoceptors were determined in the same hearts. (Modified from Böhm et al. 1988c)

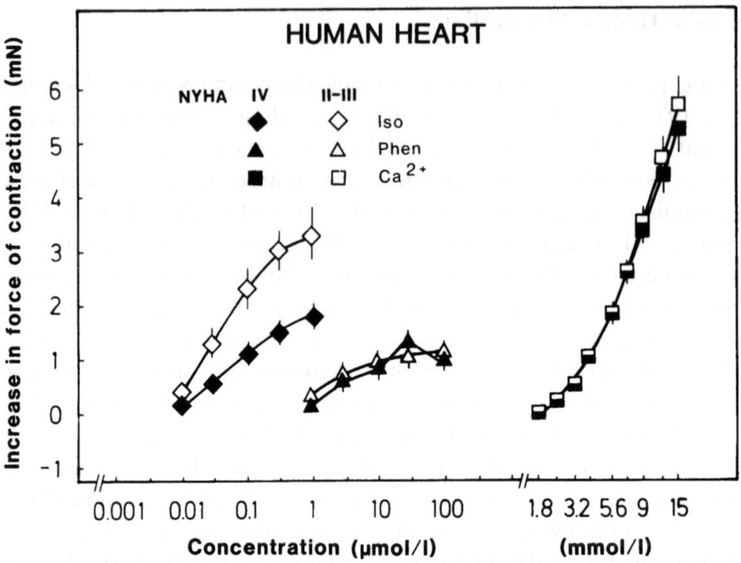

Fig. 6. Concentration–response curves for the effects of isoproterenol (*Iso*, 0.01–1 μmol/l), phenylephrine in the presence of 1 μmol/l propranolol (*Phe*, 1–100 μmol/l), and Ca^{2+} (1.8–15 mmol/l) in electrically driven (1 Hz) papillary muscle strips from patients with severe *(NYHA IV)* and moderate *(NYHA II–III)* heart failure. *Ordinate:* Increase in force of contraction in mN. *Abscissa:* Drug concentration in μmol/l or mmol/l. The predrug values were as follows. □ : 1.6 ± 0.1 mN (n = 8, from 5 hearts); ◆: 2.0 ± 0.4 mN (n = 9, from 5 hearts); △ : 1.9 ± 0.2 mN (n = 12, from 8 hearts); ▲: 1.6 ± 0.2 mN (n = 15, from 7 hearts); □ : 1.4 ± 0.1 mN (n = 20, from 10 hearts); ■ : 1.4 ± 0.1 mN (n = 21, from 8 hearts). (Modified from Böhm et al. 1988c)

effect was smaller than the efficacy and potency of β-adrenoceptor-mediated effects. To summarize, in the human heart, the number of α-adrenoceptors and of α-adrenoceptor-mediated effects is small and, hence, α-adrenoceptors might be of minor physiological importance for the regulation of myocardial force of contraction.

Influence of Aging on β-Adrenoceptors

In the aged myocardium, there is a reduced positive inotropic effect of catecholamines (Lakatta et al. 1975; Lakatta and Yin 1982) and a reduction in the β-adrenoceptor stimulated adenylate cyclase activity (Kusiac and Pitha 1983). Since these alterations are similar to those observed in the failing myocardium, it is worthwhile investigating whether aging has an influence on the loss of cardiac β-adrenoceptors in the failing human heart. The relation between age and the number of β-adrenoceptors is summarized in Figs. 7 and 8. There was no correlation between the number of β-adrenoceptors and the age of patients in either moderately (Fig. 7) or severely (Fig. 8) failing myocardium. There was no significant difference in the number of ß-adrenoceptors in groups of young and old

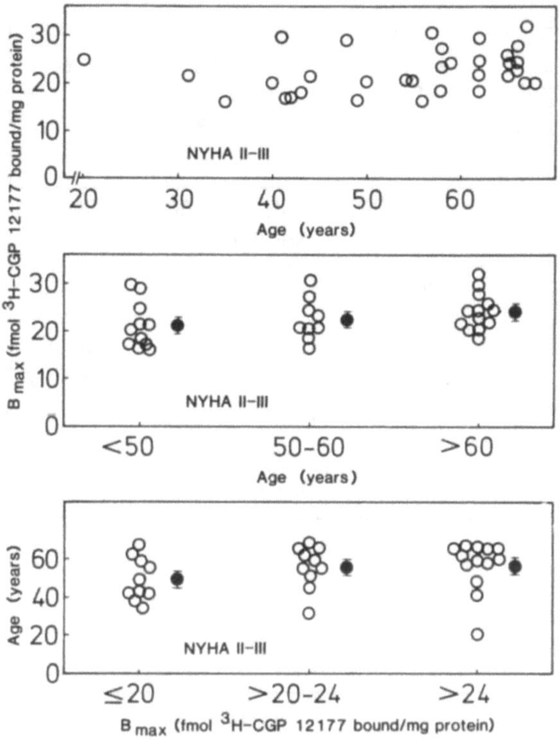

Fig. 7. Cardiac β-adrenoceptors in myocardial membranes from patients with moderate *(NYHA II–III)* heart failure in relation to age. (Böhm and Feiler, unpublished data)

patients. Moreover, the age of patients with more or less pronounced β-adrenoceptor downregulation did not differ. Thus, in failing human hearts with various stages of the disease, no contribution of age to β-adrenoceptor downregulation can be reliably detected.

Age- and Disease-Related Alterations in Spontaneous Hypertension of the Rat

In order to elucidate whether disease-related alterations mask the effect of aging, cardiac β-adrenoceptors were studied in myocardium from young and old SHRs and control rats (WKs). This approach allows the detection of alterations due to aging, since young and old normal animals can be compared whereas in the above-mentioned studies only diseased human myocardium was investigated. Moreover, SHRs have increased norepinephrine levels in the heart and, hence, as in human heart failure cardiac β-adrenoceptors are exposed to excessive agonist stimulation. Figure 9 shows a typical radioligand binding experiment in myocardial membranes from WKs and SHRs. There is a reduction in the number of cardiac β-adrenoceptors in SHRs. Figure 10 summarizes the data in old and young SHRs and WKs. In WKs, there is a decline in the number of β-adrenoceptors in 12-month-old animals. In young and old SHRs there is a reduction in cardiac β-adrenoceptors

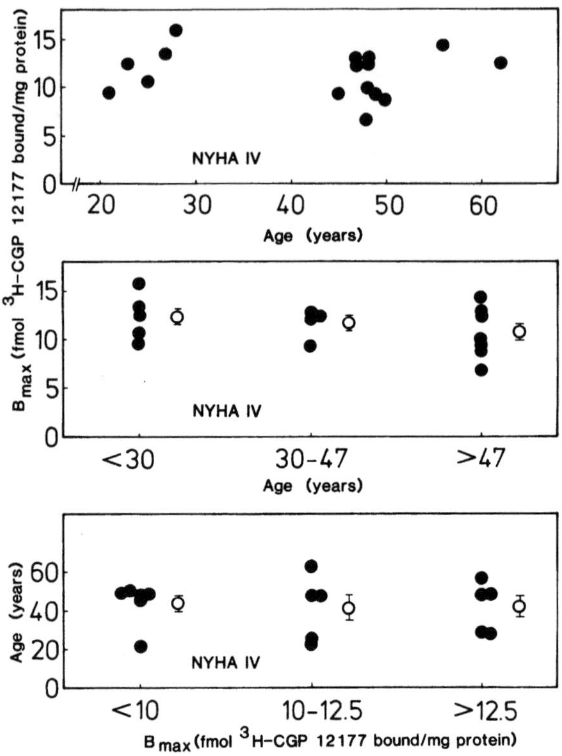

Fig. 8. Cardiac β-adrenoceptors in myocardial membranes from patients with severe *(NYHA IV)* heart failure in relation to age. (Böhm and Feiler, unpublished data)

compared to the normotensive controls. However, in the hypertensive animals, a further decline at 12 months could not be observed. To summarize, there is a β-adrenoceptor downregulation in young and old SHRs. Moreover, aging reduces the number of β-adrenoceptors in WKs, but in the presence of hypertensive cardiomyopathy no further decline in the number of β-adrenoceptors can be observed.

Summary and Conclusions

In the failing human heart, there is a reduction in the number of β-adrenoceptors and a reduction in the positive inotropic effect of β-adrenoceptor agonists and phosphodiesterase inhibitors. The density of human cardiac α-adrenoceptors and

Fig. 10. Density of cardiac β-adrenoceptors in myocardial membranes of 12-week- and 12-month-old spontaneously hypertensive rats *(SHR)* and Wistar-Kyoto rats *(WK)* as controls. *Ordinate:* Density of cardiac β-adrenoceptor in fmol ^{3}H-CGP 12 177 bound/mg protein. (Böhm and Feiler, unpublished data)

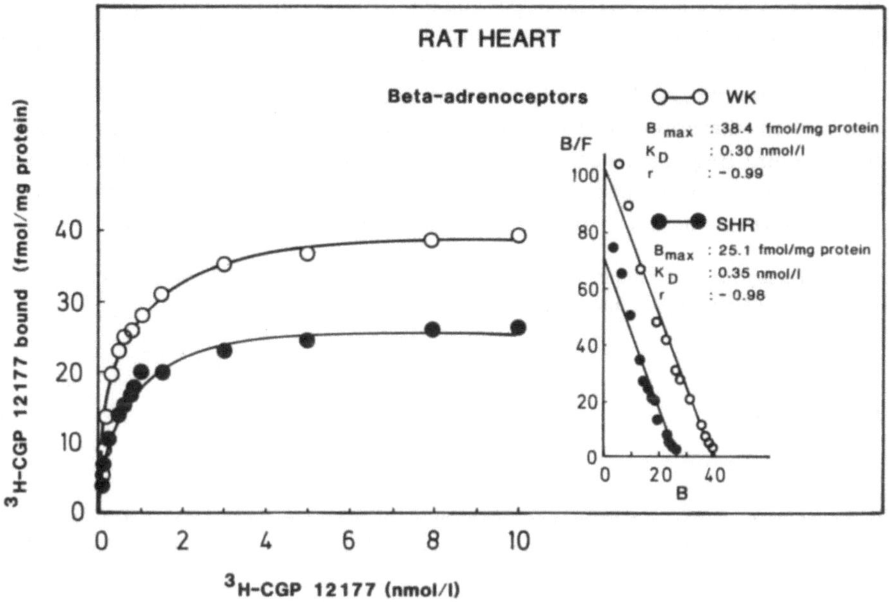

Fig. 9. Specific binding of ^{3}H-CGP 12 177 to membranes of left ventricles from Wistar rats *(WK)* and spontaneously hypertensive rats *(SHR)*. Specific binding is defined as total minus nonspecific binding as measured in the absence and presence of 10 μmol/l (−)-propranolol and is expressed as fmol/mg protein. *Inset*: Scatchard plot of ^{3}H-CGP 12 177 bound per mg protein was plotted as a function of the ratio (B/Fx10^{-6}) of bound ^{3}H-CGP 12 177 to free ^{3}H-CGP 12 177 (nmol/l). The intercept with the ordinate is the maximal number of binding sites (B_{max}); the slope is the apparent affinity (K_D). (Modified from Böhm et al. 1988d)

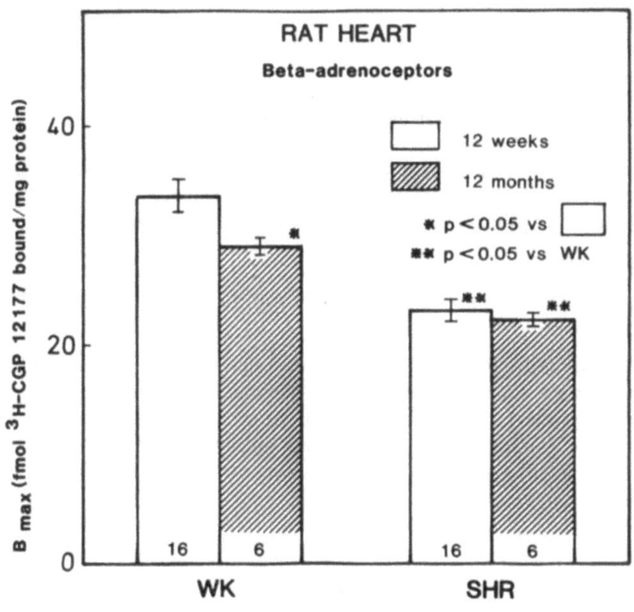

the positive inotropic effect produced by their stimulation are very small and most likely of minor physiological importance in the human heart. In diseased human and rat myocardium, a contribution of aging to β-adrenoceptor downregulation could not be observed. These findings indicate that in the presence of disease, age-related alterations of β-adrenoceptors cannot be detected. However, since heart failure frequently occurs in the elderly, the loss of β-adrenoceptors might be of clinical importance in these patients regardless of whether it is induced by heart failure or whether a primary alteration of the aging heart is leading to failure.

Acknowledgement. The studies were supported by the Deutsche Forschungsgemeinschaft and Friedrich-Baur-Stiftung, Munich, FRG.

Discussion

Klotz

In our diseased preparation there is downregulation for receptors, as you mentioned. Is there a possibility of restoring the activity of the receptors by adding, for instance, dibutyryl cyclic AMP or another cyclic nucleotide?

Böhm

We investigated te response to forskolin and dibutyrate cyclic AMP, both acting beyond the coupling processes mediated by GS. Both increased the force of contraction similarly in the normal heart and in the failing heart, indicating that the defect is located between the receptor and the catalytic subunit, possibly involving signal transduction. A reduction in GS does not occur. An increase in GI, which is involved in the inhibition of the adenylate cyclase, occurs in dilated cardiomyopathy and amounts in our hands to about 40%.

Hofecker

I think Lakatta pointed to the fact that in old age the adaptation of the heart to stronger demands functions differently than in young individuals and that the Frank-Starling mechanism becomes increasingly important. Did you find the same in rats?

Böhm

We have not looked at the Frank-Starling mechanism. But if the sympathetic nervous system cannot act, the heart uses this physiological mechanism. The point is that in aged patients there may be heart failure and not specifically age-related alterations. Therefore, one cannot distinguish between the alterations occurring as a consequence of increased sympathetic outflow in heart failure and primary alterations which are related to age.

Beischer

What about noradrenaline concentrations in blood in relation to age?

Böhm

I'm not aware of any study dealing with that topic. But if the concentration were to be lower in elderly patients, one could not find out whether it is an alteration of the aged heart or whether it is a primary defect or alteration of the sympathetic nervous system. Moreover low concentrations of noradrenaline would explain an increased density of β-adrenoceptors. In the failing heart, the downregulation of β-adrenoceptors is most likely induced by increased noradrenaline levels.

References

Aass H, Skomedal T, Osnes J-B et al. (1986) Noradrenaline evokes an α-adrenoceptor-mediated inotropic effect in human ventricular myocardium. Acta Pharmacol Toxicol 58: 88–90

Böhm M, Beuckelmann D, Brown L et al. (1988a) Reduction of beta-adrenoceptor density and evaluation of positive inotropic responses in isolated, diseased human myocardium. Eur Heart J 9: 844–852

Böhm M, Diet F, Feiler G, Kemkes B, Kreuzer E, Weinhold C, Erdmann E (1988b) Subsensitivity of the failing human heart to isoprenaline and milrinone is related to beta-adrenoceptor downregulation. J Cardiovasc Pharmacol 12: 726–732

Böhm M, Diet F, Feiler G, Kemkes B, Erdmann E (1988c) α-Adrenoceptors and α-adrenoceptor-mediated positive inotropic effects in failing human myocardium. J Cardiovasc Pharmacol 12: 357–364

Böhm M, Beuckelmann D, Diet F, Feiler G, Lohse MJ, Erdmann E (1988d) Properties of cardiac alpha- and beta-adrenoceptors in spontaneously hypertensive rats. Naunyn-Schmiedebergs Arch Pharmacol 338: 383–391

Bristow MR (1984) Myocardial beta-adrenergic-receptor downregulation in heart failure. Int J Cardiol 5: 648–652

Bristow MR, Ginsburg R, Minobe W et al. (1982) Decreased catecholamine sensitivity and beta-adrenergic-receptor density in failing human hearts. N. Engl J Med 307: 205–211

Brodde O-E, Motomura S, Endoh M, Schümann HJ (1978) Lack of correlation between the positive inotropic effect evoked by α-adrenoceptor stimulation and the levels of cyclic AMP and/or cyclic GMP in the isolated ventricle strip of the rabbit. J Mol Cell Cardiol 10: 207–219

Brückner R, Meyer W, Mügge A, Schmitz W, Scholz H (1984) α-Adrenoceptor-mediated positive inotropic effect of phenylephrine in isolated human ventricular myocardium. Eur J Pharmacol 99: 345–347

Brückner R, Mügge A, Scholz H (1985) Existence and functional role of alpha$_1$-adrenoceptors in the mammalian heart. J Mol Cell Cardiol 17: 639–645

Chidsey CA, Harrison DC, Braunwald E (1962) Augmentation of the plasma noradrenaline response to exercise in patients with congestive heart failure. N Engl J Med 267: 650–654

Cohn JN, Levine TB, Olivari MT et al. (1984) Plasma noradrenaline as a guide to prognosis in patients with chronic congestive heart failure. N Engl J Med 311: 819–823

Colucci WS, Leatherman GF, Ludmer PL, Gauthier DF (1987) β-Adrenergic inotropic responsiveness of patients with heart failure: studies with intracoronary dobutamine infusion. Circ Res 61 [Suppl I]: 82–86

Feldman MD, Copelas L, Gwathmey JK et al. (1987) Deficient production of cyclic AMP: pharmacologic evidence of an important cause of contractile dysfunction in patients with end-stage heart failure. Circulation 75: 331–339

Fowler MB, Laser JA, Hopkins GL, Minobe W, Bristow MR (1986) Assessment of the β-adrenergic receptor pathway in the intact failing human heart: progressive receptor down-regulation and subsensitivity to agonist response. Circulation 74: 1290–1302

Gilman AG (1984) G proteins and dual control of adenylate cyclase. Cell 36: 577–579

Ginsburg R, Bristow MR, Billingham ME, Stinson EB, Schroeder JS, Harrison DC (1983) Study of the normal and failing isolated human heart: decreased response of failing heart to isoproterenol. Am Heart J 106: 535–540

Guarneri T, Filburn CR, Zitnik GS, Roth GS, Lakatta EG (1980) Contractile and biochemical correlates of beta-adrenergic stimulation of the aged heart. Am J Physiol 239: H501–H508

Head RJ, Cassis LA, Robinson RL, Westfall DP, Stitzel RE (1985) Altered catecholamine contents in vascular and nonvascular tissues in genetically hypertensive rats. Blood Vessels 22: 196–204

Kunos G (1977) Thyroid hormone-dependent interconversion of myocardial α- and β-adrenoceptors in the rat. Br J Pharmacol 59: 177–189

Kunos G, Ishac EJ (1987) Mechanism of inverse regulation of α_1- and β-adrenergic receptors. Biochem Pharmacol 36: 1185–1191

Kunos G, Vermes-Kunos I, Nickerson M (1974) Effect of thyroid state on adrenoceptor properties. Nature 250: 779–781

Kusiak JW, Pitha J (1983) Decreased response with age of the cardiac catecholamine sensitive adenylate cyclase system. Life Sci 33: 1679–1686

Lakatta EG, Yin FCP (1982) Myocardial aging: functional alterations and related cellular mechanisms. Am J Physiol 242: H927–H941

Lakatta EG, Gerstenblith G, Angell CS, Shock NW, Weisfeldt ML (1975) Diminished inotropic responses of aged myocardium to catecholamines. Circ Res 36: 262–269

Mügge A, Reupcke C, Scholz H (1985) Increased myocardial α_1-adrenoceptor density in rats chronically treated with propanolol. Eur J Pharmacol 112: 249–252

Packer M (1988) Neurohormonal interactions and adaptations in congestive heart failure. Circulation 77: 721–730

Pfeffer MA, Pfeffer JM, Frohlich ED (1976) Pumping ability of the hypertrophying left ventricle of the spontaneously hypertensive rat. Circ Res 38: 423–429

Reuter H (1983) Calcium channel modulation by neurotransmitters, enzymes and drug. Nature 301: 569–574

Schmitz W, Scholz H, Scholz I, Steinfath M (1987) Increase in IP3 precedes α-adrenoceptor induced increase in force of contraction in cardiac muscle. Eur J Pharmacol 140: 109–112

Scholz J, Schäfer B, Schmitz W et al. (1988) Alpha-1 adrenoceptor-mediated positive inotropic effect and inositol triphosphate increase in mammalian heart. J Pharmacol Exp Ther 245: 327–335

Schümann HJ, Endoh M, Wagner J (1974) Positive inotropic effects of phenylephrine in the isolated rabbit papillary muscle mediated both by α- and β-adrenoceptors. Naunyn-Schmiedebergs Arch Pharmacol 284: 133–148

Schümann HJ, Endoh M, Brodde OE (1975) The time course of the effect of β- and α-adrenoceptor stimulation by isoprenaline and methoxamine on the contractile force and cAMP level of the isolated rabbit papillary muscle. Naunyn-Schmiedebergs Arch Pharmacol 289: 291–302

Yamada S, Ishima T, Tomita T, Hayashi M, Okada T, Hayashi E (1984) Alteration in cardiac alpha and beta adrenoceptors during the development of spontaneous hypertension. J Pharmacol Exp Ther 228: 454–460

Drug Treatment of Hypertensive Geriatric Patients

R. D. Kennedy[1]

The management of hypertension in the elderly and old has remained controversial for over 30 years. It has been one of those areas where geriatricians have frequently found themselves in conflict with the attitudes of the general internist. Moreover, the success of national programs aimed at detecting and lowering blood pressure has had a major effect on both the profession's and the public's attitude to this problem, particularly in the United States.

The extrapolation of results from community studies and intervention trials involving younger age groups has been a not uncommon feature in determining the medical management of high blood pressure in the old. Fortunately, with several trials now completed or underway, dealing specifically with hypertension and intervention in the elderly and old, soon we should be in a better position to make treatment decisions based on valid evidence.

Blood pressure can be regarded as a continuum, with increasing risk at increasing levels (Pickering 1972) and also in the elderly with increasing risk when the pressure falls below certain levels. As a result, the determination of normal and abnormal is somewhat arbitrary and is also complicated by the fact that reduction of blood pressure from levels just above those accepted generally as normal may result in some slight improvement in mortality and morbidity, but only for a very small number of patients over a lengthy period at increased expense, and the risk of side-effects.

The prevalence of hypertension varies in reported populations. There is no doubt that raised blood pressure is a risk factor for cerebrovascular disease and to a lesser extent coronary artery disease in both sexes with advancing years. This is more marked for blacks than whites, and for the industrialized rather than nonindustrialized societies.

The prevalence of hypertension varies in reported populations. The National Health and Nutritional Examination Study in the United States between 1976 and 1980 reported that 44% of whites and 60% of blacks aged 65–74 years had pressures in excess of 160/95 mmHg. Using 140/90 as a threshold, the prevalence increased to 63% of whites and 76% of blacks. Again, this does not deal with the population under consideration today, and the prevalence for the over-65s may be even higher (Miller 1973).

---

[1] Albert Einstein College of Medicine, Geriatric Division, Montefiore Medical Center, 111 East 210 Street, New York, N.Y. 10467, USA

Gerontology
Ed. by D. Platt
© Springer-Verlag Berlin Heidelberg 1989

Recent years have seen a major change as the focus on elevated blood pressure in the elderly has swung from the diastolic to the systolic level. The effect of age alone on pressure shows a rise in diastolic pressure in early adulthood in Westernized societies, with a peak at 45–50 years and then a slight fall with advancing years. However, systolic pressures continue to rise with age. As a result, there is increasing concern at the significance of isolated systolic hypertension in the elderly.

In the Systolic Hypertension in the Elderly Program (SHEP), the prevalence of isolated systolic hypertension (⩾160 mmHg) rose markedly from 7% for those aged 60–69 years to 20% for those aged 80 or more, while diastolic pressure ⩾90 mmHg fell from 19% to 13 % for the same age groups (Hulley et al. 1986) (Table 1).

Whom Should We Treat?

This remains highly complex. It depends on the age and race of the patient, the presence of concomitant physical and mental disorders, lifestyle, probable level of compliance, use of other medications, and the physician's attitude.

Patients with target organ involvement resulting from persistently elevated pressures clearly require medication in most instances. However, most elderly people with raised blood pressure or isolated systolic hypertension are symptomless. In hypertensive patients, death from myocardial infarction occurs two or three times more frequently than death from stroke. Intervention studies in middle-aged and "young" elderly, up to 75 years, have demonstrated that benefit occurs in the prevention of nonfatal strokes, but little in preventing morbidity and mortality from coronary heart disease. In assessing intervention, we should not regard all elderly ofer 65 years as a homogeneous group, for this is not validated by the few trials available.

The results of the European Working Party on High Blood Pressure in the Elderly (EWPHE) indicate the need for such analysis (Amery et al. 1985). The

Table 1. Blood pressure distribution at screening visit – Systolic Hypertension in the Elderly Program. [Reprinted with permission from the American Geriatrics Society, "Systolic hypertension in the elderly program (SHEP). The first three months." By Julley et al. Journal of the American Geriatrics Society 34: 101–105, 1986]

Age	Number on treatment	Not on Treatment			
		Number	SBP ⩾160 mmHg and DBP <90 mmHg	DBP ⩾90 mmHg	All others
60–69	4367	8004	7%	19%	73%
70–79	4773	6506	13%	15%	72%
>80	1428	2116	20%	13%	67%
Total	10568	16626	11%	17%	72%

Table 2. Desired qualities for an antihypertensive drug

Efficacy
Lowers blood pressure consistently and moderately
No tolerance with prolonged use
Reverses specific pathological mechanism
Safety
Minimal adverse reactions, especially serious
Minimal side-effects
Few biochemical effects
Efficacy minimally influenced by aging process
Convenience
Long dose interval
Low cost
Few drug interactions
Treats other concomitant diseases
Ease of administration

overall results showed a significant reduction in cardiovascular mortality for subjects over the age of 60. This was thought to be due to reduction in cardiac mortality and a nonsignificant decrease in cerebrovascular mortality. There was also a decrease in severe but not mild congestive heart failure. However, there was no reduction in overall mortality and this trial showed attenuation of benefit from treatment with advancing age. In particular little or no benefit from treatment was demonstrated in patients over the age of 80 years, particularly in females.

The Systolic Hypertension in the Elderly Program presently underway has as its primary objective to assess whether long-term administration of antihypertensive medication to elderly subjects with isolated systolic hypertension reduces the combined incidence of fatal and nonfatal stroke. Subjects enrolled are 65 years or more, the follow-up period is a minimum of 4 years, and drugs used are chlorthalidone at a starting dose of 12.5 mg daily with 0.05 mg reserpine once daily added if required, or atenolol.

What to Treat With?

The pharmacokinetics of antihypertensive drugs alter with age. Thus for the elderly, the ideal antihypertensive agent does not exist. The desirable qualities listed in Table 2 indicate why. The last 5 years have seen a plethora of new drugs for the management of hypertension and changes in treatment attitude. The previously widely accepted and simple form of stepped care can now be very involved. Many drugs can now be given in much lower doses than was previously customary. For example, diuretics can be given at a quarter of the former dose and not every day. While the range of drugs now available is great, it should be remembered that not all of them have been subject to controlled trials in an elderly population with particular respect to efficacy, side-effects, and drug interactions.

Diuretics

Due to proven efficacy as in the EWPHE and other trials, the thiazide diuretics remain the most used of this group but the reduction in daily dosage, or a dosage schedule on alternate days or even less, with still satisfactory blood pressure control, has meant that many of the problems of diuretic-induced hypokalemia or more rarely hypomagnesemia no longer occur. In the long term, the side-effects of thiazides may be a disadvantage for selected groups, for example the diabetic patient. The tendency for hyperuricemia, hyperglycemia, and hypercholesteremia may restrict their use in the elderly diabetic patient with coronary artery disease.

Problems of urinary frequency or incontinence will influence the use of diuretics. Indapamide, a thiazide with only mild diuretic effect but proven antihypertensive activity and lessened sid-effects, may then be of value. Diuretic-induced hyponatremia is common and if associated with overt neurological disturbances can be a dangerous problem. It has been reported more often in elderly female obese hypertensives who have other associated problems such as tube feeding, hypoglycemic drugs, diarrhea, and stroke (Asnouri 1986). Where potassium-sparing diuretics are used, reversible kidney failure may occur, especially in conjunction with administration of nonsteroidal anti-inflammatory agents or hypovolemia (Lynn et al. 1985).

The antihypertensive effects of thiazides appear to be as pronounced in older adults with low renin levels as in those with normal levels. Ambulatory EKG monitoring has shown a high prevalence of arrhythmias in hypertensives who are treated with diuretics. This appears to be benign, as the complexes are usually atrial or ventricular premature beats and do not appear to be associated with any increase in complex supraventricular or ventricular premature contractions, or frequency of abnormalities. If the diuretics at low dose do not control the pressure, other medications in conjunction with the diuretic or on their own should be considered rather than a dose increase, which often results in an increase in side-effects with no better blood pressure control.

β-Blockers

The indications and contraindications for β-blockers are much clearer than formerly. Reduced sensitivity of β-adrenergic responses, age-related reduction in renin activity, and diminished cardiac performance are all given as reasons for diminished effectiveness of β-blockers in elderly hypertensives, but in practice they are rare. Most would agree that the appropriate β-blocker for treating hypertension should be cardioselective, with once daily administration. There are several to choose from. Unlike nonselective β-blockers, these are less associated with side-effects such as limb coldness, male sexual dysfunction, and bronchospasm.

Atenolol 50 mg daily or metoprolol 100 mg once daily is usually sufficient. Metoprolol is thought to lower blood pressure by diminishing the peripheral vascular resistance, whereas atenolol appears to act by reducing the cardiac workload through a lower heart rate and cardiac output.

Labetolol should also be considered as first-line therapy. As well as β-blokkade, it possesses postsynaptic-α_1-blockade. It is valuable for the patient with a slow heart rate because of its intrinsic sympathomimetic activity. In low doses it is well tolerated, and produces minimal adverse side-effects in the presence of arterial insufficiency or left ventricular dysfunction.

Several double-blind trials have compared the efficacy of thiazide diuretics and cardioselective β-blocking agents. Most have shown minimal if any differences in efficacy between the two groups. When given together they usually show a definite synergistic effect which can be of value in the poorly controlled hypertensive.

Despite the formidable list of side-effects and contraindications, diuretics or β-blockers remain the most popular first line of therapy. The cardioprotective and antianginal action of β-blockers and the diuretic effect of thiazides are specific actions that may contribute to improved health in the appropriate patient. However, there should be a clear awareness of their limitations and adverse metabolic and biochemical effects in specific situations, as well as their lack of influence on coronary artery disease in hypertensives.

Other Drugs

Calcium channel blockers are increasingly used in the elderly as monotherapy. They have different modes of action and side-effects. An advantage is that they are not associated with any metabolic or electrolyte abnormalities. In addition, they may exert a cardioprotective action through the anticalcinotic effect on the myocardium and vascular smooth muscle. Of this group, nifedipine has been associated with fluid retention, edema, and orthostatic hypotension. It can be given as a slow release capsule, allowing for once or twice daily administration. However, it must be used with care in the setting of left ventricular dysfunction or conduction disorders.

Angiotensin converting enzyme (ACE) inhibitors are also advocated as initial drug therapy for hypertension in the elderly, despite low renin levels. In the kidneys, these drugs reduce efferent arteriolar resistance, and they are of value in diabetes mellitus and other causes of glomerulosclerosis. Captopril, enalapril, and others of this group can be very effective but, due to renal excretion, require close monitoring of renal function. The age-associated fall in glomerular filtration rate (GFR) often requires a reduction in dose, dosage interval, or both. With a GFR of less than 20 ml/min, the dosage interval may be as long as 48 – 108 h. When these drugs were given at the manufacturer's previously suggested doses, renal failure and hyperkalemia were a not infrequent occurrence in the very old.

This suggests renovascular disease and is associated with accelerating or resistant hypertension, such as renal artery stenosis (Heal et al. 1980; Ying et al. 1984). The starting dose for captopril should be 6.25 mg and for enalapril 2.5 mg daily or twice daily according to renal function, increasing to achieve maximum effect at about 4 weeks after starting therapy. Reduction of ACE sensitivity may occur with time, requiring dosage changes (Lees and Reid 1987).

Vasodilators such as hydralazine and minoxidil may effectively lower the blood pressure, but particularly with hydralazine, there may be associated reflex tachycardia, increased myocardial work, and diminishing efficacy due to drug tolerance. The α-adrenergic receptor blocker prazosin hydrochloride is an effective antihypertensive agent in a twice daily dose of 1 mg or more as required. However, the tendency to cause severe postural hypotension on the first dose may limit its use.

Reserpine appears to have enjoyed a modified comeback in the treatment of high blood pressure. The action of reserpine appears to be both central and as a peripheral adrenergic blocker. Because of major side-effects such as parkinsonism and depression it fell into disrepute. However, in a much lower dose, it has several advocates. Now it is given in 0.05–0.1 mg daily for its antihypertensive effect. In one prolonged comparative study, the effects of reserpine were compared with those of methyldopa and diuretic; there were significantly fewer compliance problems in the reserpine group and mean diastolic blood pressure was maintained at a satisfactory lower level for up to 3 years and mean systolic blood pressure for 2 years (Applegate et al. 1985).

The central α-adrenergic agonist *clonidine* effectively lowers the blood pressure at a low dosage. Its side-effects include somnolence, dry mouth, hypotension, sometimes confusion, and occasionally rebound hypertension if the drug is suddenly discontinued. It can now be given as a patch once or twice weekly allowing for satisfactory control. A major disadvantage, however, is that 10%–20% of those using clonidine patches may develop contact dermatitis, thus limiting its use (Tuck et al. 1988).

Methyldopa is the oldest drug in this group still frequently used in the elderly. With problematic side-effects of depression, altered hepatic enzymes, drowsiness, and dramatic orthostatic hypotension, it has little place in the modern treatment of the elderly with raised blood pressure. However, it may be difficult to disestablish therapy which has apparently been successful over many years.

Side-effects

Cardiovascular and renal changes of aging may reduce tolerance to antihypertensive drugs. The normal compensatory responses to drug-induced orthostatic hypotension may be impaired due to changes in baroreceptor-mediated reflexes and sympathetic activity. Defective renal salt and water conservation may render the patient liable to marked diuretic-induced natriuresis and diuresis. The pharmacokinetics of most antihypertensive drugs alter with age, and dose for dose, adverse reactions are more common in the old. Reduction in cerebral or myocardial blood flow may occur, with reduction in mean cerebral pressure.

The age-related diminution of the GFR has a major influence on the incidence of side-effects, including renal failure, orthostatic hypotension, and the possibility of too severe a fall in cerebral blood flow, resulting in transient ischemic attacks or strokes. In addition, if there is chronic renal failure the problem worsens. Yet good pressure control improves the GFR. Thus all drugs excreted by the kidneys require close monitoring.

Side-effects are also related to the number of medications taken. A cross-national comparison between the United States and Scotland showed a 2.5:1 ratio of antihypertensive medication with a 26%:15% ratio of adverse drug reactions (Lawson and Jick 1976).

Nondrug management of hypertension in the elderly continues to evoke interest. Most such treatments have only limited practicality. Dietary control of obesity and salt has in the past been held as a major self-help measure. The recent report of the Inter-Salt Cooperative Research Group found that in all nonprimitive centers, urinary sodiumexcretion was related to the slope of the blood pressure with age (Intersalt 1988). Potassium excretion was negatively correlated with blood pressure in individual subjects after adjustment had been made for confounding variables. Ethylalcohol intake and body mass index also showed strong and significant independent relationships with blood pressures in individual subjects. Thus lower sodium intake in later years might have an effect on blood pressure and therefore cardiovascular mortality. However, the magnitude of this change would be small. Taking body weight, alcohol ingestion, and potassium excretion into account, to achieve a reduction in blood pressure of 2.2 mmHg systolic or 0.1 mmHg diastolic would require reducing the sodium intake by 100 mmol/day. This seems an awfully small gain for a pretty miserable diet. Interestingly, vegetarians appear less subject to essential hypertension, and the substitution of a vegetarian for an omnivorous diet has been associated with blood pressure reduction (Rouse and Beilin 1984).

Effects of Treatment

The effects of treatment have been fairly well defined in the elderly up to the age of 75 or 80, and comprise a reduction in the morbidity and mortality from cerebrovascular disease in hypertensives. The European trial also showed a significant reduction in the cardiovascular mortality up to the age of 80. However, we still await definitive advice on the management of hypertension, particularly isolated systolic hypertension, in those aged 80 and over.

We also have some guidance as to the limits that we should attempt to achieve by lowering blood pressure. Cruickshank and colleagues, when evaluating the effect of atenolol in a population of mean age 53.6, found that (and this has also been noted in the Framingham study and elsewhere) when diastolic blood pressure was lowered below 85 mmHg, the incidence of death from myocardial infarction started to rise, especially in those with myocardial ischemia (Cruickshank et al. 1987; Anderson 1978).

Meyer and colleagues followed the clinical and cognitive course over 22 months of a group of patients with multi-infarct dementia and compared them with age-matched normals and patients with Alzheimer's disease (Meyers et al. 1986). The hypertensive patients with multi-infarct dementia showed improved cognition and clinical course when their systolic blood pressure was controlled but this had to be maintained within the 135–150 mmHg range. If systolic pressure was reduced below this level, patients with multi-infarct dementia showed deterioration in cognitive ability. They also noted that the risk of cerebrovascular events increased with diminishing cerebral blood flow, and cigarette smoking had an additive deleterious effect. The danger of excessive lowering of both diastolic and systolic pressures needs to be fully appreciated. However, there is argument as to the significance of this effect in a hypertensive population in comparison to normotensives who are untreated. Therefore, there is no clear indication what diastolic level to aim for in the elderly. The 85/90 mmHg range appears reasonable, especially as the benefit of a further decrease is onyl minimally, if at all, associated with incremental benefit.

In summary, the antihypertensive drug used must be chosen after full evaluation of the patients' needs and other illnesses. Furthermore, the limitations and risks of treatment must be clearly understood. There is considerable literature on the morbidity and mortality associated with ill-considered therapy.

Most drugs that reduce blood pressure can also reduce left ventricular hypertrophy, which is held to be desirable. Antihypertensives that do not, include diuretics and direct vasodilators such as hydralazine, which increases cardiac work due to reflex tachycardia.

Obviously β-blockers are inappropriate in the setting of congestive heart failure. Hydralazine is inappropriate in the setting of coronary artery disease. Medications causing biochemical upset having an influence on other parthological processes should be given only after careful consideration; these include diuretics and β-blockers. Other medications may have an effect on drug efficacy, e.g., nonsteroidal anti-inflammatory drugs may diminish the antihypertensive effect of diuretics, ACE inhibitors, and hydralazine (Brown et al. 1986).

Monotherapy or first-line treatment is no longer limited to diuretics or β-blockers. Several studies in the elderly have shown the efficacy of calcium channel blockers and ACE inhibitors as monotherapy. Cost or compliance regarding dosage schedule will also require consideration in deciding which drug to use.

A final comment on treatment. We need to be as aware of when to stop treatment as when to start it. This applies particularly in the elderly, who are often maintained on medication when the condition requiring it has resolved. In a study to determine the effect of withdrawing medication in a population with controlled mild to moderate hypertension, tow-thirds were normotensive at the end of 1 year and 50% at the end of 2 years. Of those available for follow-up at the end of 3 years, half were still drug free and normotensive. It was concluded that approximately 25% of elderly patients could discontinue their antihypertensive medication and remain normotensive for at least 1 year (Alderman et al. 1985). They may include the group suffering from "white coat hypertension," recently rediscovered (Pickering et al. 1988).

In all of our deliberations on the appropriate treatment for our patients, a major factor in the decisions on whether to institute therapy and which agent to use is how our intervention will affect the quality of life of the individual. We have little information on this in regard to older people but there is some evidence to show that male hypertensives up to the age of 65 on captopril show a better sense of well-being and fewer side-effects and a generally higher quality of life than those on either propanolol or methyldopa (Croog et al. 1986).

The effect of specific medication on the quality of life may conversely be disastrous. Thus, the risk – benefit equation may be altered, particularly for the very old. Antihypertensive therapy in the old demands continuity of close monitoring.

Discussion

Blaschke

You've outlined the fact that we now have a range of choices for treating hypertension in older as well as younger patients. I'm just concerned about how we are going to design studies in order to generate clinically useful data which can help decide between different therapies (for example, a calcium channel blocker or a diuretic in older patients). What do you see as the requirements for studies in this area?

Kennedy

That's very difficult, because to be meaningful we are going to require huge numbers in terms of recruitment unless we specifically focus on one study group and exclude a large number of others. I think basically we are going to look at large trials like SHEP and break them down to see what the subgroups give us in some of those areas. But to cope with all the different drugs coming through is going to be a very major problem.

Brocklehurst

I certainly agree with Dr. Kennedy about the nontreatment of people over the age of 80. I think that's one important point that has to be made, and as he said, it derives partly from the diminished effectiveness of treatment with advancing age in the European working party study. They in fact showed no benefits at all over the age of 80. There has, as most people will know, been an interesting recent study published from Finland, which was first reported about 5 or 6 years ago in the Lancet, I think, and produced a good year of confirmatory correspondence. That study showed that over the age of 85 the higher your blood pressure, the longer you are likely to live. And the recent study showed, I think without any doubt, that longevity beyond 85 is directly correlated with a higher rather than a lower blood pressure. I think this was not simply because the people with the lowest blood pressures may have been dying at the time that the blood pressure was measured, which one might assume is a possibility. Rather I feel that the finding is a reality, and I think it relates to some of the things your mentioned, like the fact that vigorous hypotensive treatment in very old people can produce strokes and so on. I was, however, a little surprised that you recommend a single diastolic hypertension as a criteria for treatment because certainly the European working party showed that only systolic hypertension was related to diminished symptoms when it was treated.

Beischer

You still recommend the thiazides and the β-blockers as the drugs of first choice? Is this justified in the light of what we heard this morning? A worse glucose tolerance and a higher risk of nonenzymatic glycosylation can be caused by both of these groups of drugs and this could be a greater danger than a help, couldn't it?

Kennedy

I think that appropriate trials will examine this question. On theoretical grounds there are many reasons for not giving thiazides. The MRC trial on mild to moderate hypertension showed that thiazides were better than β-blockers in preventing stroke in a middle-aged to elderly population. These results have got to be looked at with the newer agents to see if they can perform better. At the moment we have no drug that seems to prevent all the risk factors when treating hypertensive patients. You can take your thiazide and have a better chance of not having a stroke or you can take your β-blocker and improve the chance of not having a myocardial infarction but have a poorer chance of avoiding a stroke. I guess the best thing to do is to stop smoking. There is also the major issue of the different age groups. Certainly, on theoretical grounds it would seem that β-blockers, especially the older ones, and thiazides do not have a secure place in therapy, given the availability of newer agents.

Medvedev

What do you think about American media recommendations to take aspirin as a kind of universal method against stroke and so on? Because it was advertised in many papers – *Newsweek* for example – and I think many people just started to take it.

Kennedy

I have a large practice of patients over the age of 80. I've considerable difficulty persuading many of them that they might be a little bit better off if their blood pressure was not 105/70. And this is partly due to the effects of the publicity about hypertension for the younger and middle aged, which of course is perfectly valid. So here is one difficulty. On the other hand there is often unawareness of the major risks of hypertension, so that's got to be remembered as well. We don't want a population which sails along blithely without being too much aware of what the risks of having high blood pressure or excessive treatment might mean. There is a happy medium and I don't think either European or American society has reached it.

Brocklehurst

I come back to one small question. In relation to the angiotensin-converting enzyme inhibitors you said that the GFR should be measured first of all. Do you think that is absolutely essential?

Kennedy

No – unless there is an indication of renal failure, in which case I think it advisable to know the GFR before embarking on these medications, which can be highly dangerous in the setting of renovascular disorders. If the GFR is normal I would start on the lower doses suggested, with decent time intervals between doses, and monitor what happens with BUN, creatinine levels, or creatinine clearance in special circumstances.

References

Alderman MH, Davis TK, Gerber LM (1985) Step-down therapy for hypertension. Results of a community based program. Postgrad Med 77 (7): 89–92, 96–99

Amery A, Brixco P, Clement D et al. (1985) Mortality and morbidity results from the European Working Party on High Blood Pressure in the Elderly trial. Lancet I: 1349–1354

Anderson TW (1978) Re-examination of some of the Framingham blood pressure data. Lancet II: 1139–1141

Applegate WB, Carper ER, Kahn SE, Westbrook L, Linton M, Barker MG, Runyan JW (1985) Comparison of the use of reserpine versus alpha-methyldopa for second step treatment of hypertension in the elderly. J Am Geriatr Soc 33: 109–115

Asnouri OS (1986) Severe diuretic induced hyponatremia in the elderly. A series of eight patients. Arch Intern Med 146: 1355–1357

Brown J, Dollery C, Valdes G (1986) Interaction of nonsteroidal anti-inflammatory drugs with anti-hypertensive and diuretic agents: control of vascular reactivity by endogenous prostanoids. Am J Med 81 (Suppl 2B): 43–47

Croog SH, Levine S, Testa MA et al. (1986) The effects of anti-hypertensive therapy on the quality of life. N Engl J Med 314: 1657–1664

Cruickshank JM, Thorp JM, Zacharies FJ (1987) Benefits and potential harm of lowering high blood pressure. Lancet I: 581–584

Heal RC, Brogden RN, Speight TM (1980) Captopril: a preliminary review of its pharmacological properties and therapeutic efficacy. Drugs 20: 409–452

Hulley SB, Feigal D, Ireland C, Kuller LH, Smith WM (1986) Systolic hypertension in the elderly program (SHEP). The first three months. J Am Geriatr Soc 34: 101–105

Intersalt (1988) An international study of electrolyte excretion and blood pressure: results for 24 hour urinary sodium and potassium excretion. Br Med J 297: 319–328

Lawson DM, Jick H (1976) Drug prescribing in hospitals: a international comparison. Am J Public Health 66: 644–648

Lees KR, Reid JL (1987) Age and the pharmacokinetics and pharmacodynamics of chronic enalapril treatment. Clin Pharmacol Ther 41: 597–602

Lynn KL, Bailey RR, Swainson CP, Sainsbury R, Low WI (1985) Renal failure with potassium sparing diuretics. NZ Med J 98: 629–633

Meyer JS, Judd BW, Tawakina T, Rogers RL, Mostel KF (1986) Improved cognition after control of risk factors for multi-infarct dementia. JAMA 256: 2203–2209

Miller HW (1973) National Center for Health Statistics. Plan and operation of the national health and nutritional examination survey, United States 1971–73. Vital and health statistics, series 1 Nos. 10a, 10b, US Department of Health, Education and Welfare, Publications No. 73–1310, US Government Printing Office, pp 1–46

Pickering G (1972) Hypertension and definitions: national histories and consequences. Am J Med 52: 570

Pickering TG, James GO, Boddie C, Harshfield GA, Blank S, Laragh JH (1988) How common is white coat hypertension? JAMA 259: 225–228

Rouse IL, Beilin LJ (1984) Vegetarian diet and blood pressure. J Hypertens 2: 231–240

Tuck ML, Griffiths RF, Johnson LE, Stern N, Morley JE (1988) UCLA grand rounds: hypertension in the elderly. J Am Geriatr Soc 36: 630–643

Veterans Administration Cooperative Study Group on Antihypertensive Agents (1967) Effects of treatment on morbidity in hypertension. JAMA 202: 1028–1034

Veterans Administration Cooperative Study Group on Antihypertensive Agents (1970) Effects of treatment on morbidity in hypertension II. JAMA 213: 1143–1182

Ying CY, Tifft CP, Gavras H, Chobonian AV (1984) Renal revascularization in the azotemic hypertensive patient resistant to therapy. N Engl J Med 31: 1070–1075

β-Blockade in the Elderly

F. W. Lohmann[1]

Today, β-blockade is an indispensable principle of therapy in cardiovascular diseases, in particular in coronary heart disease and arterial hypertension. Both clinical pictures are found especially often in elderly people, i.e., from the 60th to the 65th year of life. Consequently, administration of β-blockers is a frequent clinical necessity, especially in elderly patients.

Besides observance of the absolute contraindications to β-blockade (manifest heart failure, high degree atrioventricular blockade, syndrome of the sick sinoatrial node, obstructive disorder of ventilation), which naturally occur at a raised frequency in old age, further specific criteria must be observed:

1. In old age, the number or density of β-receptors and/or activity of the action-mediating adenyl cyclase system is reduced (Brodde 1988).
2. In elderly people, the distribution spaces for drugs have become smaller. In addition, the renal and hepatic clearance function is reduced (Platt 1988). Both aspects make it necessary to administer β-receptor blockers at a lower dose initially and overall in the elderly than in younger people in order to avoid side-effects. When the effect on the clinical picture is not sufficient, a combination therapy should be administered at a very early stage.
3. Especially elderly patients with cardiovascular diseases display disorders of carbohydrate and lipid metabolism as causative or enhancing factors. Since besides the cardiovascular target indication, β-receptor blockers can automatically influence metabolic functions controlled via catecholamines, it is important or even necessary to take these interrelationships into account in the administration of β-receptor blockers (Lohmann 1984, 1986, 1987a, b, 1988a, b)

Table 1 shows the influence of the sympathetic nervous system on metabolic processes. In particular, the different regulation via β_1- or β_2-receptors is pointed out. In clinical application of β-blockers, a distinction must be made between the mainly β_1-selective and the nonselective (mixed) β-blockers. The therapeutic effect is associated with the blockade of mainly β_1-receptors, which predominante up to 90% in the heart. Nonselective (mixed) β-receptor blockers, which occupy β_1- and β_2-receptors to an equal extent, have no additional therapeutic advantages, but restrict the subjective and objective tolerance of β-blockade owing to the

[1] Krankenhaus Neukölln, Rudower Str. 48, D-1000 Berlin 47 / FRG

Gerontology
Ed. by D. Platt
© Springer-Verlag Berlin Heidelberg 1989

Table 1. Influence of the sympathetic nervous system on metabolic processes (Lohmann 1988a)

Metabolic process	Sympathetic receptors		
	α	β_1	β_2
Insulin secretion	∅	(+)	+
Glycogenolysis			
Liver	+	(+)	+
Muscle		(+)	+
Free faty acids and glycerol (= lipolysis)	(+)	+	(+)
Renin secretion		+	(+)
T_4 to T_3		(+)	+
Secretion of parathormone, calcitonin, glucagon		(+)	+

∅, inhibition, +, activation.

unnecessary inhibition of organ functions controlled via β_2-receptors. This applies in particular to carbohydrate and lipid metabolism (Lohmann 1984, 1987a, 1988a).

In connection with carbohydrate metabolism, the influence on insulin secretion and glycogenolysis (chiefly in skeletal musculature) will be commented on below.

The insulin reserve (which can be activated inter alia via β_2-receptors) undergoes a relevant restriction under mixed β-blockade, so that for example in metabolically healthy subjects the glucose tolerance test has an erroneously pathological result, whereas this test is unimpaired under β_1-selective blockade. In patients with type II diabetes mellitus, who can be treated with a diet or in addition with an oral antidiabetic, a clinically relevant decompensation of carbohydrate metabolism may occur in this way under mixed β-blockade in situations of stress (infection, operation, etc.). For this reason, such diabetics should be treated with a β_1-selective blocker when there is an indication for β-blocker treatment. In this connection, it is also to be mentioned that the hyperglycemic effect of saluretics (e.g., hydrochlorothiazide) can be potentiated in patients with type II diabetes mellitus by the additional administration of a mixed β-receptor blocker (e.g., propranolol), so that the combination of a thiazide saluretic with a mixed β-receptor blocker has an unfavorable effect in patients with type II diabetes mellitus. The β_1-selective receptor blockers are thus also to preferred in this connection.

The inhibition of glycogenolysis in the skeletal musculature (which can be activated via β_2-receptors) with mixed β-blockade is generally of major clinical importance. With sustained physical exercise, a performance-limiting hypoglycemia with possibly paradoxial circulatory regulation (rise in blood pressure, fall in pulse rate) may thus occur in consequence of the resulting glycose consumption and lack of fresh supply. With use of equipotent doses of β_1-selective blockers and a mixed β_1, β_2-blocker (pindolol), we found a pronounced and significant fall in the blood sugar even into the hypoglycemic range in hypertensive patients during ergometric exercise in the steady state over 30 min with mixed β-receptor blockade with pindolol alone. The fresh rise in the blood sugar in hypoglycemia of different etiology in is naturally also impeded under mixed β-blockade.

For this reason, nonselective β-blockers are to be regarded as contraindicated today in patients with diabetes mellitus requiring insulin (type I) because of the raised risk of hypoglycemia. Under mixed β-blockade, the adaptation of the body both to a raised energy requirement during sustained physical exercise and in the situation of hypoglycemia owing to inhibited glycogenolysis is thus disturbed. Such unfavorable effects on the carbohydrate metabolism can be avoided by use of a β_1-selective blocker. In this connection, it is significant both with regard to carbohydrate metabolism and to energy metabolism in general that the cellular potassium homeostasis may be disturbed under mixed β-receptor blockade: a greater rise in the potassium level under physical exercise as well as a delayed fall in the potassium level in the recovery phase, since the reuptake of potassium into the cell takes place with mediation of β_2-receptors. For this reason, a pretreatment with a mixed β-blocker also appears to be exceedingly unfavorable in the therapy for a possible diabetic coma.

In mixed β-blockade, there is a greater suppression of catecholamine-induced lipolysis with consequent pronounced reactive alterations of lipoproteins and the metabolism of which is moreover disturbed owing to a reduced enzyme activity (e.g., of lipoprotein lipase). The consequence of this is a rise in triglycerides corresponding to an increase in the very low density lipoproteins and a fall of the anti-atherogenically active high density cholesterol. On the other hand, β_1-selective blockers have less and moreover only temporary effects on lipoproteins, and can therefore also be administered in patients with primary hyperlipoproteinemia. In this connection, Table 2 shows the behavior of the lipoproteins under chronic therapy with the β_1-selective blocker metoprolol and the calcium-antagonist verapamil in the intraindividual comparison in 18 hypertensive patients after 6 weeks' duration of treatment in each case. There were no significant alterations of the lipoproteins either under metoprolol or under verapamil. This means that in long-term therapy with β_1-selective blockers noteworthy potentially unfavorable alterations of the lipoproteins are not to be expected, so that the discussion on a possible induction of arteriosclerosis-promoting alterations by lipoproteins under chronic β-blockade is unnecessary in use of β_1-selective blockers. In this connection, it is worth mentioning that the alterations in the lipoproteins occurring under therapy with saluretics can be largely reversed or avoided by β-blockade. A cardioprotection of the same extent has been demonstrated in the context of secondary prevention after myocardial infarction under a β_1-selective blockade and under nonselective β-blockade. These results as well as the clinical experience elsewhere hence indicate that the therapeutic effect of β-blockers clearly outweighs a possible atherogenic effect in the respective cardiovascular target indication. On the other hand, an intrinsic sympathomimetic activity (ISA) of the β-blocker has proved to be unfavorable in this connection, since this property of the ISA more or less cancels the cardioprotective action of a β-blockade. Since up to 90% of β_1-receptors are to be found in the heart, the mainly β_1-selective

Table 2. Lipoproteins before and after 6 weeks of treatment with metoprolol (M) and verapamil (V) in 18 hypertensive patients (Lohmann 1988a)

	VLDL			HDL			LDL		
	∅	M	V	∅	M	V	∅	M	V
Mean value	208.6	214.2	172.1	41.3	40.1	47.1	152.5	148.9	143.0
± SD	146.1	101.8	83.8	12.3	11.8	12.9	38.7	33.1	20.8

Overall, no significant differences. ∅, before therapy.

blockers are virtually able to lower the myocardial oxygen consumption (above all under exercise) and thus to exert a cardioprotective effect. For this reason, the predominantly β_1-selective agents without ISA should be administered preferentially in elderly people in order to avoid negative effects on carbohydrate and lipid metabolism and to enable simultaneous cardioprotection (Lohmann 1986; Schreiber et al. 1988).

Besides the reduction of cardiac work and thus of myocardial oxygen consumption, this cardioprotection is brought about under β-blockade in particular in that there is a prolongation of the respective duration of diastole owing to the lowering of the resting and exercise heart rate and thus an improved myocardial blood flow even in ischemic areas. This is significant in particular for elderly hypertensive patients, since in principle patients with arterial hypertension may already display a relevant restriction of the functional coronary reserve even when the coronary angiogram is still normal, but elderly hypertensive patients nearly always display a more or less clinically significant coronary heart disease. An asymptomatic resting bradycardia even of 50 beats per minute due to therapy is not serious in this connection so long as the PQ time remains normal in the ECG and the pulse rate rises adequately in exercise. From the cardiac point of view, such a resting bradycardia under β-blockade is indeed to be regarded as benefical especially in elderly patients for the reasons described above (Lohmann 1988b).

This is why β-blockers appear to be generally suitable for administration both in coronary heart disease and in arterial hypertension alone or as a component of a combination therapy. However, they appear to be especially suitable and appropriate for elderly patients, since of all the substances available in these indications the β-blockers are most effectively able to reduce the myocardial oxygen consumption (especially under exercise) in accordance with the decrease in the pressure frequency product (systolic blood pressure times pulse rate) and thus to take into consideration the restricted coronary reserve (Schreiber et al. 1988).

In observation of the absolute contraindications, β_1-selective blockers without ISA possess an excellent global tolerance with a limiting rate of side-effects of only about 4% even in elderly patients. In a practical study (Platt 1984) in more than 1500 patients with arterial hypertension and an age of over 60 years, the rate of discontinuation of β_1-selective blockade with atenolol was indeed only 3.1%. Thus β_1-selective blockers without ISA are today the agents of choice in monotherapy and in combination therapy with nitrates and/or calcium antagonists of the nifedipine type in stable and instable angina pectoris, especially in elderly patients. They can also be used effectively in arterial hypertension in elderly people, at best in an early combination with a low-dose saluretic or another indirect vasodilator (e.g., nifedipine). In a recently published randomized double-blind study on hypertensive patients between 60 and 75 years old (Wikstrand et al. 1986) it could be shown that an antihypertensive therapy with 100 mg metoprolol once a day and possibly additional administration of 12.5 mg hydrochlorothiazide displayed a better subjective and objective tolerance combared to saluretic therapy with 25 mg and 50 mg hydrochlorothiazide on its own, with an equally effective and certain lowering of blood pressure. It was shown that by the combined treatment with β-blocker/saluretic a good lowering of blood pressure could be attained in up to 80% after 8 weeks (diastolic blood pressure equal to or less than 95 mmHg). It is also to be emphasized that hypopotassemia and a rise in the uric acid level in the serum occurred more frequently under treatment with hydrochlorothiazide alone than under the β-blocker/saluretic combination treatment with a lower dose of the single agents. At all events, an excessive saluretic therapy should be avoided especially in elderly hypertensive patients, since cerebrovascular complications are possible owing to hypovolemia and hemoconcentration. In a double-blind randomized comparative study in elderly hypertensive patients, the β_1-selective blocker bisoprolol indeed showed a better tolerance compared to nifedipine, with an equally good blood pressure-lowering action (Amabile and Serradimigni 1987).

An increase in the anthihypertensive potency is achieved with the triple combination of β-blocker/saluretic/vasodilator.

Since besides their vasodilatatory action, calcium antagonists of the verapamil type in addition have an antitachycardiac or antiarrhythmic action on the atrium and the atrioventricular node, they should not be combined with a β-blocker in order to avoid in particular possible high degree disorders of atrioventricular transmission. In this connection, a report is important in which a patient who received timolol eyedrops because of a glaucoma, developed a pronounced bradycardia owing to the additionally administered verapamil; this bradycardia was reversible after switching the verapamil medication to nifedipine (Pringle 1987).

In contraindication of a β-blockade or its intolerance, nitrates and/or calcium antagonists in coronary heart disease and the group of indirect vasodilators, if necessary in combination with a low dose saluretic, are the alternative therapy in arterial hypertension. However, it is emphasized once more that a cardioprotective action comparable to that achieved with the β-blockers has not yet been demonstrated for these drugs. β-Blockers with simultaneous and additional vasodilatory action are likely to constitute a perspective both in coronary heart disease and in arterial hypertension. The double point of action (cardiac and cardiac afterload) of such agents with the possibility of a low dosage makes such drugs appear favorable, especially for elderly patients. Appropriate studies will have to decide on this.

To summarize, β_1-selective blockers without an intrinsic sympathomimetic action are very suitable and especially appropriate for monotherapy and in particular for early combination therapy at a low dosage for treatment of cardiovascular target indication in elderly people provided that the absolute contraindications to β-blockade are not present.

Discussion

Platt

What do you think about the treatment of hypertension with reserpine, as Professor Kennedy mentioned in his paper?

Lohmann

I Think we no longer need this substance because the quantity and quality of side-effects are much more unfavorable than with the described new therapeutic regime. Professor Kennedy says depression and Parkinson's disease side-effects of reserpine and similar substances which influence the central nervous system. Furthermore reserpine has no effect on the blood pressure under working conditions and therefore no cardiac protective capacity. I think the substance was necessary as an initial form of medical treatment of hypertension, but today we have more selective and better therapeutic possiblities.

Hager

How do you control elderly patients who thake beta-blockers for the first time – I mean to prevent, for example, congestive heart disease?

Lohmann

Especially in elderly people one has to look for the mentioned contraindications. It is necessary to decide whether a patient is suitable for beta-blockade or not. Clinical investigations, including additional ray examinations of the chest, provide a reliable means of deciding whether the patient can tolerate the beta-blocker. And especially initially a low dose should be given. The patient should be seen 1 or 2 days after the commencement of this low dose, and asked how he feels. In this way I believe potential problems can be avoided.

References

Amabile G, Serradimigni A (1987) Comparison of bisoprolol with nifedipine for treatment of essential hypertension in the elderly: comparative double-blind trial. Eur Heart J 8 [Suppl M]: 65–69

Brodde OE (1988) Die Rolle adrenerger alpha- und beta-Rezeptoren in der Pathogenese von Hypertonie und Herzerkrankungen. Internist 29: 397–413

Lohmann FW (ed) (1984) Die klinische Bedeutung der Beta-1-Selektivität. Verlag für angewandte Wissenschaften, München

Lohmann FW (1986) Zur Therapie der arteriellen Hypertonie mit Beta-Rezeptorenblockern. Nieren- und Hochdruckkrankheiten 15: 8–14

Lohmann FW (ed) (1987a) Die Bedeutung der Beta-1-Selektivität für Klinik und Praxis. Walter de Gruyter, Berlin

Lohmann FW (1987b) Kombinationstherapie des Hochdrucks im Alter. Med Welt 38: 935–939

Lohmann FW (1988a) Betablocker, Kohlenhydrat- und Lipidstoffwechsel im Alter. Med Welt 39: 858–860

Lohmann FW (1988b) Hochdrucktherapie. In: Platt D (ed) Pharmakotherapie und Alter. Springer, Berlin Heidelberg New York

Platt D (1984) Beta-Blocker in der Geriatrie. MMV Medizin, München

Platt D (1984) Pharmakotherapie und Alter. Springer, Berlin Heidelberg New York

Pringle SD (1987) Severe bradycardia due to interaction of timolol eye drops and verapamil. Br Med J 294: 155–157
Schreiber P, Nehm K, Kähler H, Lohmann FW (1988) Vergleich der antihypertensiven Wirkung und Wirkungsdauer des Beta-Rezeptorenblockers Metoprolol und des Kalziumantagonisten Verapamil. Herz/Kreisl 20: 104–114
Wikstrand J, Westergren G, Berglund G et al. (1986) Antihypertensive treatment with metoprolol or hydrochlorothiazide in patients aged 60 to 75 years. Report from a double-blind international multicenter study. JAMA 255: 1304–1310

The Aging Human Cerebral Cortex: Morphometry of Areal Differences and Their Functional Meaning

H. HAUG[1]

Introduction

The description of the aging human brain centers on the biological or physiological aspects of the aging process. All pathological changes, including presenile dementia, have been omitted from our own examination.

Even today, some scientists are still of the opinion that increasing numbers of neurons will be lost during life. This belief is founded research published about 30 years ago, the basis of which was the work of Brody (1955). Brody himself expressed this view in vague terms because his statistical basis was too small for a definite statement. However, subsequent interpretations by other scientists and in the press have created the conviction that neurons are lost throughout life.

About 20–30 years ago, these interpretations led to the common opinion that the dementia of aging people begins at 40 years. In some firms in the USA, the managers over 40 were dismissed. However, the lack of experience of the younger managers caused problems for their firms. After only a few years this nonsense was totally stopped and, as the reader will know, an elderly man was elected president of the USA.

The brain is made up of several parts. The functionally most important structure is the gray matter, consisting of a large number of nerve cells and their connections. The latter are established by means of a network of long extensions like axons and dendrites and special contacts through the synapses. One nerve cell, depending on its size, can have hundreds to many thousands of such connections. The other substance is white and contains the fiber connections between the different grays.

There are many levels of gray matter for basic functions, most of which operate without the individual being aware of them. The highest functions in the human brain are found in the cortex cerebri, with locations for all those functions which are connected with consciousness and mind. In the areas of the cortex we find various functions of the higher nervous activities, like sensory analysis, higher analysis of sensory input, speech, and motor output, for motivation and inhibition of our behavior. One can distinguish between about 40 areas having specific

[1] Institute of Anatomy, Medical University of Lübeck, Ratzeburger Allee 160, D-2400 Lübeck 1 / FRG

Gerontology
Ed. by D. Platt
© Springer-Verlag Berlin Heidelberg 1989

cytoarchitectonic structures (Brodmann 1909; Vogt and Vogt 1926; Economo and Koskinas 1925).

Analysis of this very complex organ is complicated. However, in recent decades procedures have been evolved to achieve results regarding functional aspects of these structures. The measuring of histological sections is called morphometry. The data obtained can be transformed to three-dimensional magnitudes by stereology, which was nearly unknown 30 years ago.

Stereology in connection with sensitive morphometric equipment is able to estimate three-dimensional sizes at all levels from macroscopy to electron microscopy. The following results have been gained with such procedures (Haug 1986).

The Aim of Investigations

The following points have an influence on the morphometric brain morphology:

1. The secular acceleration of the body size leads to concomitant increases in brain volume over successive generations.
2. Modern procedures allow estimates not only of the whole brain weight but also of the volume fraction of the various parts of the brain. With the help of stereology, it is possible to determine whether various parts of the brain undergo changes in size at the same rate.
3. The effect of shrinkage during preparative procedures can be accurately examined in order to correct the morphometric data evaluated and achieve precise results for neuron density and size.
4. The synaptic level will be examined by means of electron microscopy.

Results gained through animal research can be transferred to human aging with caution. Some psychological investigations have also opened up new vistas on human brain aging that relate to our morphological results.

All efforts to enlarge our knowledge on aging require sensitive techniques and large quantities of material. This means that future investigations of aging in the human brain will lead to increasing expense. Both the high variability of human brain structures and changes of the tissues during preparation affect results of studies on the aging process.

Material and Procedures

Some remarks on material and methods are necessary. The macroscopic report on the different age-related changes in the various parts of the human brain is based on over 30 human brains from individuals 20–100 years old.

Morphometric analysis of neurons was performed on over 150 human brains of a similar age span without any sign of neuropathological change. A total of nearly 300 individual evaluations of cortical areas and the striatum were made. Each individual evaluation resulted in measurements of 1500–2000 neurons for all layers. It should be noted that each cell was measured over a drawing mirror of a microscope with a computerized digitizer (Haug 1979).

In order to examine alterations of neuron densities and size we used parts with different functions. A total of four cortical areas (Brodmann 1909) and one subcortical griseum were measured (Fig. 1):

1. Area 6 in the frontal lobe, which has an extrapyramidal function and has recently been designated the „supplementary motor area" by Eccles (1982).
2. Area 11 in the orbital section of the frontal lobe, which is a typical human area of the cerebral cortex and is linked with psychosocial functions.
3. Area 7 in the convexity of the parietal lobe, which is related to sensory and especially speech analysis.
4. The projection area 17, or visual cortex, which lies in the occipital lobe and performs the first analysis of visual input.
5. The corpus striatum, which is one of the important centers for the performance of movement.

The influence of procedures on the results is important, since a remarkable change of the volume can be observed during the preparation of the tissue from the removed brain to the stained histological sections. We have systematically

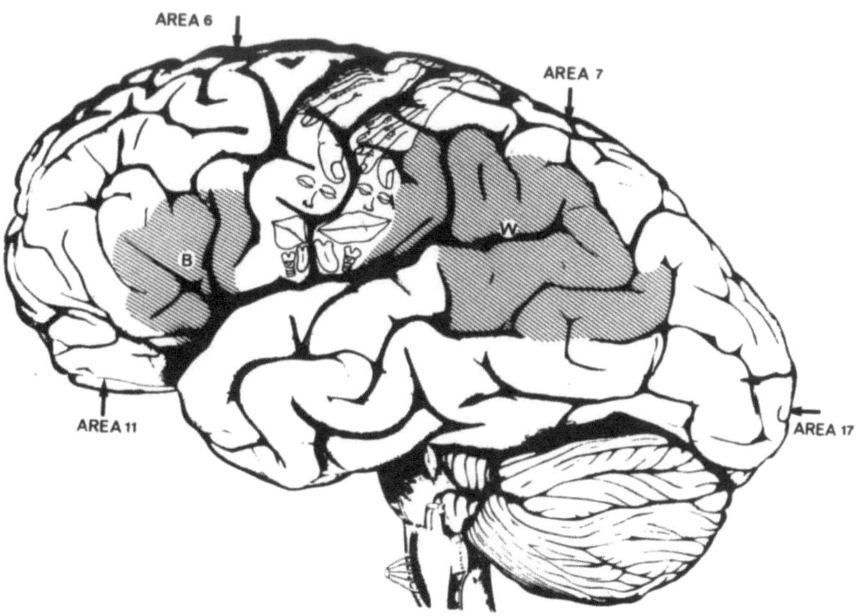

Fig. 1. The lateral aspect of the human brain. The cortical areas which we have estimated are indicated. *B* = Broca's motor speech area. *W* = Wernicke's sensory speech area

measured this change and found that the shrinkage of the tissue is dependent on age in some procedures (Haug 1980; Eggers et al. 1984a; Sass 1982).

Figure 2 shows the size of the volume changes during embedding using methylbenzoate as an intermediate. The shrinkage of the brain tissue belonging to a younger person is more pronounced than that of tissue from an older individual, probably because of the different water content.

The more pronounced shrinkage of younger tissue tends to yield higher neuron densities in the stained slide. The difference in shrinkage during embedding between tissue taken from individuals of 20–75 years amounts to about 15%. Consequently, we observe a 15% lower density of neurons in microscopic images of the aged individuals in spite of the fact that the neuron densities are in reality very similar.

That shrinkage during embedding is age dependent was unknown to early investigators, who probably correctly counted the amount of neurons but erroneously postulated a neuron loss which was, in fact, caused by differences in the shrinkage of brain tissue. This fact shows that many findings can be influenced by the complex reaction of the tissue as a whole. Therefore, results may be falsified if all aspects of the preparative changes are not taken into account.

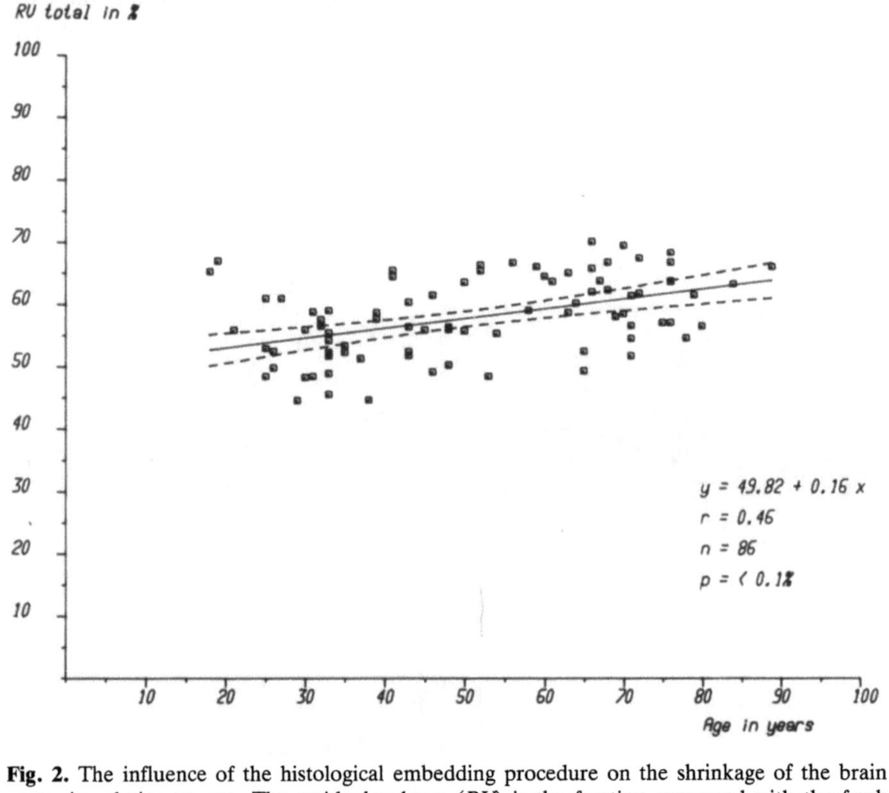

Fig. 2. The influence of the histological embedding procedure on the shrinkage of the brain parts, in relation to age. The residual volume (*RV*) is the fraction compared with the fresh volume. Embedding involved the use of methylbenzoate

Macroscopic Findings

Secular acceleration is the increase of human body size from generation to generation. Developmental acceleration refers to the accelerated development of a single individual, leading to earlier maturity. The latter process is probably caused by increased standards of living. The increase in height due to secular acceleration amounts to about 1 mm per year, meaning that the mean body height is presently 10 cm greater than 100 years ago. Human body size remained constant between the birth of Christ and about 1750 A.D. (Haug 1984a).

The larger the body, the larger the brain. Therefore, brain weight also increases by an average of 0.6 g per year. This means that taking secular acceleration into account, the brain weight of one generation is proportionately greater than that of the preceding generation as measured in their youth.

We have calculated the fraction of the generational difference in brain weights due to secular acceleration , showing that the mean human brain weight is constant up to the 60th year of age. Figure 3 contains the human brain weight on the ordinate. The dotted lines correspond to the means of 22000 brains examined in different transverse estimations. The straight lines show the theoretical longitudinal development of the mean human brain weight, which is constant up to the 60th year of age. After the 65th year we can observe a real loss in human brain volume. In the eighties this loss amounts to about 6% and is statistically significant (Haug 1984b).

Furthermore, our results demonstrate that the onset of brain volume loss is highly divergent. For instance, one can find extremely high brain weights in very old individuals. This means that the onset and rate of macroscopic aging events in the human brain differ widely from individual to individual.

Turning to the aging of the various parts of the brain, with the help of newer morphometric procedures we have measured the size of different regions of the

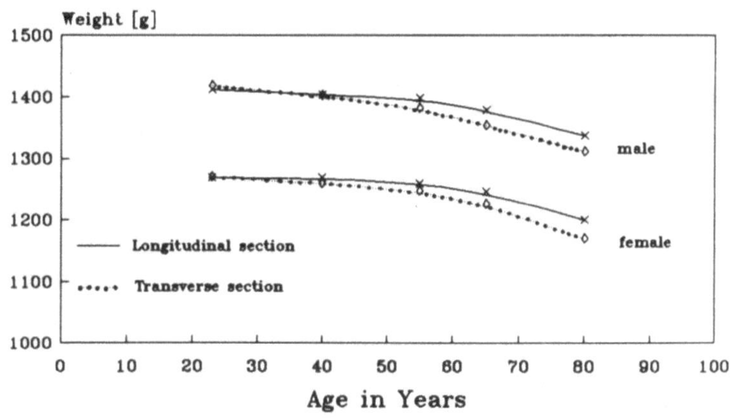

Fig. 3. The influence of secular acceleration on the brain weight in aging. The *straight lines* exhibit the change during individual life (longitudinal section) while the *dashed lines* show values estimated within a short time (transverse section)

Table 1. The changes of volume in the human brain during aging; the average brain volume at age 20–40 equals 100%

	Age		
	20–40 years	75–85 years	Change during aging
Entire brain	100.0	94.0	– 6%
Cerebral cortex	45.2	44.4	– 2%
Frontal cortex	9.0	8.1	– 10%
Lateral cortex	17.0	16.8	– 1%
White matter	36.4	32.3	– 11%
Corpus striatum	1.73	1.55	– 12%

Cerebral cortex without allocortex. Frontal cortex withour precentral area and medial part. Lateral cortex includes convexity and depth of the lateral fissure of the parietal, occipital, and temporal lobes. Corpus striatum includes nucleus caudatus and putamen.

brain. Our results are expressed in percentages due to the large variability of brain size. Calculations of the entire brain size were based on our results of the effects of secular acceleration (Eggers et al.1984b, Haug 1984b). Table 1 shows the most important results. The entire brain of an 80-year-old is, on average, 6% smaller than that of a 30-year-old. However, the entire cerebral cortex diminishes by only about 2% while the frontal cortex does so disproportionately, by 10% . On the other hand, the regions involving sensory and speech functions in the parietal and occipital lobes do not change their size. The corpus striatum and the white matter, in particular the connecting fibers, also decrease in size, by 11%–12%.

To summarize: The various regions of the brain undergo different macroscopic alterations during aging. This also applies to the cerebral cortex, where the frontal cortex shrinks strongly during aging, whereas the parieto-occipital cortex does not change in size.

Microscopic Findings

The morphometry of the number and size of neurons in the aging cortex must take into account the high variability within a population. Therefore, our estimates are based on measurement of at least 50 brains in respect of each area. In Fig. 4 the density of neurons in $1000/mm^3$ is expressed on the ordinate and the age on the abscissa. All results of microscopic morphometry are corrected for fresh or unfixed brain. In this case the density of neurons does not decrease during aging.

It is striking that some areas show an increase in neuron density per mm^3 with age (Haug et al. 1983,1984). This is true primarily of area 6, the supplementary motor cortex. On the other hand, we found that macroscopically this area decreases markedly in size. The increase in density is connected with the decrease in volume. This question will be discussed further. The higher sensory area 7 has

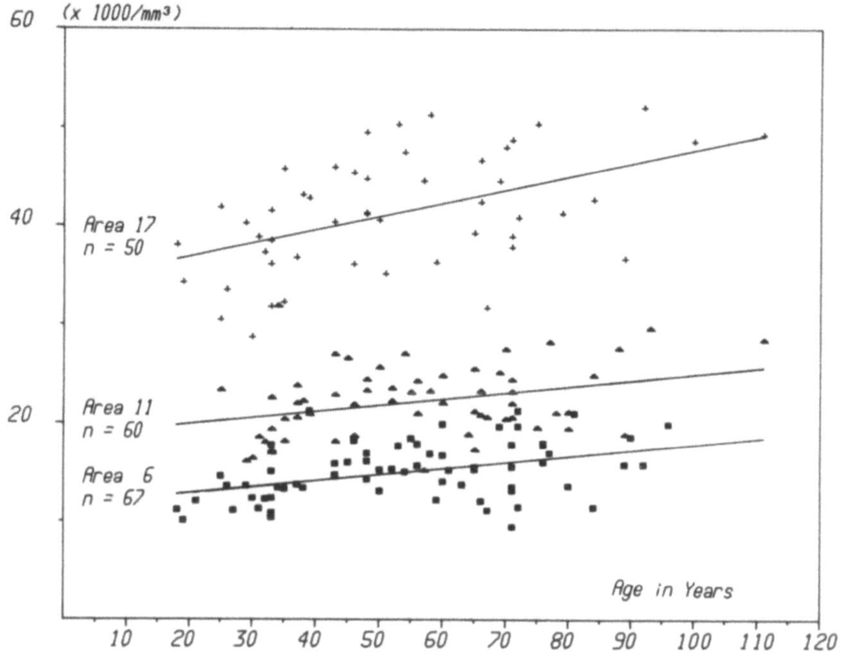

Fig. 4. Density of neurons in areas 6, 11, and 17 (visual cortex) during aging. The increase is due to the shrinkage of the entire area during aging

a pattern similar to that of the psychosocial area 11.A small increase in neuron density with age can be observed in all areas.

Figure 5 shows quite different tendencies in perikaryon size between the three areas. The supplementary motor cortex, area 6, exhibits a striking degree of diminution of neuron size during life, while the visual area 17 shows a smaller, though still statistically significant, reduction in size. A first glance at area 11 with its psychosocial functions reveals similarities to area 6. However, the decrease in neuron size does not occur continuously. Perikaryon size remains nearly constant up to 60–65 years, when it strongly decreases.

The parietal cortex area 7, not demonstrated in Fig. 5, performs superior sensory functions and reveals a relatively small and steady decrease in nerve cell size until old age, with a shrinkage amounting to about 10% of the original volume. The motor area 6 has a mean volume decrease of 30%–35%, whereas the psychosocial area 11 is diminished by between 10% and 30%.

Figure 5 does not demonstrate how the different neuron sizes contribute to the reduction in mean projection area. This is demonstrated by the size distribution graphs. Figure 6 shows the overall neuronal size distribution for 12 size classes. The total number of cells analyzed for each curve corresponds to 100%. The curves depict three age groups. The distance between the curves expresses the size differences between the perikaryon projection areas. The right lines and signs concern those aged below 45 years, the middle ones those ages between 45 and

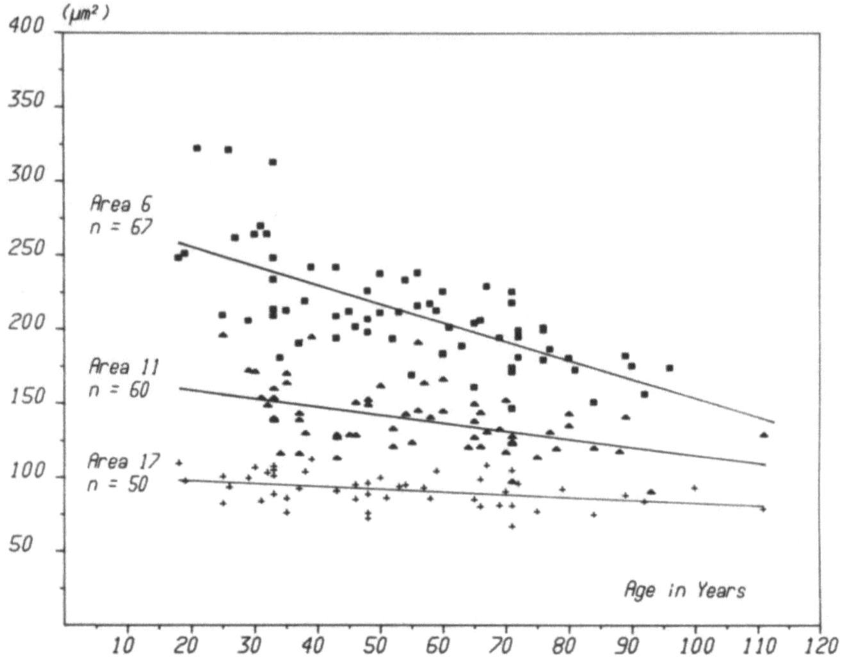

Fig. 5. The mean area of perikarya in areas 6, 11, and 17 during aging (for details see text)

65 years, and the left ones all individuals over 66 years. The curves lying more to the right are based on larger cell size distribution than those on the left. Areas 7 and 11 are based on classes with 34 μm^2, while area 6 has a basis of 46 μm^2 (Haug 1985).

The large distances separating the age curves for area 6 mean that the cell sizes diminish continuously between the three age groups in all size classes. By contrast the age curves for area 7 show only a very small decrease in size during the aging process. Area 11 exemplifies another pattern. Cell sizes remain nearly unchanged up to the 65th years of age, after which a distinct decrease in size can be observed. This accords with the behavior of mean sizes. The visual cortex (not shown) with its small cells shows a slight but continuous diminution of cell sizes during life. The graphs demonstrate that the decrease in various cell sizes in one area is similar.

We did not find remarkable differences in shrinkage for the various sizes of neurons within one area. Similar observations have been made by Uemura and Hartmann (1978).

Our examinations involve the various layers of the cerebral cortex. Though some smaller differences can be observed, they have no implications for our view of the aging process.

The results on neuron densities and the volume of the cerebral cortex make it possible to calculate the total number of neurons in the individual cortex. The

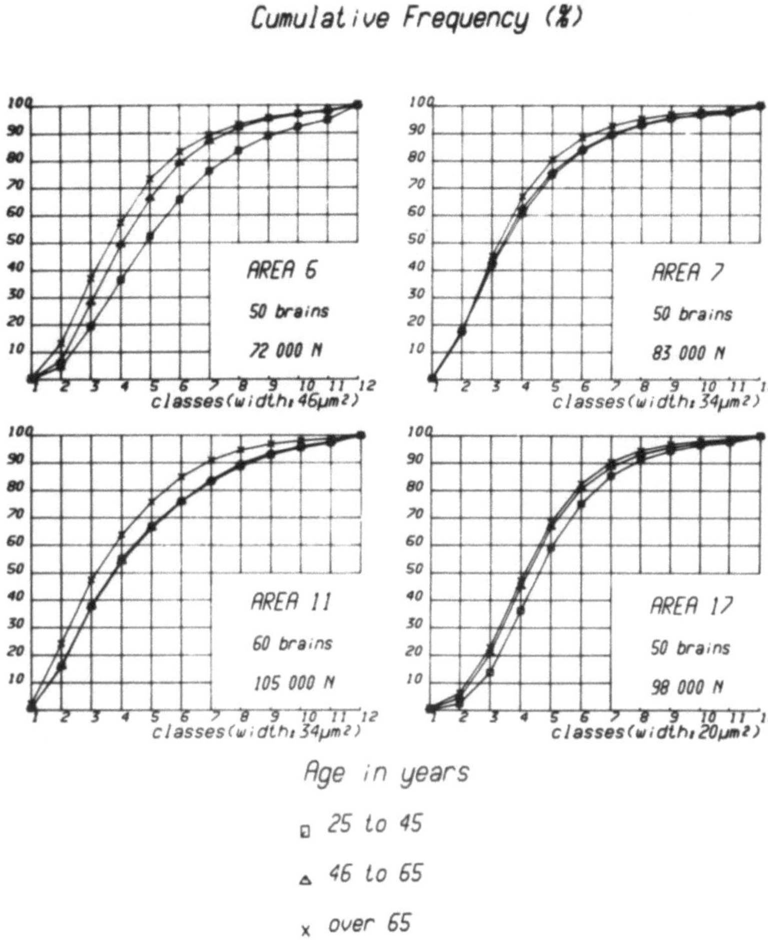

Fig. 6. The size distribution of the neurons in the estimated areas for three age groups. The curves represent sum frequencies (for details see text)

volume occupied by the cortex amounts to about 47.5% of that of the total brain. This percentage increases with aging to nearly 50%, because during aging the cortex does not shrink to the same degree as the other brain parts.

Figure 7 shows the total number of neurons in individual human cortices in ten billions. The abscissa depicts age and shows that the number of neurons varies considerably between individuals. It should be noted that only those brains for which values were based on two or more areas have been used. The mean number of neurons in the human cortex cerebri totals 13.9 billions, with a range between 10 and 20. We cannot discern any tendency for the number of neurons to diminish with age, but it must be stated that the decrease in brain size is counterbalanced by an increase in neuron density. Otherwise the number of neurons demonstrates a clear dependence on brain size (Haug 1985).

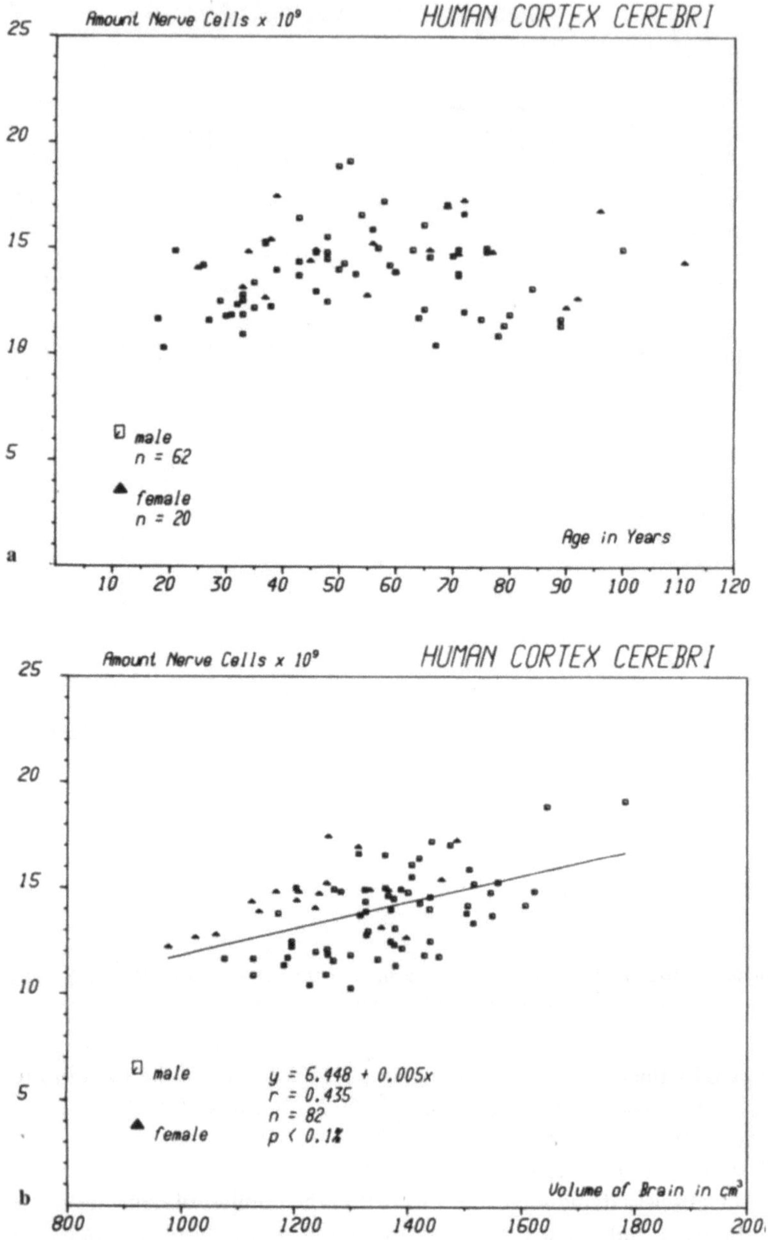

Fig. 7. The total number of neurons in the individual cerebral cortices of humans in relation to **a** age and **b** brain size. Males are represented by *squares* and women by *triangles*

An interesting point should also be mentioned in respect of this graph. The female values marked by triangles are arranged among the male values and show no tendency to deviate from the mean value of the males. This point is remarkable, because on average females have smaller brains (about 100–150 ccm) than males. The statistically significant higher neuron density of the areas in the females compensates for this smaller brain size (Haug 1985).

The corpus striatum, the volume of which can be easily measured, shows an interesting behavior. Eggers et al. (1987) found that the total volume of the striatum decreases with age. On the other hand they demonstrated that the neuron

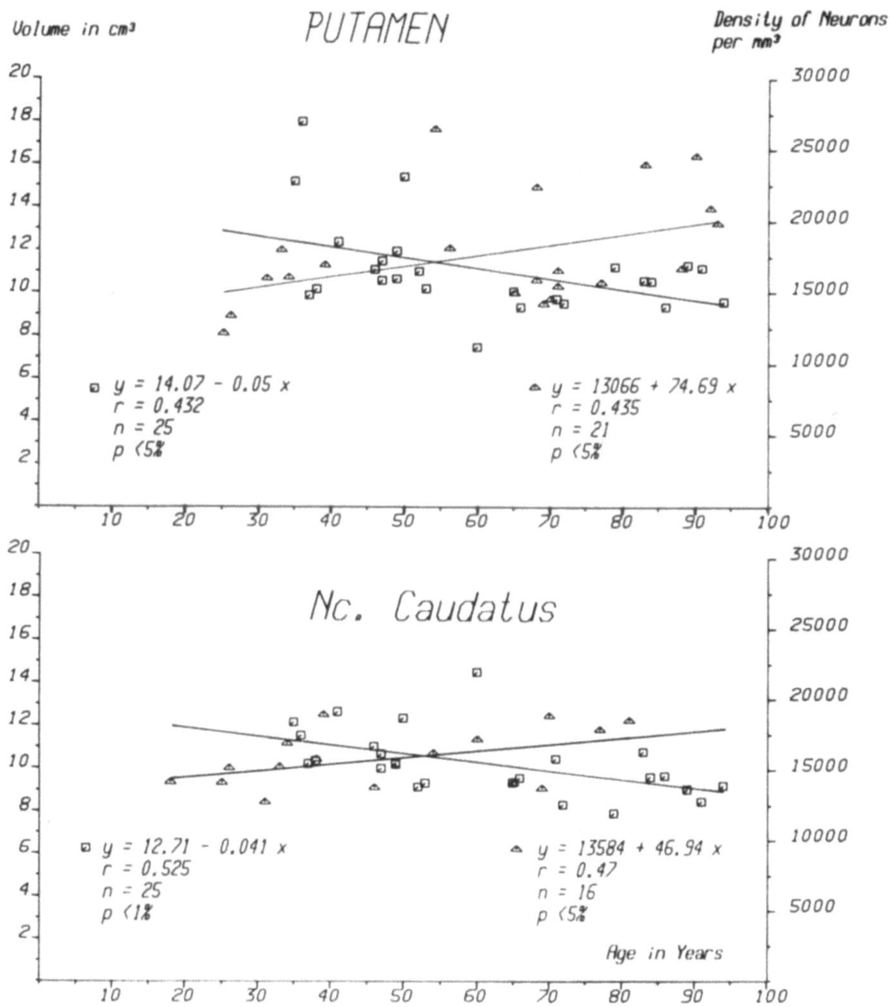

Fig. 8. The human corpus striatum and aging. The *right-hand y-axis* shows the neuron density and the *left-hand y-axis* the volume of both parts of the corpus striatum. The slopes of both regressions are similar, but they are positive in the density and negative in the volume. (Eggers et al. 1987)

density increases. Both processes have about the same slope but in reverse directions. Figure 8 demonstrates impressively that the neurons do not disappear though the gray diminishes in size. However, they show a distinct shrinkage in size, like in area 6.

The following statement may be made in respect of the neurons: The total number of neurons in the human cerebral cortex and corpus striatum does not change during the aging process, if all pathological material is excluded. However, this result need not be representative for all regions of the brain or the cortex.

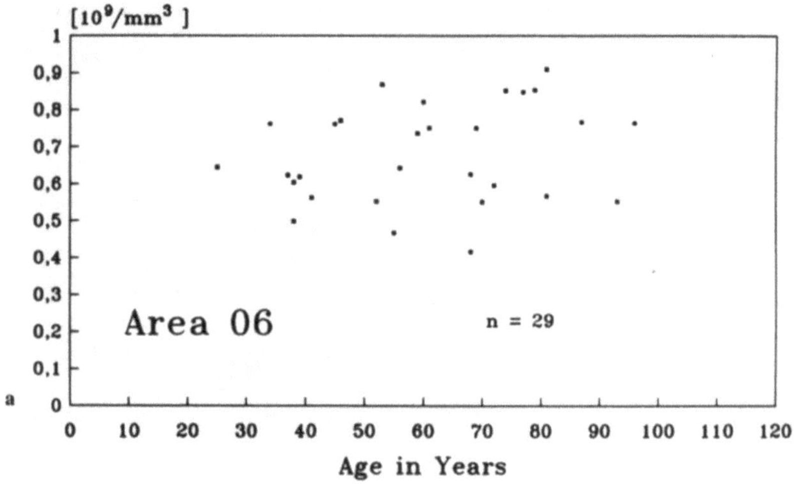

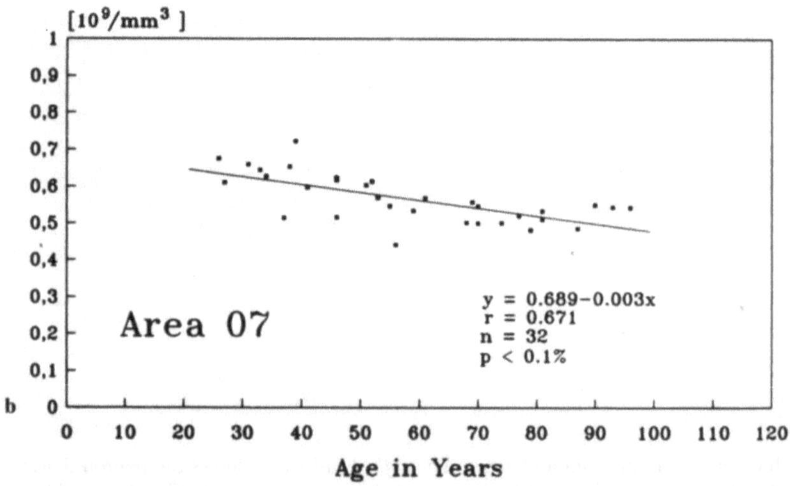

Fig. 9. The results of the evaluation of synaptic densities in areas 6 (**a**) and 7 (**b**) (After Haug et al., in press)

Futhermore, it is probable that pathological material reveals degeneration, as, for example, reported by Terry et al. (1987) in Alzheimer's disease.

Electron Microscopic Findings

At the ultrastructural level it is possible to stain the switching structures called synapses in the human brain with a special procedure for electron microscopy, instead of the autolysis of other ultrastructural components. The use of ethanolic phosphotungstic acid (EPTA) after Bloom and Aghajanian (1968) allows the synapses to be seen as long as fixation of the brain occurs within 96 h of death (Muser, in preparation). With the help of stereological procedures the real density of synapses can be estimated.

Figure 9 shows our results regarding areas 6 and 7 (Haug et al. in press.). Area 7, which displays only small changes at the macroscopic and microscopic levels, exhibits a distinct decrease in synaptic density during aging. This demonstrates that the number of synapses decreases in this area. While the number of neurons does not decrease, the number of synapses per neuron must diminish. On the other hand Fig. 9 shows that the number of synapses in area 6 is highly variable but does not diminish. However, this result also exhibits a decrease in the number of synapses per neuron, because the neuron density increases in accordance with the decrease in volume of the area.

The electron microscopic results show that at this level the aging process proceeds independently of the high stability in the number of neurons. This fact provides a possible explanation why the functional use of cortical structures inhibits the involution usually associated with aging. Synapses are dynamic structures which can be partially lost during life but on the other hand are rebuilt if their use is demanded (Eccles 1979: Cotman and Nieto-Sampedro 1984; Sirevaag and Greenough 1988). This behavior of synaptic structures can explain the clinical observation that rehabilitation of elderly people leads to a distinct improvement of psychological abilities in some cases (Lehrl and Fischer 1986).

Our own investigation as well as those of Huttenlocher (1978, 1979) and Uemura (1985) demonstrates that the density of synapses decreases slightly with higher age. However, in many cases elderly people live in an impoverished situation before their death. This might lead to a loss of synapses, in combination with restrictions imposed by ill health.

Conclusion

These and other results have led to new insights into the morphological and functional changes taking place in the human brain during the aging process. The main results are summarized in Fig. 10 and Table 2.

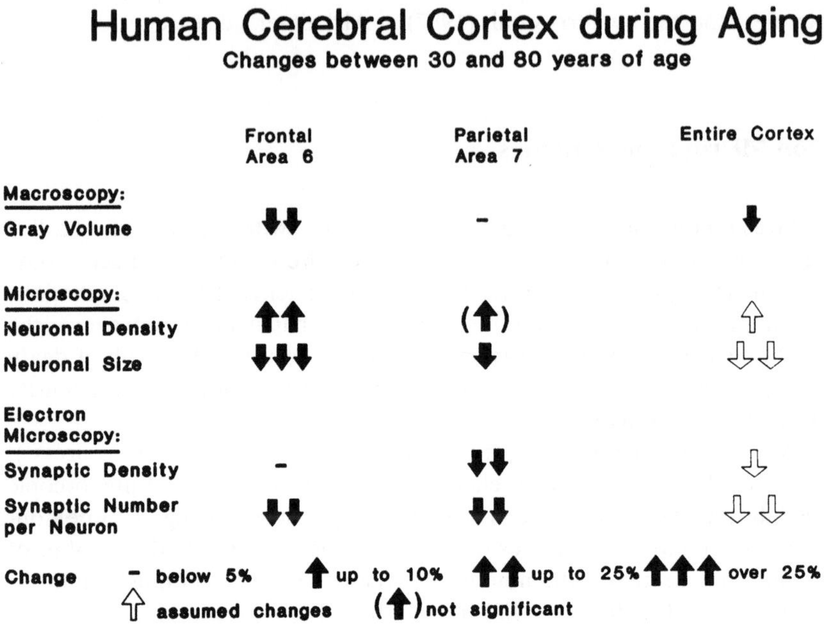

Fig. 10. Composition of our results in areas 6 and 7 for the different levels of investigation (for details see text)

Table 2. Results of the investigation on brain aging

Macroscopy:	1. Diminution of brain after the 60th year 2. High individual variability 3. High local variability
Microscopy:	1. No loss of neurons in the cortex 2. Shrinkage of neuronal perikarya with local variability 3. A minor loss of synapses
Reaction of grays:	1. Area 6: early, large, significant 2. Area 7: very little change 3. Area 11: after 60 – 65 years, significant 4. Area 17: little change

1. Morphometric results of macroscopy and light microscopy show that up to 60–65 years of age no or only small changes in the human cerebral cortex can be observed, with the exception of the supplementary motor cortex. It should be pointed out that this is a statistical statement, meaning that, on average, the onset of morphological age changes in the human cortex may be expected around the 60–65th year of age. In the individual case such changes may begin earlier or later. The time of onset and speed of aging probably depend on a genetic program.

Haug

The standard deviation in respect of the brain is much smaller than the variation between individuals: there is a local variation of about 5% and an interindividual variation of 20%.

Linke

And what is the technique, how do you do it?

Haug

We performed measurements with a semiautomatic system and in part with an automatic system by tracing the outline of the nerve cells on a digitizer board over a drawing mirror on the microscope. We have a special program in our system.

Platt

What about the constant level of the nerve cells? Do the constant values refer to the six areas you looked at, or to the total brain? If they refer only to the six areas, you can't exclude the possibility that the other areas show either increases or decreases.

Haug

That's totally unknown. But we have selected locations with different functions. I think we have a certain overview of the brain. But it's actually possible that some parts of the cortex deviate from these results.

Frenzel

What is the exact explanation for the increase in the volume density of nerve cells – a smaller extracellular space or a loss of dendrites?

Haug

As far as we know it's a loss of dendrites, and axons as well.

Klotz

I would like to make a comment concerning one of your figures. There was no decline in the cell numbers with aging. Looking at the points, there seems to be a U-shaped curve. Thus, there might be some increase during maturation. This increase might occur until 40 – as you said, using and training does a lot to the brain – whereas afterwards there is a decline, giving a biphasic effect.

Haug

I must admit that this question is not solved. With the usual statistical procedure we cannot find a clear result. I think there are too few results for a definite statement.

Kidd

I am very interested in this paper; I knew that somebody, someday would show an increase in neuronal density. I'm very pleased by this because I feel that although some people have been counting neurons for quite a long time they change their minds in the most disconcerting way. Not Brody, but others. But they did not dare to publish an increase in density.

In fact biochemists, for example Dr. Bowen, a colleague of Professor Davidson in London, estimate enzymes and neurons *per lobe* or *per brain* and not per unit volume. And the only way you can talk about neurons being lost in normal aging (or any kind of aging) is *per brain*. Shrinkage must be allowed for; I think this is really an important point. Now it's true that some people say that the brain doesn't shrink statistically, but I think most people who deal with these brains say that they do shrink.

Well, Professor Haug has provided evidence in the normal brain that there is shrinkage, so I think that this is a particularly interesting paper from that point of view because the real thing is (I would have thought) a loss of synapses – and this is what you addressed in the end. Whether the synapses are lost because the cell body that carries those synapses has died or has not died, it's the synapses that matter; these are the things that we are actually using. It's quite possible to count neurons which appear to be normal but in fact have lost their dendrites, or part of them. The Golgi preparations of Scheibel show this; he shows specimens in which neurons appear to have lost their dendrites and yet they would be counted in an ordinary Nissl preparation.

Haug

I can count the synapses in the electron microscopical level, but I cannot estimate the dendrites. If there is a definite loss of synapses there will be a loss of some dendrites and axon terminals at the same time. The number of synapses only represents the changing situation.

Kidd

But this is the trouble, I am about to start to do some Golgi preparations as Scheibel did and I intend to measure them. There are difficulties with Golgi staining, but in a good preparation you can see the spines on the dendrites.

Haug

I have not performed a Golgi preparation. I did not have enough time for that. I have carried out a large-scale enquiry and I am now working on the capillaries and the basement membrane, an evaluation which is not yet finished. I was of the opinion that other scientists, especially the English circles around Barry (London), are more acquainted with dendrites and they would make these investigations.

Barrows

We have repeatedly failed to show a decrease in the total DNA of the brains of rats with age. Since it has been shown by Frank that the DNA/nucleus of brain remains constant with age, total DNA is a reasonable index of total cell numbers. Therefore, our data reported on rats agree with yours found in man.

Kidd

What I say to my students is that numbers cannot go up in the adult. We accept that they must go down but what Professor Haug is saying is that the statistical variation is so great that it is impossible to detect the change. It can't be very large.

Haug

I should point out that in his newer investigations on the human nuclei of the brain stem, Brody has never found a decrease in cell number. In addition the cortex cerebri is a very complicated structure and a highly developed technique is needed to evaluate it.

References

Bloom FE, Aghajanian GK (1968) Fine structural and cytochemical analysis of the staining of synaptic junctions with phosphotungstic acid. J Ultrastruct Res 22: 361–375

Brodmann K (1909) Vergleichende Lokalisationslehre der Großhirnrinde. JA Barth Leipzig (Reprint 1985)

Brody H (1955) Organization of the cerebral cortex. III. A study of aging in the human cerebral cortex. J Comp Neurol 102: 511–556

Connor JR, Beban SE, Hopper PA, Hansen B, Diamond MC (1982) A Golgi study of the superficial pyramidal cells in the somatosensory cortex of socially reared old adult rats. Exp Neurol 76: 35–45

Cotman CW, Nieto-Sampedro M (1984) Cell biology of synaptic plasticity. Science 225: 1287–1294

Diamond MC, Johnson RE, Protti AM, Ott C, Kajisa L (1985) Plasticity in the 904-day-old male rat cerebral cortex. Exp Neurol 87: 309–317

Eccles JC (1979) Synaptic plasticity. Naturwissenschaften 66: 147–153

Eccles JC (1982) The initiation of voluntary movements by the supplementary motor area. Arch Psychiatr Nervenkr 231: 423–441

Economo v C, Koskinas GN (1925) Die Cytoarchitektonik der Hirnrinde des erwachsenen Menschen. Springer, Wien Berlin

Eggers R, Haug H, Örün C (1984a) Präparative Einflüsse auf das Schrumpfungsverhalten und das mikroskopische Bild von Gehirngewebe. Verh Anat Ges 78: 529–531
Eggers R, Haug H, Fischer D (1984b) Preliminary report on macroscopic age changes in the human prosencephalon. A stereologic investigation. J Hirnforsch 25: 129–139
Eggers R, Haug H, Kunkel M (1987) Altersveränderungen des Volumens des menschlichen Corpus striatum und seiner Nervenzelldichte. Anat Anz Jena 163: 149
Fischer B, Lehrl S (1983) Vierte Klausenbacher Gesprächs-Runde. Biologische und informationspsychologische Grundlagen des zerebralen Jogging. Gunter Narr, Tübingen
Haug H (1979) The evaluation of cell-densities and of nerve-cell-size distribution by stereological procedures in a layered tissue (cortex cerebri). Microsc Acta 82: 147–161
Haug H (1980) Die Abhängigkeit der Einbettungsschrumpfung des Gehirngewebes vom Lebensalter. Verh Anat Ges 74: 699–700
Haug H (1982) Möglichkeiten der Stereologie (Methodik, Anwendung und Probleme). Acta Histochem 26: 321–325
Haug H (1984a) Der Einfluß der säkularen Akzeleration auf das Hirngewicht des Menschen und dessen Änderung während der Alterung. Gegenbaurs Morphol Jahrb 130: 481–500
Haug H (1984b) Macroscopic and microscopic morphometry of the human brain and cortex: a survey in the light of new results. Brain Pathol 1: 123–149
Haug H (1985) Are neurons of the human cerebral cortex really lost during aging? A morphometric examination. In: Traber J, Gispen WH (eds) Senile dementia of the Alzheimer type. Springer, Berlin Heidelberg New York, pp 150–163
Haug H (1986) History of neuromorphometry. J Neurosci Methods 18: 1–17
Haug H, Barmwater U, Eggers R, Fischer D, Kühl S, Sass N-L (1983) Anatomical changes in aging brain: morphometric analysis of the human prosencephalon. Aging 21: 1–12
Haug H, Kühl S, Mecke E, Sass N–L, Wasner K (1984) The significance of morphometric procedures in the investigation of age changes in cytoarchitectonic structures of human brain. J Hirnforsch 25: 353–374
Haug H, Knebel G, Lodd M (in press) Die Dichte der Synapsen im menschlichen Cortex. Eine Untersuchung zur Alterung der Areae 6 und 7. Verh Anat Ges
Huttenlocher PR (1978) Synaptic density in human cerebral cortex – development changes and effects of aging. Neurology 4: 375
Huttenlocher PR (1979) Synaptic density in human frontal cortex – development changes and effects of aging. Brain Res 163: 195–205
Lehr U (1983) Die Beziehungen zwischen den Generationen – Konflikte und Kooperation. Z Gerontol 16: 197–199
Lehr U (1988) Gerontopsychologie. In: Asanger R, Wenninger G (eds) Handwörterbuch Psychologie. Psychologie-Verlag Orion, München, Weinheim pp 231–238
Lehrl S, Fischer B (1986) Individuelle Informationshygiene: Berücksichtigung der großen zwischenmenschlichen Unterschiede. Geriatrics-pregeriatrics-rehabilitation 2: 133–147
Muser C (in preparation) The influence of the time between death and fixation on the morphometry of cortical synapses of the rat.
Sass N-L (1982) The age-dependent variation of the embedding-shrinkage of neurohistological sections. Mikroskopie (Wien) 39: 278–281
Sirevaag AM, Greenough WT (1988) A multivariate statistical summary of synaptic plasticity measures in rats exposed to complex, social and individual environments. Brain Res 441: 386–392
Terry RD, DeTeresa R, Hansen LA (1987) Neocortical cell counts in normal human adult aging. Ann Neurol 21: 530–539
Uemura E (1985) Age-related changes in the subiculum of *Macaca mulatta:* synaptic density. Exp Neurol 87: 403–411
Uemura E, Hartmann HA (1978) RNA content and volume of nerve cell bodies in human brain. I. Prefrontal cortex in aging normal and demented patients. Neuropathol Exp Neurol 37: 487–496
Vijayashankar N, Brody H (1977a) Aging in the human brain stem. A study of the nucleus of the trochlear nerve. Acta Anat 99: 169–172

Vijayashankar N, Brody H (1977b) A study of aging in the human abducens nucleus. J Comp Neurol 173: 433–438
Vogt C, Vogt O (1926) Die vergleichende architektonische und vergleichende reizphysiologische Felderung der Großhirnrinde mit besonderer Berücksichtigung der menschlichen. Naturwissenschaften 14: 1190–1194

The Amyloidosis of Alzheimer's Disease

M. Kidd[1] and M. Landon[2]

Introduction

Alzheimer's disease is a brain-limited amyloidosis: one of a number of such disorders which we have suggested can be seen as protein storage diseases (Landon et al. 1987), a concept that draws parallels with the accumulations of carbohydrates and complex lipids in the well understood storage diseases where catabolic enzymes are reduced or missing.

Amyloid is a generic term used to describe pathological deposits of insoluble protein filaments which are usually extracellular and are identifiable by specific staining properties, the most characteristic being birefringence when stained with Congo red. Production of amyloid occurs in a number of distinct hereditary and acquired human and animal syndromes in which specific proteins are partially degraded to form deposits which are either systemically distributed or, less commonly, limited to a single organ. For recent reviews see Glenner (1980a, b), Husby and Sletten (1985), and Landon et al. (1987). An account of age-related non-cerebral amyloid [R.P. Linke] is found in this volume.

In Alzheimer's disease the definitive lesions are the senile plaques in the neuropil and the intraneuronal neurofibrillary tangles; both of these have the staining properties of amyloid (including argyrophilia and birefringent congophilia) although the paired helical filaments characteristic of the tangles are morphologically distinct from all other amyloid filaments (Kidd 1963). However, the parsimonious principle that only one chemical type of amyloid occurs in one disease has not yet been demonstrated for the paired helical filaments. In addition, the accumulation of cerebrovascular amyloid (congophilic angiopathy) in many cases of this disease has taken on greater significance from the protein chemical advances reviewed here. We will present the morphological information available for each form of cerebral amyloid under separate headings but the chemical information will draw together the common features of the extracellular amyloid.

None of the three types of amyloid deposition associated with Alzheimer's disease is unique to this disorder; all are found at low levels in normal ageing. Both senile plaque and tangle numbers have been correlated with loss of cognitive function (Wilcock and Esiri 1982) although a threshold level of plaque concentra-

Departments of Human Morphology[1] and Biochemistry[2], University of Nottingham Medical School, Queen's Medical Centre, Nottingham NG7 2UH, UK

Gerontology
Ed. by D. Platt
© Springer-Verlag Berlin Heidelberg 1989

tion must usually be achieved before noticeable dementia is apparent (Blessed et al. 1968). Non-demented elderly people may exhibit a brain-limited intramural vascular amyloid (Tomlinson 1979), which has been related to plaque incidence (Mandybur 1986).

All three types of amyloid deposit are found in significant amounts in the brain in essentially all cases of Down's syndrome over 40 years of age (Wisniewski et al. 1985). This, together with the chemical data reviewed here, had suggested chromosome 21 as the site of the gene coding for the amyloid precursor protein; this prediction was confirmed in the recent series of reports following the successful cloning of the amyloid precursor protein cDNA and proof of the location of the gene on this chromosome (Kang et al. 1987; Goldgaber et al. 1987; Tanzi et al. 1987; St. George-Hyslop et al. 1987; Robakis et al. 1987).

Morphology of the Amyloid in Senile Plaques

The classical senile plaque is spherical, 50–200 μm in diameter, and consists of an extracellular core of amyloid fibrils surrounded by an argyrophilic rim of dystrophic neurites (hence the designation "neuritic") which contain paired helical filaments and abnormal organelles, together with normal glial processes (Kidd 1964; Terry et al. 1964). A number of studies have identified immunoreactive material in the neuritic elements of the plaque periphery, indicating that a variety of neurons of different neurotransmitter types contribute to the lesion.

As noted later, significant amounts of extracellular amyloid are present in the plaque periphery. Not all plaques contain cores and those without have been called "primitive" plaques (Wisniewski and Terry 1976), which can vary in size from the smallest, only observable with the electron microscope, to some as large as the classical variety. Finally, a "burnt out" plaque (Wisniewski and Terry 1976) is a core without peripheral cellular involvement and the name again presumes a stage in development: the terminal state.

The core of the plaque in Alzheimer's disease most often consists of bundles of filaments apparently radiating from a central point, giving a stellate appearance. Less regularly organised "amorphous" cores also occur and this type may predominate in Down's syndrome (Allsop et al. 1986c). The stellate appearance of a plaque core is an unusual form of amyloid deposition but not unique to the brain; "sunflower" (Vital and Vital 1984) and "star-like" (Mancardi and Mandybur 1983; Mori et al. 1985) as well as "stellate" (Sorensen et al. 1964; Tischler and Compagno 1979; Osamura et al. 1982; Westermark et al. 1976) are descriptions that have been given to paracrystalline arrays of different chemical forms of amyloid deposited near to or at the initial site of secretion in a variety of locations in a number of amyloidoses.

The filament bundles present in senile plaques and cerebrovascular amyloid resemble those of most other amyloids and show the characteristic features of 8–10 nm diameter uniform filaments which are poorly defined with conventional electron-dense stains. Negatively stained cerebral amyloid filaments have been described as pairs of helically wound 6 nm protofilaments (Merz et al. 1983).

Morphology of Cerebrovascular Amyloid

The accumulation of cerebrovascular amyloid (congophilic angiopathy) is not an invariable occurrence in Alzheimer's disease; when present, cerebrovascular amyloid is found with the light microscope (using the Congo red stain) to lie in cortical arteriolar walls. On the evidence of serial sections in electron microscopy it has been suggested that the senile plaques are usually traceable to amyloidotic vessels (Miyakawa et al. 1982).

Protein Chemistry of Plaque and Cerebrovascular Amyloid

Since accumulations of pathological proteins in vivo indicate an inability to degrade a precursor to its constituent amino acids it is perhaps no surprise that amyloids have always proved to be intractable materials for the protein chemist; difficulties of extraction have been common, giving low yields of material of uncertain purity. The amyloid present in the brain has proved to be especially difficult to study; a sparse distribution of amyloid often precludes most valid Alzheimer brains as source material; the exceptional heavily affected brain (perhaps one or two in 100) is the key to any preparative procedure.

The original studies on plaque cores exploited the stability of their paracrystalline organisation in purification methods where disruption of tissue and protease treatments leave the cores intact (Allsop et al. 1983; Kidd et al. 1985b). Reproducible amino acid compositions clearly established the unusual nature of the core amyloid (Allsop et al. 1983); in particular, a level of valine higher than that of almost any known protein composition, and also a low value for threonine were indications of this uniqueness. This protein also proved to be insoluble in most protein solvents.

The most significant advance towards fuller characterisation came from the isolation of the amyloid protein from deposits in the walls of leptomeningeal vessels (Glenner and Wong 1984a). Here a conventional amyloid extraction and isolation method yielded a "β-protein" from which a unique partial amino acid sequence was obtained; it was immediately apparent that this protein had an amino acid composition very similar to that found for cores and a common structure was proposed (Kidd et al. 1985a; Allsop et al. 1986a). It was subsequently confirmed that the two proteins were identical by the independent isolation of cores, their disruption using formic acid and the determination of the same partial amino acid sequence for "A_4" protein (from the molecular size of 4 kd) (Masters et al. 1985b); in contrast to β-protein, where a single sequence was found, core protein had N-terminal length heterogeneity. A_4 will be the term used here for

Table 1. Amino acid sequence of cerebral amyloid in Alzheimer's disease

5 10 15
Asp-Ala-Glu-Phe-Arg-His-Asp-Ser-Gly-Tyr-Glu-Val-His-His-Gln-
20 25 30
Lys-Leu-Val-Phe-Phe-Ala-Glu-Asp-Val-Gly-Ser-Asn-Lys-Gly-Ala-
35 40
Ile-Ile-Gly-Leu-Met-Val-Gly-Gly-Val-Val-Ile-Ala-Thr

The complete amino acid sequence of plaque core protein. N-terminal sequence determination on intact core protein (residues 1–36 except 32, 33) and on two CNBr cleavage products (residues 36–42 and 36–43): it was completed and confirmed by the cDNA sequence (Kang et al. 1987). A proportion of the isolated material terminated at residue 42.

Sequence data in order of publication:
Cerebrovascular amyloid (meningeal vessels) from Alzheimer's disease (Glenner and Wong 1984a); residues 1–24 identified (except 11 = Gln).
Cerebrovascular amyloid (meningeal vessels) from Down's syndrome (Glenner and Wong 1984b); residues 1–24 identified.
Plaque core protein from Alzheimer's disease (Masters et al. 1985b); residues 1–28; 12% started at residue 1, 64% at residue 4, 16% at residue 8, 8% at residue 9. The same sequence was found for Down's syndrome (Masters et al. 1985a) with 22% starting at residue 1, 45% at residue 4, 33% at residue 8. Residues 27, 28 erroneously given as Ser, Ala in both sequences.
Cerebrovascular amyloid (meningeal vessels) from Alzheimer's disease and Down's syndrome (Wong et al 1985); residues 1–28 in each case (except residue 11 = Gln in Alzheimer's disease).
Cortical microvessel amyloid from Alzheimer's disease (Pardridge et al. 1987): residues 1–10; 61% started at residue 1, 39% at residue 2: another fraction was not amenable to sequence determination.
Neurofibrillary tangle (paired helical filament) protein from Alzheimer's disease (Masters et al. 1985a): residues 1–15 (N-terminal heterogeneity seen).
Neurofibrillary tangle protein from Guamanian parkinsonism-dementia (Guiroy et al. 1987); residues 1–15 (some N-terminal heterogeneity seen).

this protein common to plaque cores and cerebrovascular amyloid. Application of the same extraction procedures to meningeal vessels from Down's syndrome also revealed the same protein (Glenner and Wong 1984b) while plaque cores from Down's syndrome yielded the same amino acid sequence and N-terminal heterogeneity (Masters et al. 1985b) to complete the pattern of identity in the two diseases. All of the sequence data are summarised in Table 1 and the protein chemical data are summarised in Table 2.

A number of methods, similar in principle to the original one, have been described for plaque core isolation (Selkoe et al. 1986; Roher et al. 1986; Gorevic et al. 1986), the products appearing to show only minor differences. The use of a protease to produce bond cleavage permitted sequence determination (Masters et al. 1985b) while the inability of Selkoe et al. (1986) to obtain a sequence for plaque core protein might be interpreted in the light of the observations of Pardridge et al. (1987), who used cortical micro-vessels to obtain the same partial sequence as for A_4 protein, but with evidence for a partially blocked N-terminus. Amino acid compositions of bulk plaque cores (columns F and G in Table 2) compare very favourably with the calculated composition of an equimolecular mix of 42 and 43 residue sequences (column A in Table 2).

Table 2. Comparison of amino acid compositions (mole %) of isolated vessel and plaque core amyloids with that calculated from the known sequence

	A	B	C	D	E	F	G
Asp	9,4	11,1	3,9	5,9	9,4	9,3	7,8
Thr	1,2	1,4	2,6	1,5	0,7	2,7	1,5
Ser	4,7	5,4	7,2	6,5	7,5	6,5	4,8
Glu	9,4	11,2	12,1	12,3	11,4	10,0	11,2
Pro	0,0	Trace	1,7	1,0	0,7	Trace	2,0
Gly	14,1	15,2	18,3	17,0	15,2	17,5	15,0
Ala	9,4	7,9	8,5	9,3	9,7	7,7	9,0
Cys	0,0	Trace	–	–	Trace	1,0	–
Val	14,1	11,7	11,2	13,0	9,2	9,3	12,8
Met	2,4	2,5	0,2	0,1	2,5	1,8	1,9
Ile	7,1	3,9	3,9	3,5	4,3	4,8	6,7
Leu	4,7	6,3	6,4	5,4	7,0	7,0	6,6
Tyr	2,4	2,1	2,6	2,1	2,8	3,6	2,4
Phe	7,1	7,0	6,2	6,9	6,0	5,5	5,4
His	7,1	5,9	6,1	6,6	5,2	4,3	5,2
Lys	4,7	5,4	4,5	4,7	5,5	5,4	5,3
Arg	2,4	2,9	4,5	4,3	2,7	4,4	2,3

A: Theoretical composition calculated from cDNA sequence on the basis of equal amounts of 42 and 43 residue materials (Kang et al. 1987).
B: Cerebrovascular (meningeal) amyloid (Glenner and Wong 1984b): β_2 fraction from reverse-phase HPLC – sequence obtained (see Table 1) from this material.
C: Cerebrovascular (cortical) amyloid (Pardridge et al. 1987): fraction 2 from reverse-phase HPLC – sequence obtained (see Table 1) from this material.
D: Cerebrovascular (cortical) amyloid (Pardridge et al. 1987): fraction 1 from reverse-phase HPLC – no sequence obtained from this material.
E: Plaque core protein (Masters et al. 1985b): A_8 from size-dependent HPLC – sequence obtained (see Table 1) from this material.
F: Plaque cores – bulk material (Selkoe et al. 1986).
G: Plaque cores – bulk material (Allsop et al. 1983).

The publication which first elucidated the sequence of the full length cDNA encoding the putative intact amyloid precursor (Kang et al. 1987) also further illuminated its protein chemistry. Yields of 44% for the amino acid derivatives obtained from sequence determinations on plaque cores and data indicative of a total sequence of at most 42 or 43 amino acid residues compatible with the cDNA sequence indicate a major single protein of around 4 kd present in the starting material.

The vessel amyloid deposits in Alzheimer's disease are the most similar of the three forms to that of non-cerebral amyloidosis, including the codeposition of P component (Westermark et al. 1982; Rowe et al. 1984), which is absent from plaques (Westermark et al. 1982; Kidd et al. 1985b) and tangles (Westermark et al. 1982).

It is a tribute to the protein chemists that such large increases in knowledge have accrued so rapidly despite the small amounts of intractable material that have been available for analysis.

The Immunochemistry of A_4 Amyloid Deposits

Immunochemical data using antisera (Masters et al. 1985a; Wong et al. 1985) or monoclonal antibodies (Allsop et al. 1986b) raised against synthetic peptides representing part of the sequence of A_4 protein fully support the basic identity of cerebrovascular and plaque core amyloid.

Immunohistochemical studies also show a surprising abundance of A_4 reactivity in the plaque periphery (Allsop et al. 1986b). Since, in the latter study at least, the monoclonal antibody used does not stain the paired helical filaments, the stain must have reacted with extracellular A_4. Previously a picture of all of the amyloid coalescing into a core as the plaque enlarges was accepted, but it is now clear that in the majority of cases most plaques have significant amounts of amyloid in the periphery, often in the absence of a developed core; on this basis relating amyloid merely to the core of the plaque substantially underestimates the total amount of plaque-related amyloid in the diseased brain. It is noteworthy here that the separated amorphous plaque cores of Down's syndrome show amyloid fibrils intermingled with cellular material (Allsop et al. 1986c).

A_4 Amyloid Precursor Protein

Identification of the full length cDNA encoding the precursor for A_4 amyloid showed that it consisted of 695 amino acid residues (Kang et al. 1987); in comparison with other precursor product relationships in the amyloidoses this precursor is unusually large and its amyloid product is relatively small. A number of features of this sequence show similarities with cell-surface receptor integral membrane proteins; that is, there is a large N-terminal extracellular region and a small C-terminal intracellular region linked by a short hydrophobic sequence compatible with spanning a membrane. The A_4 sequence of 42 or 43 amino acids extends towards the N-terminus from about half way across the putative transmembrane sequence (Kang et al. 1987).

Two recent developments are noteworthy. First: the identification of alternative forms of the precursor; insertion of a 56 amino acid (Ponte et al. 1988; Tanzi et al. 1988) or a 75 amino acid (Kitaguchi et al. 1988) additional region, in each case with similarities to Kunitz protease inhibitor sites, shows that functionally distinct precursors occur. Second: immunohistochemical evidence of A_4 synthetic peptide binding sites (Allsop et al. 1988); this suggested proteolytic release of an active ligand from an A_4 precursor molecule, which was linked by these authors to structural similarities between the A_4 precursor and epidermal growth factor precursor. The latter is also an integral membrane protein with a large extracellular domain (from which epidermal growth factor is released proteolytically), a single membrane-spanning region and a small intracellular domain. Cleavage of the putative ligand derived from A_4 precursor would be from the extracellular region just adjacent to the transmembrane sequence (Allsop et al. 1988) as found with epidermal growth factor formation.

At present it is not possible to understand the implications of different precursor forms and further work is necessary to establish the functions of these molecules. It will be of great interest to see whether amyloidogenesis is restricted either to certain tissue sites of the many already established for A_4 precursor or to specific precursor forms or, indeed, whether both constraints apply together; perhaps an understanding of the deposition of A_4 protein in plaques, cerebral vessels or elsewhere will follow from the unravelling of these early data.

Gaps in the Protein Chemical Data

At present the excitement of the work on the cDNA sequence and its implications has overshadowed the protein chemistry; it should be noted, however, that there are still questions outstanding. It is important to know if the protein present at all sites is identical; while the same precursor-product relationship is indisputable, the fine detail of potentially complete or partial N-terminal blocking and overall size remains to be adduced unequivocally, together with any contribution from post-mortem changes. Significantly many of the same questions remain unanswered for other amyloids and it is a frustration that current methodology cannot conveniently provide the answers; a full understanding of the post-translational and degradative events leading to amyloid accumulation may provide a means of attacking the amyloidoses through rational therapy.

The Morphology of Neurofibrillary Tangles

The paired helical filament (PHFs) of the tangles are unique structures and since no animal model of Alzheimer's disease is yet known, are peculiar to man. The term neurofibrillary degeneration introduced by Alzheimer is misleading, since work in the last 20 years casts doubt on the implication of a major content of neurofibrils in the tangles. Kidd first observed that the constituent filaments of the tangles were paired and helical or twisted and named them "paired helical filaments" (Kidd 1963); later authors proposed "twisted tubules" after this helical nature was accepted. At the time it was felt necessary to avoid the term "double helix" to preclude any suggestion of a resemblance to the double helix of DNA. The helix was described (Kidd 1963) as being composed of two axially opposed helical filaments of diameter approximately 10 nm, with a complete period of 160 nm, that is, the half-period (an axial rotation of 180°) was 80 nm in length, and the sense of the helix was right-handed. Later in that year it was stated that the neurofibrils composing the tangles "are thus apparently not different in structure from those of the normal cell body" (Terry 1963). In 1964, fuller accounts were published, including descriptions of the ultrastructure of the plaques, and again (Kidd 1964) evidence of a double helix was deduced from electron micrographs of these structures viewed at different angles in randomly oriented sections, while others (Terry et al. 1964) described elongated structures which they considered to be "twisted tubules". The description "twisted tubule" (which seems to have implied intermittent twists in the length of a tubule) was widely used in the ensuing years until 1976, when using X-ray images of wire models and micrographs of tilted specimens evidence was presented that these were, in fact, PHFs (Wisniewski et al. 1976b). The half-period of a double helix gives the appearance of an intermittent twist, although this feature is better described as a cross-over (Wischik et al. 1985). Since, in three dimensions, a helix is uniform throughout its length, it is only when seen from a particular viewpoint that there appears to be a constriction where the images of the two strands cross each other.

The first electron micrographs of negatively stained PHFs had an ambiguous appearance, in some areas showing clear PHFs but in others regions of regularly arranged subunits which could be helically wound flattened tubules (Kidd 1970). It was not until recent years that image analysis of negatively stained PHFs indicated that the individual filaments of the pair are ribbon-like arrays of "globular" domains (Wischik et al. 1985; Crowther and Wischik 1985), and that the sense of the helix was left-handed. A four-stranded helix has been deduced from extracted, negatively stained PHFs (Wisniewski et al. 1984; Allsop et al. 1986a), which could suggest that the PHFs are pairs of cerebral amyloid filaments. An eight-stranded helix had also been deduced from thin sections (Wisniewski and Wen 1985) but the image analysis studies suggested that this appearance could be caused by lining-up of the "globular" domains of the subunit, and the existence of protofilaments was rejected (Crowther and Wischik 1985). It remains possible that image analysis of the ultrastructure of other cerebral amyloid filaments might reveal that these too have "globular" domains. Recently X-ray diffraction patterns from PHFs and plaque cores indicative of cross-β structures have been obtained (Kirschner et al. 1986).

Tangles of other filaments can occur in the neuron perikaryon but are morphologically distinct from PHFs, closely resembling normal structures. Accumulations of neurofilaments have been described as part of the "axon reaction" in neurons with severed axons, both in light and electron microscopy (Evans and Gray 1961). The type of non-helical tangle most relevant to Alzheimer's disease is that of experimental aluminium encephalopathy (Klatzo et al. 1965), which has been quoted a number of times as a possible model for the human disease. In this syndrome, produced by intracerebral insertion of various inorganic aluminium compounds, abnormally massive tangles are observed (larger than those of the axon reaction), albeit mainly in spinal cord and brain stem rather than cerebral cortex, and there are no plaques. The ultrastructure of these tangles (still here a reasonable name) shows that they are composed of apparently normal neurofilaments, although electron microprobe analysis has shown that they contain a marked amount of aluminium (Terry and Pena 1965). Use of this syndrome as an informative model for Alzheimer's disease is limited by the fact that plaques and PHFs are absent from the brain in this animal condition and are also absent from aluminium-induced human dialysis encephalopathy (Burks et al. 1976). Straight, unpaired filaments have occasionally been found in the tangles of Alzheimer's disease (Anderton et al. 1982), but their importance is obscure. On the other hand, evidence has been presented which shows that there is an abnormal accumulation of aluminium compounds in the plaques and the tangles of Alzheimer's disease, so that independently of the morphological differences from the animal model, aluminium intoxication is considered by some to be an important possibility as a cause of the dementia of Alzheimer's disease – the most comprehensive histochemical data being published recently (Candy et al. 1986).

The Chemistry of Neurofibrillary Tangles

Protein chemical and immunochemical approaches to the paired helical filaments of tangles have provided conflicting pictures of their chemical make-up. Each approach has its own limitations; protein chemistry has lacked a source of pure protein since even the best preparations contain significant amounts of contaminating material; on the other hand immunochemistry has provided only qualitative observations on tangles in situ or, less often, on partially purified (i.e. SDS extracted) PHFs.

Immunohistochemical data have built up a picture of tangles in situ as structures with a heterogeneous protein content, a view supported by more limited observations on the partially purified PHFs. Some reduction of the number of proteins (or epitopes thereof) contributing to tangles has recently emerged from assessment of the cross-reactivities of a number of monoclonal antibodies that react with tangles (Ksiezak-Reding et al. 1987; Nukina et al. 1987). Anti-neurofilament (NF) and anti-microtubule associated protein 2 (MAP2) monoclonal antibodies also react with another MAP, tau; these antibodies apparently recognise phosphorylated epitopes common to the different proteins. This leads to a simpler notion that one of the group – tau protein – (or certain phosphorylated epitopes of tau) not normally seen in the perikaryon is present in tangles in situ and in part-purified PHFs.

Similarities between the amino acid compositions of plaque core protein, cerebrovascular amyloid (subsequently both were shown to contain A_4 protein, as described above) and PHF preparations led to the proposal that the same protein was present in all three structures (Kidd et al. 1985a; Allsop et al 1986a); this suggestion for PHFs appeared to be given strong support by subunit characterisation and protein sequence data showing identity with A_4 protein (Masters et al. 1985a), albeit on the usual preparation known to contain contaminants. However, in addition to the purity problem, a lack of quantitation of some of the findings led some to believe that the observations were made merely on contaminating plaque or vessel amyloid; these doubts have been partially eliminated by publication of essentially identical chemical data on the PHFs isolated from a case of Guamanian parkinsonism-dementia (Guiroy et al. 1987), where tangles are found in the absence of plaques.

Immunochemical observations give only weak support for the presence of A_4 protein sequences in tangles; a single report of an antiserum, raised against residues 1-11 of A_4 protein, reacting with tangles (Masters et al. 1985a) is at odds with a number of negative observations (Wang et al. 1985; Allsop et al. 1986b; Coria et al. 1987).

While few immunochemical observations on tangles can be considered definitive, it is possible to simplify the picture further by experiment; some observations have been made on extracellular of "ghost" tangles which very often appear to show restricted immunoreactivities in comparison with intracellular tangles; a progression from a more heterogeneous intracellular structure to a "purer" extracellular (paired helical filament only?) form is a possible interpretation that requires more intensive investigation of the extracellular tangle. Nonetheless, the earlier suggestion of identity of tangle protein and cerebral amyloid cannot easily be supported at present.

The emergence of tangles may or may not be the primary event in Alzheimer's disease; nevertheless, interest in their mechanism of production is important. This interest appears to have been given a major impetus from the identification of the multifunctional protein ubiquitin as a component closely associated with tangles (Cole and Timiras 1987; Mori et al. 1987; Perry et al. 1987). Ubiquitin is a small protein showing little change between animal groups, and appears to label cytoplasmic proteins which are due for destruction. Further interest in ubiquitin arises from its very recent identification in a number of proteinaceous inclusions in both neurons and other cell types in a variety of diseases (Lowe et al. 1988), as shown in Table 3.

It is clear from Table 3 there is a pattern of association of filaments and ubiquitin, in a range of intracellular proteinaceous inclusion bodies which has been extended to include the membrane-bounded bodies of the granulovacuolar

Table 3. Pathological features showing ubiquitin immunoreactivity from a variety of diseases

Disease	*Pathological feature*	*Associated protein*
Alzheimer's disease	Neurofibrillary tangle[a]	Paired helical filaments
	Plaque neurites[a]	Paired helical filaments
	Granulovacuolar degeneration	None identified
Parkinson's disease	Brain stem Lewy body	Neurofilament protein[b]
	Cortical Lewy body	Neurofilament protein
Pick's disease	Pick body	Mainly 15-nm straight filaments, makeup unknown
Cerebellar astrocytoma	Rosenthal fibre	Glial fibrillary acidic protein[b]
Alcoholic liver disease	Mallory body	Cytokeratin[b]
Cytoplasmic body myopathy	Cytoplasmic body	Desmin

All observations are originally from Lowe et al. (1988) except for the following:
[a] Cole and Timiras (1987), Mori et al. (1987), and Perry et al. (1987) which were confirmed by Lowe et al. (1988).
[b] Peripheral filaments with amorphous core. Ubiquitin stains periphery where named protein occurs.

degeneration of Alzheimer's disease (Lowe et al. 1988). This represents a new compartment for ubiquitin, which has previously been most closely linked to cytoplasmic events although it is known to be attached to histones in the nucleus and is also now being seen associated with certain receptors on the cell surface (Rechsteiner 1987).

It now seems apparent that the formation of tangles and other inclusion bodies involves cytoskeletal events and a fundamental role for ubiquitin; these early observations look like providing the basis both for methods for investigation of what may be key events in neuronal degeneration and also for model systems that could be helpful in assessing therapeutic intervention in Alzheimer's disease and in related disorders.

Other Syndromes with Plaques, Tangles or Cerebrovascular Amyloid

While the amyloidosis of the transmissible subacute encephalopathies is known to consist of a separate protein, plaques and tangles of PHFs may be found in a range of other human diseases, which has encouraged one of us to propose the term "Alzheimer's syndrome" to cover such a response of the brain to a range of different primary stimuli (Kidd 1981; Kidd et al. 1985b).

Down's syndrome has been mentioned above and will not be considered further here. Dementia pugilistica or post–traumatic dementia arises often in an earlier age group than even the presenile type of Alzheimer's disease, but is characterised by the general absence of amyloid plaques with an abundance of tangles (Wisniewski et al. 1976a). A similar exhibition of tangles in the absence of plaques is found in Guam–Parkinson dementia, which disease is regarded as genetic in origin (Wisniewski et al. 1979).

Some Speculations on the Generation of Alzheimer Amyloid

The appearance of the plaque core as a stellate body, characteristic of amyloid deposits at sites of secretion, suggests that here is another such site. Some support for this is given by observations of coated pits (cell membrane sites of protein absorption or secretion) on the cells adjacent to these deposits (Roher et al. 1988), although these authors were unable to identify the cells concerned. Macrophages have been similarly suggested to secrete into the cores (Terry et al. 1964), by analogy with their activity in secondary amyloidosis; unpublished observations by one of us seemed to suggest neurons or their processes as the source, but again this was not certain. It is, of course, of great importance to identify these cells unequivocally. The finding of ubiquitin in association with the PHFs suggests that the protein of these structures is to be degraded; it would be easy to suggest that failure of the degradation system would lead to the PHF protein being expelled to form the extracellular amyloid. A neurogenic theory of the expression of the amyloid (espoused by Beyreuther and Masters and their colleagues) would run contrary to the older theory of a haematogenous origin for the amyloid precursor (on the basis of the observation of vascular amyloid). It is still possible that the cerebral amyloid may deposit in the arteriolar walls from outside, that is, from the brain parenchyma, while it could pass out to the serum through the capillaries. Finally, since the precursor (or precursors) of this abnormal protein appears to be a normal protein, it is important to establish its normal function. AA protein of secondary amyloidosis is a normal acute phase inflammatory protein (although its function is not known further than this); it may be that Alzheimer amyloid is the deposit from overproduction of a normal reactive protein in abnormal circumstances.

Summary

Amyloid is found in the Alzheimer's diseased brain in three sites: in the senile plaques, often in arteriolar walls and also apparently in the neurons as neurofibrillary tangles. Recent protein chemical observations indicate that the amyloid of the plaque cores and the vessel walls is the same protein composed of 42–43 and 39 amino acids respectively, with an unusual amino acid composition and sequence. Molecular biological observations indicate that this protein (encoded by a normal gene on chromosome 21) is derived from alternatively spliced mRNAs coding for 695, 751 or 770 residues. All of the precursors have sequences suggesting a plasma membrane protein with a trans-membrane portion and a small cytoplasmic region, while the larger forms also contain the characteristic sequence of a protease inhibitor. On the other hand, the neurofibrillary tangles still present an enigma, in that there is no agreement that this intracellular proteinaceous material is another product of the same precursor or that they are composed of neurofilaments, although they do contain ubiquitin, which has interesting implications.

Acknowledgement. The authors are grateful to the Wellcome Trust for financial support.

References

Allsop D, Landon M, Kidd M (1983) The isolation and amino acid composition of senile plaque core protein. Brain Res 259: 348–352

Allsop D, Landon M, Kidd M (1986a) Cerebral amyloid and Alzheimer's syndrome. In: Glenner GG, Osserman E (eds) Amyloidosis, Plenum, New York, pp 723–732

Allsop D, Landon M, Kidd M, Lowe JS, Reynolds GP, Gardner A (1986b) Monoclonal antibodies raised against a subsequence of senile plaque core protein react with plaque cores, plaque periphery and cerebrovascular amyloid in Alzheimer's disease. Neurosci Lett 68: 252–256

Allsop D, Kidd M, Landon M, Tomlinson A (1986c) Isolated senile plaque cores in Alzheimer's disease and Down's syndrome show differences in morphology. J Neurol Neurosurg Psychiatry 49: 886–892

Allsop D, Wong CW, Ikeda S, Landon M, Kidd M, Glenner GG (1988) Immunohistochemical evidence for the derivation of a peptide ligand from the amyloid β-protein of Alzheimer disease. Proc Natl Acad Sci USA 85: 2790–2794

Anderton BH, Breinburg D, Downes MJ et al. (1982) Monoclonal antibodies show that neurofibrillary tangles and neurofilaments share antigenic determinants. Nature 298: 84–86

Blessed G, Tomlinson BE, Roth M (1968) The association between quantitative measures of dementia and of senile changes in cerebral grey matter of elderly subjects. Br J Psychiatry 114: 797–811

Burks JS, Alfrey AC, Huddleston J, Norenberg MD, Lewin E (1976) A fatal encephalopathy in chronic haemodyalysis patients. Lancet i: 764–768

Candy JM, Klinowski J, Perry RH et al. (1986) Aluminosilicates and senile plaque formation in Alzheimer's disease. Lancet i: 354–356

Cole GM, Timiras PS (1987) Ubiquitin-protein conjugates in Alzheimer's disease. Neurosci Lett 79: 207–212

Coria F, Castano EM, Frangione B (1987) Brain amyloid in normal aging and cerebral amyloid angipopathy is antigenically related to Alzheimer's disease β-protein. Am J Pathol 129: 422–428

Crowther RA, Wischik CM (1985) Image reconstruction of the Alzheimer paired helical filament. EMBO J 4: 3661–3665

Evans DHL, Gray EG (1961) Changes in the fine structure of ganglion cells during chromatolysis. In: The cytology of nervous tissue. Taylor and Francis, London, pp 71–74

Glenner GG (1980a) Amyloid deposits and amyloidosis. The β-fibrilloses, part 1. N Engl J Med 302: 1283–1292

Glenner GG (1980b) Amyloid deposits and amyloidoses. The β-fibrilloses, part 2. N Engl J Med 302: 1333–1343

Glenner GG, Wong CW (1984a) Alzheimer's disease: initial report of the purification and characterization of a novel cerebrovascular amyloid protein. Biochem Biophys Res Commun 120: 885–890

Glenner GG, Wong CW (1984b) Alzheimer's disease und Down's syndrome: sharing of a unique cerebrovascular amyloid fibril protein. Biochem Biophys Res Commun 122: 1131–1135

Goldgaber D, Lerman MI, McBride OW, Saffiott U, Gajdusek DC (1987) Characterization of chromosomal localization of a cDNA encoding brain amyloid of Alzheimer's disease. Science 235: 877–880

Gorevic PD, Goni F, Pons-Estel B, Alvarez F, Peress NS, Frangione B (1986) Isolation und partial characterization of neurofibrillary tangles and amyloid plaque core in Alzheimer's disease: immunohistological studies. J. Neuropathol Exp Neurol 45: 647–664

Guiroy DC, Miyazaki M, Multhaup G et al. (1987) Amyloid of neurofibrillary tangles of Guamanian parkisonism-dementia and Alzheimer disease share identical amino acid sequence. Proc Natl Acad Sci USA 84: 2073–2077

Husby G, Sletten K (1985) Chemical and clinical classification of amyloidosis. Scand J Immunol 23: 253–265

Kang J, Lenaire HG, Unterbeck A et al. (1987) The precursor of Alzheimer's disease amyloid A4 protein resembles a cell-surface receptor, Nature 325: 733–736

Kidd M (1963) Paired helical filaments in electron microscopy of Alzheimer's disease. Nature 197: 192–193

Kidd M (1964) Alzheimer's disease: an electron microscopical study. Brain 87: 307–320

Kidd M (1970) (Discussion) In: Wolstenholme GEW, O'Connor M (eds) Alzheimer's disease. Churchill, London, pp 202–203

Kidd M (1981) Animal models of Alzheimer's syndrome. Gerontology 27: 107

Kidd M, Allsop D, Landon M (1985a) Senile plaque amyloid, paired helical filaments and cerebrovascular amyloid in Alzheimer's disease are all deposits of the same protein. Lancet i: 278

Kidd M, Allsop D, Landon M (1985b) Senile plaque amyloid. In: Clifford Rose F (ed) Modern approaches to the dementias, part 1, Karger, Basel (Interdiscipl Topics Geront, vol 19, pp 114–126)

Kirschner DA, Abraham C, Selkoe DJ (1986) X-ray diffraction from intraneuronal paired helical filaments and extraneuronal amyloid fibers in Alzheimer disease indicates cross-β configuration. Proc Natl Acad Sci USA 83: 503–507

Kitaguchi N, Takahashi Y, Tokushima Y, Shiojiri S, Ito H (1988) Novel precursor of Alzheimer's disease amyloid protein shows protease inhibitory activity. Nature 331: 530–532

Klatzo I, Wisniewski HM, Streicher E (1965) Experimental production of neurofibrillary degeneration. I. Light microscopic observations. J Neuropath Exp Neurol 24: 187–199

Ksiezak-Reding H, Dickson DW, Davies P, Yen S (1987) Recognition of tau epitopes by anti-neurofilament antibodies that bind to Alzheimer neurofibrillary tangles. Proc Natl Acad Sci USA 84: 3410–3414

Landon M, Kidd M, Allsop D (1987) Amyloidosis with particular reference to cerebral amyloid in Alzheimer's disease and the transmissible subacute encephalopathies. Rev Neurosci 1: 101–126

Lowe JS, Blanchard A, Morrell K et al. (1988) Ubiquitin is a common factor in intermediate inclusion bodies of diverse type in man including those of Parkinson's disease, Pick's disease and Alzheimer's disease as well as Rosenthal fibres in cerebellar astrocytomas' cytoplasmic bodies in muscle and Mallory bodies in alcoholic liver disease. J Pathol 155: 9–15

Mancardi GL, Mandybur TI (1983) Solitary intracranial plasmacytoma. Cancer 51: 2226–2233

Mandybur TI (1986) Cerebral amyloid angiopathy: the vascular pathology and complications. J Neuropathol Exp Neurol 45: 79–90

Masters CL, Multhaup G, Simms G, Pottgeisser J, Martins NR, Beyreuther K (1985a) Neuronal origin of a cerebral amyloid: neurofibrillary tangles of Alzheimer‘s disease contain the same protein as the amyloid of plaque cores and blood vessels. EMBO J 4: 2757–2763

Masters CL, Simms G, Weinman NA, Multhaup, McDonald BL, Beyreuther K (1985b) Amyloid plaque core protein in Alzheimer‘s disease and Down‘s syndrome, Proc Natl Acad Sci USA 82: 4245–4249

Merz PA, Wisniewski HM, Somerville RA, Bobin SA, Masters CL, Iqbal K (1983) Ultrastructural morphology of amyloid fibrils from neuritic and amyloid plaques. Acta Neuropathol 60: 113–124

Mori H, Mori S, Saitoh Y, Moriwaki K, Iida S, Matsumoto K (1985) Growth hormone-producing pituitary adenoma with crystal-like amyloid immunohistochemically positive for growth hormone. Cancer 55: 96–102

Mori H, Kondo J, Ihara Y (1987) Ubiquitin is a component of paired helical filaments in Alzheimer‘s disease. Science 235: 1641–1644

Miyakawa T, Shimoji A, Kuramoto R, Higuchi Y (1982) The relationship between senile plaques and cerebral blood vessels in Alzheimer‘s disease and senile dementia, Morphological mechanism of senile plaque production. Virchows Arch [Cell Pathol] 40: 121–129

Nukina N, Kosik KS, Selkoe DJ (1987) Recognition of Alzheimer paired helical filaments by monoclonal neurofilament antibodies is due to cross-reaction with tau protein. Proc Natl Acad Sci USA 84: 3415–3419

Osamura RY, Watanabe K, Komatsu N, Ohya M, Kageyama N (1982) Amorphous and stellate amyloid in functioning human pituitary adenomas: histochemical, immunochemical and electron microscopic studies. Acta Pathol Jpn 32: 605–611

Pardridge WM, Vinters HV, Yang J et al. (1987) Amyloid angiopathy of Alzheimer‘s disease: amino acid composition and partial sequence of a 4,200-dalton peptide isolated from cortical microvessels. J Neurochem 49: 1394–1401

Perry G, Friedman R, Shaw G, Chau V (1987) Ubiquitin is detected in neurofibrillary tangles and senile plaque neurites of Alzheimer disease brains. Proc Natl Acad Sci USA 84: 3033–3036

Ponte P, Gonzalez-DeWhitt P, Schilling J et al. (1988) A new A4 amyloid mRNA contains a domain homologous to serine proteinase inhibitors. Nature 331: 525–527

Rechsteiner M (1987) Ubiquitin-mediated pathways for intracellular proteolysis. Annu Rev Cell Biol 3: 1–30

Robakis NK, Wisniewski HM, Jenkins EC et al. (1987) Chromosome 21q21 sublocalization of gene encoding beta-amyloid peptide in cerebral vessels and neuritric (senile) plaques of people with Alzheimer disease and Down syndrome Lancet i: 384–385

Roher A, Wolfe D, Palutke M, KuKuraga D (1986) Purification ultrastructure and chemical analysis of Alzheimer disease amyloid plaque core protein. Proc Natl Acad Sci USA 83: 2662–2666

Roher A, Gray EG, Paula-Barbosa M (1988) Alzheimer's disease: coated vesicles, coated pits and the amyloid-related cell. Proc R Soc Lond B 232: 367–373

Rowe IF, Jensson O, Lewis PD, Candy J, Tennent GA, Pepys MB (1984) Immunohistochemical demonstration of amyloid P component in cerebro-vascular amyloidosis. Neuropathol Appl Neurobiol 10: 53–61

St. George-Hyslop P, Tanzi RE, Polinsky RJ et al. (1987) The genetic defect causing familial Alzheimer's disease maps on chromosome 21. Science 235: 885–889

Selkoe DJ, Abraham CR, Podlisny MB, Duffy LK (1986) Isolation of low-molecular-weight proteins from amyloid plaque fibers in Alzheimer's disease. J Neurochem 46: 1820–1834

Sorenson GD, Heefner WA, Kirkpatrick JB (1964) Experimental amyloidosis: II. Light and electron microscopical examinations of liver. Am J Pathol 44: 629–644

Tanzi RE, Gusella JF, Watkins PC et al. (1987) Amyloid beta-protein gene: cDNA mRNA distribution and genetic linkage near the Alzheimer locus. Science 235: 880–884

Tanzi RE, McClatchey AI, Lamperti ED, Villa-Komaroff L, Gusella JF, Neve RL (1988) Protease inhibitor domain encoded by an amyloid precursor mRNA associated with Alzheimer's disease. Nature 331: 528–530

Terry RD (1963) The fine structure of neurofibrillary tangles in Alzheimer's disease. J Neuropathol Exp Neurol 22: 629–642

Terry RD, Pena CJ (1965) Experimental production of neurofibrillary degeneration. II. Electron microscopy phosphatase chemistry and electron probe analysis. J Neuropath Exp Neurol 24: 200–210

Terry RD,Gonatas NK, Weiss M (1964) Ultrastructural studies in Alzheimer's presenile dementia. Am J Pathol 44: 269–297

Tischler AS, Compagno J (1979) Crystal-like deposits of amyloid in pancreatic islet cell tumors. Arch Pathol Lab Med 103: 247–251

Tomlinson BE (1979) The ageing brain. In: Smith WJ, Cavanagh JB (eds) Recent advances in neuropathology, vol 1. Churchill-Livingston, Edinburgh, pp 129–159

Vital A, Vital C (1984) Amyloid neuropathy: relationship between amyloid fibrils and macrophages. Ultrastruct Pathol 7: 21–25

Westermark P, Natvig JB, Anders RR, Sletten K, Husby G (1976) Coexistence of protein AA and immunoglobulin light-chain fragments in amyloid fibrils. Scand J Immunol 5: 31–36

Westermark P, Shirahama T, Skinner M, Brun A, Cameron R, Cohen AS (1982) Immunohistochemical evidence for the lack of amyloid P component in some intracerebral amyloids. Lab Invest 46: 457–460

Wilcock GK, Esiri MM (1982) Plaques, tangles and dementia — a quantitative study. J Neurol Sci 56: 343–356

Wischik CM, Crowther RA, Stewart M, Roth M (1985) Subunit structure of paired helical filaments in Alzheimer's disease. J Cell Biol 100: 1905–1912

Wisniewski HM, Terry RD (1976) Re-examination of the pathogenesis of the senile plaque. In: Zimmerman HM (ed) Progress in neuropathology, vol 2. Grune & Stratton, New York, pp 2–26

Wisniewski HM, Wen GY (1985) Substructure of paired helical filaments from Alzheimer's disease neurofibrillary tangles. Acta Neuropathol 66: 173–176

Wisniewski HM, Narang HK, Corsellis JAN, Terry RD (1976a) Ultrastructural studies of neuropil and neurofibrillary tangles in Alzheimer's disease and posttraumatic dementia. J Neuropathol Exp Neurol 35: 367

Wisniewski, HM Narang HK, Terry RD (1976b) Neurofibrillary tangles of paired helical filaments. J Neurol Sci 27: 173–181

Wisniewski KE, Jervis GA, Moretz RC, Wisniewski HM (1979) Alzheimer neurofibrillary tangles in diseases other than senile and presenile dementia. Ann Neurol 5: 288–294

Wisniewski HM, Merz PA, Iqbal K (1984) Ultrastructure of paired helical filaments from Alzheimer's neurofibrillary tangles. J Neuropathol Exp Neurol 43: 643–656

Wisniewski KE, Wisniewski HM, Wen GY (1985) Occurrence of neuropathological changes and dementia of Alzheimer's disease in Down's syndrome. Ann Neurol 17: 278–282
Wong CW, Quaranta V, Glenner GG (1985) Neuritic plaques and cerebrovascular amyloid in Alzheimer disease are antigenically related. Proc Natl Acad Sci USA 82: 8729–8732

Amyloid Deposits Derived from Various Proteins – A Hallmark of Old Age

R. P. LINKE [1]

Aging can be studied in different ways. Biochemical and functional changes can be monitored in vitro using single cell suspensions or analyzed in vivo. A third approach involves the registration and analysis of age-related diseases that render old age painful, troublesome, and undesired. This third approach is adopted here. I will summarize data on the age-related distinct pathological protein deposits which were designated "amyloid" by Rudolph Virchow (1854).

Senile amyloidosis was and still is believed by many to represent a rare condition of little significance and of interest only to some specialists. In reviewing the literature and by addition of own data, I shall show that senile amyloid is widespread indeed, and that some forms are of clinical significance and a burden for health insurance systems. The burden will become even greater as the average age of individuals increases, due in part to improved consciousness of what is healthy and the associated reduction in calorie intake and avoidance of drugs such as tobacco and alcohol.

Recently, there have been three major advances in respect of amyloid: (a) amyloid deposits have been biochemically analyzed (Glenner 1980); (b) the amyloid disease of Alzheimer has been chemically identified (Glenner and Wong 1984); and (c) a new type of amyloid has attracted attention, because it leads to bone fractures and, distressingly to the physician, is in particular caused by treatment of renal failure by hemodialysis (Gejyo et al. 1985).

Diagnosis of Amyloid Deposits and Amyloidosis

The diagnosis of amyloid deposits is done on tissue sections using the alkaline Congo red staining method according to Puchtler et al. (1962). The basis of the diagnosis includes the recognition of an apple green color in polarized light (Missmahl and Hartwig 1953). Figure 1 illustrates Congo red bindings and the apple green polarization color. Electron microscopically, amyloid is fibrillar in nature with 60–80 Å thick straight and unbranched fibrils (Cohen 1967). The major secondary structure is the β-pleated sheet that is recognized by X-ray

[1] Institut für Immunologie der Ludwig-Maximilian-Universität München, Goethestr. 31, D-8000 München 2 / FRG

Gerontology
Ed. by D. Platt
© Springer-Verlag Berlin Heidelberg 1989

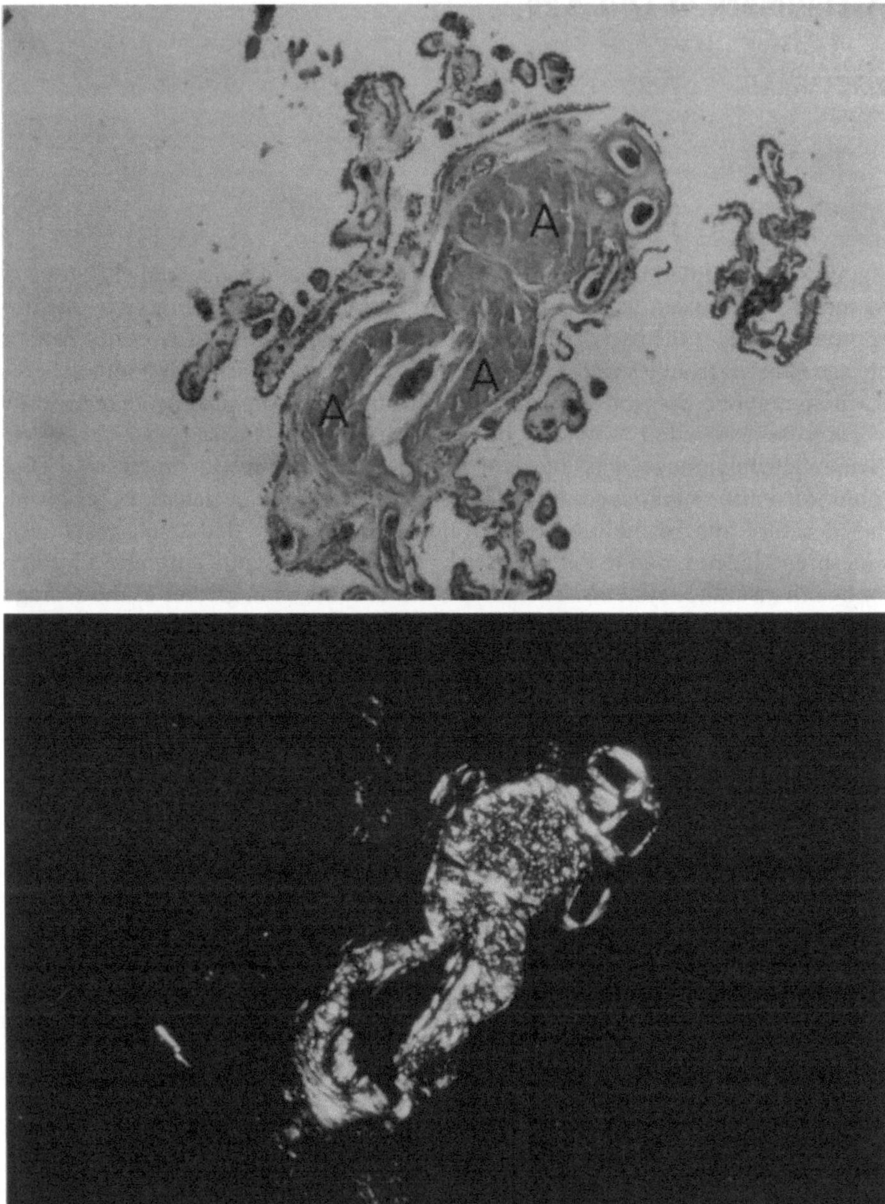

Fig. 1. Diagnosis of intravascular amyloid in an artery of the plexus choroideus. *Top:* Homogeneous masses (*A*) represent amyloid. They are stained red in original section. *Bottom:* The same section in polarized light. Material depicted above appears apple green in polarized light in original section

Table 1. Diagnosis of amyloidosis

1. Macroscopic (Rokitanski 1842)[a]
2. Staining with Lugol's solution (Virchow 1854)
3. Microscopic (Virchow 1854)
4. Metachromasia (Lubarsch 1929)
5. Aqueous Congo red (Bennhold 1922)
6. Alcoholic Congo red (Missmahl and Hartwig 1953)
7. Alkaline, alcoholic, high salt Congo red (Puchtler et al. 1962)[a]
8. Polarization microscopic (Missmahl and Hartwig 1953)[a]
9. Clinical (primary/atypical/type I – secondary/typical/type II (Lubarsch 1929)
10. Fluorescence optical (Schwarz 1970)
11. Electron microscopic (Cohen 1967)[a]
12. X-ray diffraction (Glenner et al. 1974)
13. Histochemical ($KMnO_4$ resistance) (Wright et al. 1977)
14. Morphological (perireticular-pericollagenous) Missmahl and Hartwig 1953)
15. Chemical (amino acid sequence analysis) (Benditt et al. 1971; Glenner 1980)[a]
16. Immunochemical (immunodiffusion) (Linke 1985)
17. Immunohistochemical (Linke et al. 1986a)[a]
18. Immunoelectron microscopic (Linke et al. 1983)[a]

[a] Methods decisive for the diagnosis of amyloid today.

diffraction analysis (Glenner et al. 1974). For clinical use, the Congo red staining is sufficient when the Puchtler method (Puchtler et al. 1962) is applied. So far, the diagnosis of amyloid cannot be made from serum, urine, or other body fluids. Diagnostic measures used during the last century are summarized in Table 1.

Biochemical Analysis of Amyloid Deposits

The biochemical analysis of amyloid fibrils presupposes that the ens morbi, the amyloid fibrils, can be separated from the rest of the tissue constituents. Methods have been devised for concentrating the different amyloid deposits from involved tissues (Linke 1983, 1985; Pras et al. 1968) to such a degree that the major amyloid fibril proteins might become identifiable. Solubilization of amyloid fibrils has been achieved by highly concentrated salt solutions, strong acidic, or strong alkaline solutions (Benditt et al. 1971; Glenner 1980). Separation of solubilized amyloid fibril proteins is achieved by diverse chromatographic methods such as gel filtration. In this way homogeneous proteins are obtained that can be sequenced (Benditt et al. 1971; Glenner 1980). Amino acid sequence analysis has finally identified a series of unrelated proteins (Table 2). These proteins have in common that they can form fibrillar, enzyme-resistant deposits with a β-pleated sheet structure (Glenner et al. 1974). Although the fibrils are morphologically virtually indistinguishable, based on amino acid sequence they are chemically unrelated. Structural requirements for these β-fibrils with the conformation of amyloid have

Table 2. Amyloid-forming proteins

In vivo
Immunoglobulin light chains (Glenner 1980)
Serum amyloid A (Linke et al. 1975)
Prealbumin/transthyretin (Araki 1986)
(Pro-) calcitonin (Sletten et al. 1976)
Hormone of the calcitonin gene family (Westermark et al. 1987)
Cerebral β/A4 protein (Glenner and Wong 1984; Masters et al. 1985)
Prion/SAF protein (Diringer et al. 1983; Prusiner 1982)
β_2-Microglobulin (Gejyo et al. 1985; Linke et al. 1986b)
Cystatin C (Cohen et al. 1983)
Atrial natriuretic peptide (Johannson et al. 1987; Linke et al. 1988)
Insulin, iatrogenic (Dische et al. 1988)
In vitro
Immunoglobulin light chains (Glenner 1980)
Insulin (Glenner et al. 1974)
Glucagon (Glenner et al. 1974)
Calcitonin (Kedar et al. 1976)
Parathormone (Kedar et al. 1976)
Cerebral β/A4 protein (Allsop 1986)
β_2-Microglobulin (Connors et al. 1985)

not been identified. Yet these fibrils are pathogenic by virtue of their accumulation with time: When the deposits reach a critical size in vital organs, life-threatening clinical symptoms ensue, with destruction of organs such as the kidney and heart or the central nervous system (Glenner 1980).

Chemical Heterogeneity of Amyloidosis

Chemical analysis has shown an unexpected heterogeneity of amyloid fibril proteins (Benditt and Eriksen 1971; Glenner 1980). The most important finding, however, was that each amyloid fibril protein is associated with a specific clinical syndrome. Thus, each amyloid fibril protein can be used as the marker protein of a specific disease, clinical syndrome, or group of chemically and pathogenetically related syndromes. This new nosology (Glenner 1980) of amyloid deposits and amyloidoses has led to exact antigenic definition of amyloid diseases. It has furthermore yielded pathogenetically defined disease groups that are accessible to therapeutic trials, some of which have already been successful and others of which have shown some benefits. However, no systematic attempt has been made to diagnose amyloid diseases found in old age. In order to identify the prevalence of these diseases in the aged and correlate amyloid with age-related ailments, a prospective study would be necessary.

The following amyloid syndromes have been identified so far:

Immunoglobulin light chain-derived deposits are found in B cell neoplasms such as multiple myeloma, Waldenström's disease, Bence-Jones plasmacytoma, and plasma cell dyscrasia, which is most likely not of malignant neoplastic origin. The deposits can be generalized, organ limited, or strictly localized (Glenner 1980).

Serum amyloid A protein-derived deposits (Benditt et al. 1971; Linke et al. 1975) are found without predisposing disease (uncommon), after chronic inflammation (such as viral and bacterial), or after autoimmune inflammation. It also can be found after hereditary inflammation, such as familial Mediterranean fever, Muckle-Wells syndrome, or other periodic diseases such as periodic fever. The main clinical symptoms are apparent from the kidney, although the preponderant deposits are found in spleen, liver, adrenals, and gastrointestinal tract.

Prealbumin/transthyretin-derived amyloid deposits (Costa et al. 1978; Stetten et al. 1980) are identified in two clinically distinct syndromes, i.e., hereditary amyloid polyneuropathy and senile cardiovascular amyloidosis. Both are distinct by virtue of the chemistry of the amyloid fibril proteins. While in the latter no amino acid difference was seen (Saraiva et al., in press), in the former single point mutations have been identified, whereby each point mutation defines a variant clinical syndrome (Araki 1986).

β_2-Microglobulin-derived amyloid fibrils cause severe symptoms in hemodialysis, such as carpal tunnel syndrome, osteoarthritis, periarthritis, bone fractures, and amyloid stones in kidney (Linke et al. 1986b), subcutaneous (Floege et al., 1989), or cardiac tissues (Gejyo et al. 1988).

Calcitonin-related proteins are identified in amyloid of medullary carcinoma of the thyroid (Sletten et al. 1976).

Cystatin C-derived amyloid is present in hereditary Islandic apoplexia (Cohen et al. 1983).

β/A4 protein in the brain and leptomeningeal vessels is directly associated with Alzheimer's disease and related diseases (Allsop 1986; Glenner and Wong 1984; Masters et al. 1985). The amyloidosis of Alzheimer's disease is discussed in more detail in the chapter by M. Kidd and M. Landon. We also have chemically identified this protein and have produced a rabbit antiserum against the β/A4 protein that identifies β/A4 protein in tissue sections. We use this antibody to distinguish in tissue sections Alzheimer disease and related syndromes from brain amyloid of the scrapie type, which does not stain with this antibody (Fig. 2).

SAF/PrP protein is present in all cerebral diseases of the scrapie group comprising infectious syndromes in man and animals (Diringer et al. 1983; Prusiner 1982).

A new hormone of the calcitonin gene family is found in amyloid deposits in insulinoma and in islet hyalin of patients with type II diabetes, which is of great importance in old age (Westermark et al. 1987).

Atrial natriuretic peptide is the amyloid fibril protein precursor of isolated atrial amyloidosis (Johannson et al. 1987; Linke et al. 1988).

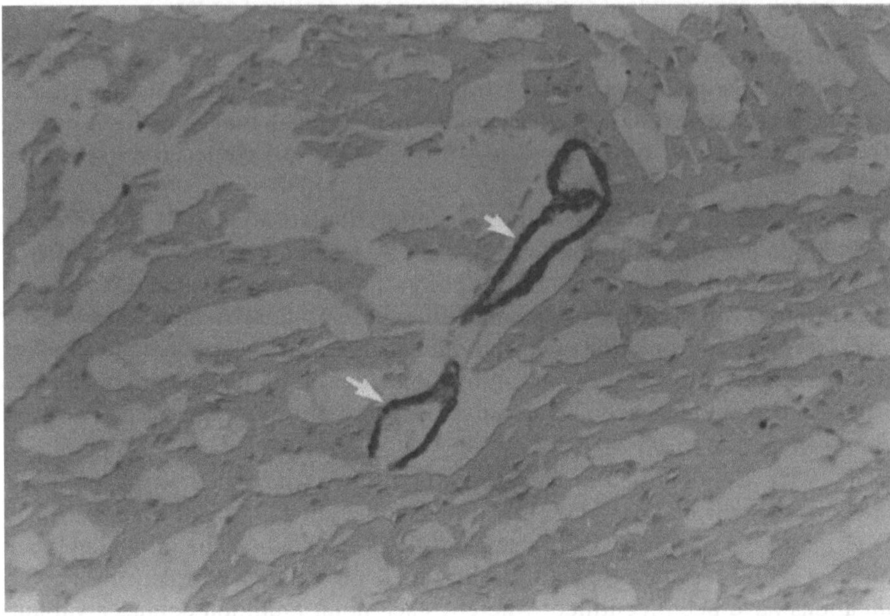

Fig. 2. Cerebral amyloid angiopathy, immunohistochemically identified with a polyclonal rabbit anti-β/A4 protein, on a formalin-fixed and paraffin-embedded brain tissue section. Dark color (arrows) in vessel walls is red-brown oxidized amino ethylcarbazol in original section. The brain tissue is damaged by freezing. Empty spaces represent the former position of ice crystals

Insulin is deposited in amyloid conformation at the site of insulin injection in patients with diabetes mellitus (Dische et al. 1988).

Prevalence of Amyloid in Old Age

The prevalence of amyloid in old age is documented by a series of independent reports (Buerger and Braunstein 1960; Hodkinson and Pomerance 1977; Pomerance 1966; Störkel et al. 1983; Wright and Calkins 1975). The overall prevalence of the different amyloid syndromes in the aged varies greatly, although all increase with age. It differs with the chemical nature of the proteins laid down as amyloid. Amyloid deposits appear in the fifth decade (ca. 5%), increase in the sixth (ca. 15%), and in the eighth decade reach approximately 80%. All individuals over 90 years old have amyloid somewhere. Exact numbers related to specific diseases will be given below. While the widespread nature of amyloid deposits is well documented, its presence is less appreciated by physicians at large because of lack of both symptoms and also of therapeutic approaches. For these reasons, the diagnosis of amyloid deposits and amyloidosis is usually made only when excessively large deposits cause severe clinical symptoms that may lead to death.

In spite of the high prevalence of amyloid in many organs in old age, there is not a single prospective report to answer the question as to how these deposits are related to age-related diseases. Retrospective studies show an association of the amount of amyloid with clinical symptoms in the cases of cardiovascular amyloidosis (Pomerance 1966; Roberts and Walter 1983; Wright and Calkins 1975), amyloidosis of the atria (Cornwell et al. 1983), which is chemically distinct from the former, and also Alzheimer's disease. Such an association may well also exist in other age-related amyloid syndromes.

Heterogeneity of Amyloid in Old Age

Since age-associated amyloid deposits belong to different clinical syndromes, the different diseases will be further characterized here and their chemical heterogeneity pointed out.

Senile Cardiovascular Amyloidosis

When it became known that senile cardiovascular amyloidosis was generalized, it was also named "senile generalized amyloidosis." In the older German literature it was also called *"Greisenamyloid"* (Pitkänen et al. 1984).

The heart is the main site of amyloid deposition. In the heart amyloid replaces muscular tissue, so that the heart usually does not increase its weight. The greatest amount of amyloid is observed in the heart. Large amounts of amyloid are also seen in pulmonary septal vessels. Less amyloid is found in the aorta, pulmonary artery, and in the form of smaller spots in many other larger arteries throughout the organism (Pitkänen et al. 1984). Very recently, we have identified cardiovascular amyloid as the major amyloid type contributing also to the carpal tunnel syndrome (Stein et al. 1987).

The prevalence over the age of 80 is above 30% (Fig. 3) (Cornwell et al. 1983; Hodkinson and Pomerance 1977; Pomerance 1966; Wright and Calkins 1975). The contribution to heart condition, digitoxin toxicity, and other age-related cardiac disturbances have not been fully evaluated. Because of its high prevalence, it can be expected that further studies will reveal a major contribution of this type of amyloid to diseases in the elderly.

The amyloid fibril protein (designated ASc_1) is derived from prealbumin/transthyretin (Sletten et al. 1980). Whether this prealbumin has amino acid substitutions is not clear at present. It represents fragments and aggregates of probably normal prealbumin (Saraiva et al., 1988). An antiserum to this type of amyloid clearly stains this amyloid type well (see Fig. 4), and it cross-reacts with amyloid in familial amyloid polyneuropathy that is also derived from prealbumin (Linke 1982), however from a prealbumin with amino acid substitutions (Araki 1986).

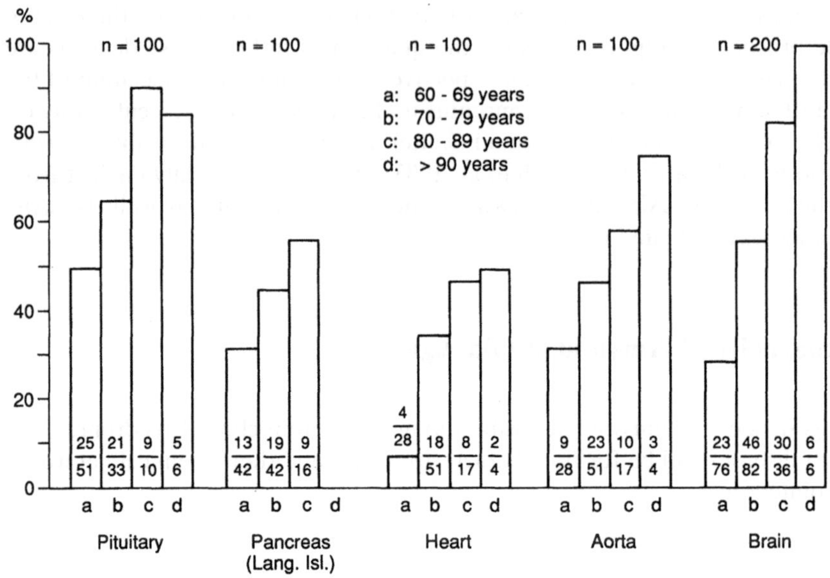

Fig. 3. Prevalence of the amyloid deposits in the age groups examined (Störkel et al. 1983)

Isolated Atrial Amyloid

Isolated atrial amyloid appears earlier in life than ASc_1; in some reports it is stated to be related to atrial fibrillation, and its prevalence is even higher than that of cardiovascular amyloidosis (Cornwell et al. 1983; Westermark et al. 1979). In fact, it is the most common type of cardiac amyloid. In the ninth decade over 90% of patients have this type of amyloid in the atria. In this case, too, the constribution of the amyloid to old age-related cardiac dysfunctions has not been clearly delineated. According to the N-terminal amino acid sequence, the amyloid fibril protein is derived from the atrial natriuretic peptide or cardiodilatin (Johannson et al. 1987; Linke et al. 1988a). The C-terminal end of this amyloid fibril protein has not yet been identified.

Islet Amyloid in Type II Diabetes

Islet hyalinosis has long been known to be associated with type II diabetes, a disease that is very common in the elderly. Islet hyalinosis has been identified as amyloid and thus type II diabetes has been recognized as an amyloidosis of old age (Westermark and Wilander 1978). Very recently, this type of amyloid was chemically identified as being derived from a new hormone that is related to the calcitonin gene family. The amyloid found in the stroma of insulinomas is of the same type (Westermark et al. 1987).

Senile Elastic Amyloid of the Temporal Artery

Senile elastic amyloid of the temporal artery has been recognized as a form separate from other types (Muckle 1986) since it does not stain with antisera against known amyloid type (Linke et al. 1988b). It is very common in the elderly. It is related to the fragmentation of the elastica interna and stains well in tissue section with an antiserum to the amyloid-P-component (Linke et al. 1988b).

Chemically Unidentified Age-Related Amyloid Diseases

There are several other forms of amyloid, the nature of which is unknown. An incomplete summary is shown in Table 3. This catalogue demonstrates the variety of different deposits. Which of them belongs to the same type can only be shown by chemical analysis and immunohistochemical examination.

Table 3. Unidentified age-related amyloid diseases

Senile aortic amyloidosis
Intervertebral disc amyloid
Pituitary amyloids (possibly several forms)
Amyloid of the parathyroid
Senile prostatic amyloid
Senile amyloid of the seminal gland
Non-ASc_1 amyloid of large vessels and lung
Senile amyloid of the temporal artery
Senile amyloid associated with arteriosclerosis
Amyloid in osteoarthritis
Amyloid in senile heart valves

Summary

This chapter has presented several important aspects of amyloid deposits and amyloidosis, which represent protein storage diseases:

1. Amyloid fibril proteins are chemically diverse. Each of the stored proteins marks a different disease with a different pathogenesis. In spite of this chemical diversity, amyloid fibrils share remarkable similarities in morphology (dimensions of amyloid fibrils), secondary structure (β-pleated sheet), and physiochemical properties (enzyme resistance).
2. Amyloid fibril proteins are altered proteins. They can be altered by proteolytic cleavage, by amino acid substitutions, and/or by conformational change that leads to severe antigenic alterations in all investigated proteins when compared with the native precursor proteins.

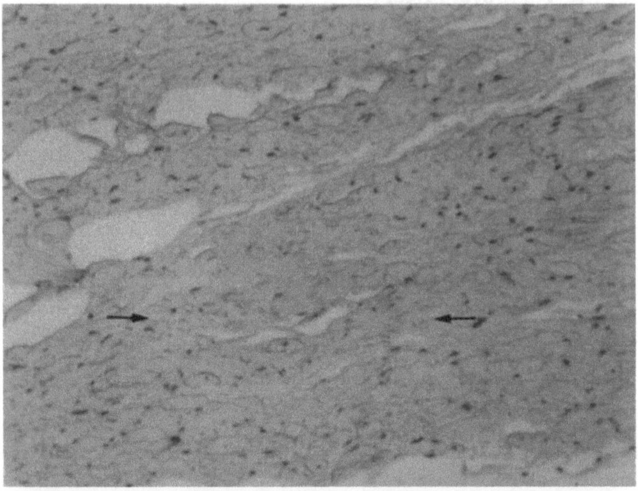

a

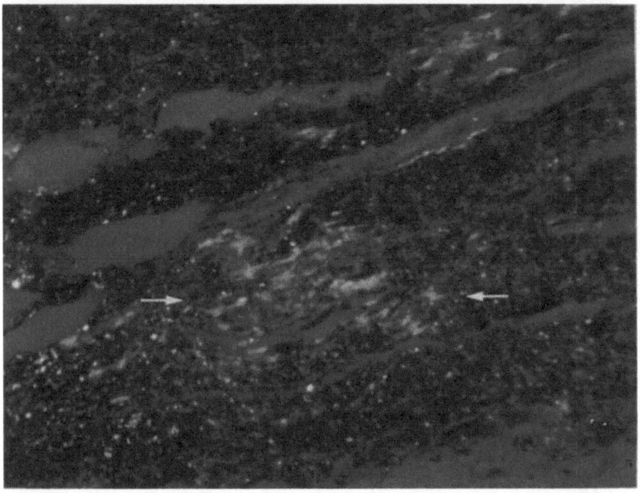

b

Fig. 4a–d. Immunohistochemical identification of cardiovascular amyloid deposits in the heart using an anti-ASc_1 antibody (Linke 1983). **a** Congo red staining; **b** same section in polarized light; **c** anti ASc_1 positive on adjacent section; **d** anti-AA, monoclonal, negative; on adjacent section

3. Amyloid fibril proteins are usually more hydrophobic than their native precursor proteins (Linke 1981).
4. Amyloid in old age is manifested in the brain, the cardiovascular system, the endocrine system (pancreas, pituitary gland, gonads), and the connective tissue system. In all cases the amyloid increases steeply with age.
5. The contribution to age-related ailments is only clear in some amyloid diseases (type II diabetes, Alzheimer's disease).

The elucidation of the mechanisms leading to these alterations still lies ahead of us.

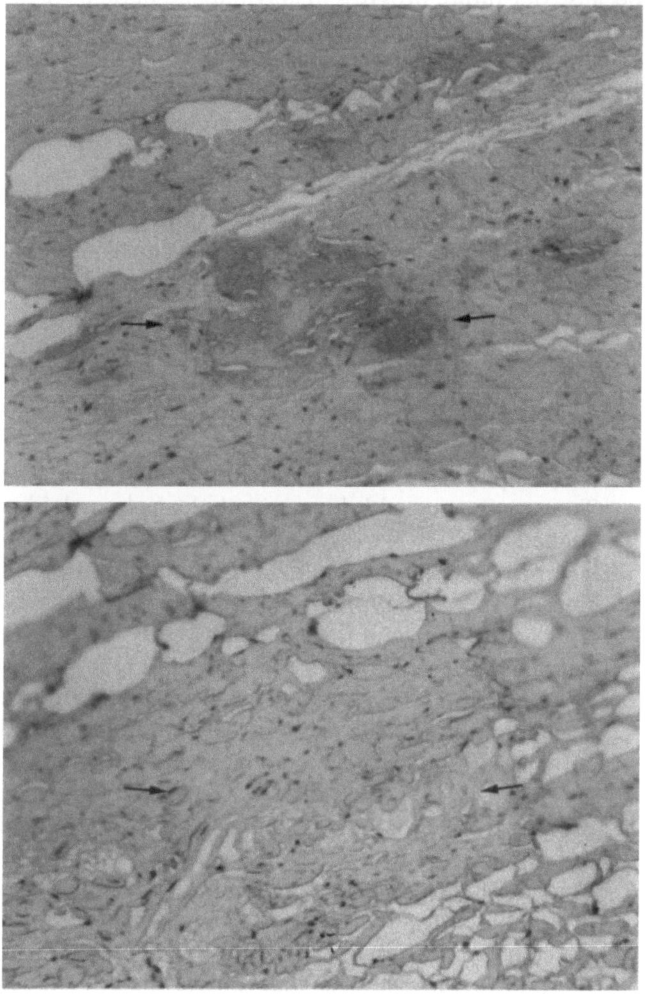

c

d

Future Research

Unlike in other countries, such as the United States, Japan, Sweden, The Netherlands, and Portugal, in Germany no concentrated effort has been made to highlight amyloidosis as *a general phenomenon*, such as cancer. There has never been a controlled effort to correlate amyloid deposits with ailments in old age. Only a few groups in Germany are working on the molecular level and only one (my own) is immediately applying the knowledge to clinical practice. Patients are too dispersed throughout the country and sometimes lack the necessary guidance.

In other countries there are specialist amyloid clinics. It should be considered whether one or more amyloid clinics should be established in Germany, too, because our future progress in amyloid and perhaps in old age research might be tremendously stimulated by such institutions. This has happened, for instance, in Japan, who within a short time has become one of the leading countries in amyloid research. An amyloid clinic in particular would be necessary to probe therapeutic trials in order to influence the insidious clinical course of most of the severe cases.

The following is a list of future aims:

1. The identification of all possible amyloid fibril proteins, including those in old age (see Table 3). Monoclonal and polyclonal antibodies need to be developed against them in order to be able to diagnose clearly the different amyloids in tissue sections.
2. The correlation of ailments in the elderly with age-related amyloid deposits, as has been done with type II diabetes.
3. The establishment of in vitro models in order to understand better the process of amyloid formation.
4. The adoption of animal for the study of important aspects of amyloidogenesis. Transgenic mice with human pathological amyloid protein genes should be studied.
5. The provision of answers to several important questions: Why does the organism synthesize proteins that finally can kill the organism itself? How does the organism prevent this happening early in life? What is missing in old age that amyloid fibril proteins of many different classes, including those found in Alzheimer's desease, type II diabetes, and cardiovascular amyloidosis, can accumulate and lead to pathological protein storage? Which of the genes cause early manifestation of amyloid that would otherwise be manifested in old age as, for instance, in hereditary Alzheimer's disease? How is it possible to prevent these protein storage diseases? More difficult, how is it possible to remove amyloid from affected organs and restore normal function?
6. The adoption of appropriate administrative measures: (a) the concentration of patients with amyloid diseases in one or a few centers in Germany to handle the course of the disease better, to start therapeutic trials in order to optimize possible therapy, and to train physicians and students; (b) supporting this effort by an aligned scientific institute.

It is important to separate normal aging from age-related diseases and to try to find the cause and a treatment of the latter. In this way one can envisage improving conditions so as to render old age more enjoyable.

Discussion

Platt

How would you explain the fact that amyloid synthesis can't be found in the liver of some species? For instance in livers of humans or of rats. Using Congo red staining we have looked at a lot of livers in individuals of a high age – 3-year-old animals or 80- or 90-year-old persons. We never found amyloid.

Linke

Amyloid has been reported in liver of several species, especially mice; it's also very common in dogs, cats, and cattle.

Platt

OK, but why not in rats?

Linke

We don't know. They seem to be very resistant.

Platt

Has anybody tried to look for amyloid synthesis after endotoxin or casein in rats?

Linke

Yes.

Platt

You can produce it in rats?

Linke

No, it was not possible. We made a big effort several years ago, by inducing osteomyelitis in rats. The osteomyelitis just healed; it could not be maintained. One can inject rats with almost any load of bacteria. Amyloidosis does not develop.

Platt

With casein?

Linke

In contrast to mice, guinea pigs, and rabbits, which develop amyloidosis, there is no effect in rats.

Platt

How would you explain that?

Linke

Some papers came out giving an explanation. To induce inflammation-induced amyloid in animals one needs the acute phase protein serum amyloid A protein (SAA). In rats the gene of SAA seems not to be present or is not transcribed. Rats seem to be less susceptible to inflammation so that after longstanding inflammation no amyloid can develop, probably due to the missing gene product SAA. Maybe rats had an advantage in evolution because of the missing protein.

Platt

If you assume that the synthesis of amyloid fibrils is possible in apo-III, which is synthesized in the liver, how is it possible that the liver can synthesize apo-III and transport it by membranes in the blood plasma, but is not able to synthesize amyloid in the cell.

Linke

We usually don't see amyloid in cells. When on rare occasions amyloid is present intracellularly, it is located in lysosomes. Here it is not synthesized but broken down after phagocytosis. The intracellular enzymatic machinery seems to be more perfect than its extracellular counterpart. It also seems to be more intelligent since it can digest almost whatever is phagocytosed. The intracellular catabolism is probably over one billion years older than the extracellular proteolytic machinery and is, thus, far more refined. Scientists estimate that approximately 70 different proteinases exist in neutrophil granulocytes and the breakdown of proteins, the variety of which may be in the order of 10 000 different proteins per cell, takes place in an ordered manner, according to Professor Bohley in Tübingen, a leading scientist on intracellular metabolism. The different proteinases have different and in part overlapping specificity. So, some cleave proteins either at the N- or the C-terminus, and others in the middle of the molecule yielding peptides. Again, other proteinases cleave at special residues only and others cleave at multiple sites. The concert of proteinases that work in a cascade fashion guarantees an ordered removal of all protein aggregates, peptides, including amyloidogenic fragments. So, we have sent to Professor Bohley amyloidogenic proteins which are easily transformed into amyloid in the test tube. When present intracellularly, they are completely digested. This result shows that amyloidogenic proteins can be more easily handled inside the cell than by extracellular enzymes. It also means that the extracellular enzymes do not suffice to prevent the generation of amyloidogenic protein fragments. So, the extracellular proteolytic machinery can be defective under certain conditions, such as old age, in the presence of specific point mutations in proteins with high β-content yielding new stable amyloidogenic intermediates due to an unusual splitting pattern and/or in the presence of connective tissue components which still have to be defined.

An imbalance can also occur with an excessive amount of substrate, as can be assumed in multiple myeloma. Due to monoclonal immunoglobulins and Bence Jones proteins one can assume a relative defect in the panel of proteinases, so that more resistant, amyloidogenic fragment intermediates can survive and can aggregate into amyloid, or into nonamyloid light chain deposit diseases.

Also, in inflammation-induced amyloid long-lasting intermediates occur, due to both an increase in serum amyloid A protein and a decrease in macrophage surface proteases that have been shown to degrade the ensuing intermediate, which seems to be similar in size to the AA protein and which is found in the amyloid deposits.

There is another point that relates to your question about rats. I think I can give an example in man. Individuals with rheumatoid arthritis have a chronic, sometimes very severe inflammatory disease. But only about 5% will develop amyloidosis, in spite of similar inflammatory severity. It's the same in smokers you know. Many smoke, but only a certain proportion of individuals succumb to lung cancer. So, people say no, it doesn't come from smoking. But that's incorrect. When an inflammatory stimulus hits a person who cannot destroy the pathogenic intermediate for genetic or other reasons, then amyloidosis may occur. In this respect rats may reside on the safer side due to their genetic setup, which includes the fact that SAA is not elevated in their acute phase response and may not be transcribed sufficiently in the first place.

Frenzel

I think it is very interesting that amyloid deposits in the atria of the elderly correspond biochemically with ANP. ANP release is increased in chronic pulmonary disease and the frequency of chronic pulmonary disease is increased in the elderly. May there be a better correlation between these atrial amyloid deposits with pulmonary disease and chronic heart insufficiency than with age?

Linke

Yes, it's possible. And this type of amyloid, which is called isolated atrial amyloid, may be found someday also in the ventricles because the ventricular muscle cells synthesize ANP in heart insufficiencies. This is speculative, because amyloid of the ANP type has not been shown in the heart other than in the atrium, so far.

Beischer

Please comment a little more on the amyloid deposit in type II diabetes. Where is it deposited? How common is it? You spoke of a hormone; how is this proven and what are the actions of this hormone?

Linke

The hormone was identified only last year by the group of Per Westermark in Sweden. Nobody knows its function. This hormone was found for the first time in amyloid deposits, and very recently it has been analyzed on the cDNA level.

Beischer

How was it proven that it is a hormone?

Linke

By homology with other hormones. If one finds a peptide that is homologue chemically one can assume that the homologue is a hormone as well. This new hormone is synthesized by beta cells besides insulin. Since insulin is amyloidogenic in vitro, an amyloid-forming peptide of insulin origin was assumed. However, by extraction and amino acid analysis, a striking difference from insulin was found, which excluded insulin as a precursor candidate for amyloid formation. And now your question is the relation to aging ...

Beischer

Is it common?

Linke

Very common.

Beischer

And where in the organ is it deposited?

Linke

It is deposited in the vicinity of B cells, in the outer rim of the islets of Langerhans. The old pathologists call it islet hyalinosis but many do not notice that it is indeed amloid. I mean you have to perform a special staining of tissue sections to identify the amyloid nature of these proteinaceous deposits.

Rauterberg

Do you think that amyloid formation may be involved in the pathogenesis of atherosclerosis?

Linke

I would not go so far as to say that amyloid is involved in the pathogenesis of arteriosclerosis, but it can be associated.

Rauterberg

It might be a smaller secondary effect.

Linke

We don't know what it is chemically, but one can sometimes find it in association with the arteriosclerotic plaques.

Greiling

I was surprised that you have shown only the protein molecule of your amyloid. I thought that this is a glycoprotein. Have you neglected the carbohydrate chains or are you sure that this protein has no carbohydrate chains.

Linke

Amyloid is not *one* protein. I've shown you a host of different amyloidogenic proteins. Immunoglobulins, which are transformed into amyloid in vivo, have five times more carbohydrate than the average immunoglobulin. So when a light chain, a lambda light chain, has a carbohydrate, it has a propensity to create amyloid. This has been shown by Sletten in Norway. Other proteins, such as the A protein, do not have carbohydrate covalently bound, except for the matrix where AA is deposited. So it's not part of the fibril. The amyloid fibril, therefore, does not have to be a glycoprotein. Sometimes it is, sometimes it is not. But I think I know what you are driving at. The amyloid deposit in tissues, as shwon to you, is not just the fibril, it's not a pure protein, it is embedded in a matrix of acid glycosaminoglycans which increase with the amount of amyloid. But whether these are unspecific or not we don't know. Whether they induce the deposition and formation of the fibril we don't yet know. Within the deposit in each different class of amyloid one can find the same types of glycosaminoglycans in high amounts.

Greiling

Yes, but I mean is it possible in the biosynthesis of these amyloid fibrils that degradation of posttranslational glycoprotein occurs? That's your opinion. But this is the second process, the addition or precipitation with glycosaminoglycans or proteoglycans.

Linke

All amyloid-forming proteins are not synthesized as such because they are insoluble. All proteins which are synthesized have to be soluble at a certain point, similar to collagen, elastin, and all those other insoluble structured proteins. And with amyloid it's just the same. They are soluble proteins at first and they become insoluble later. A structural change must occur in some way, I think. In insulin we did it by adding acid and heating it. There was a conformational change and aggregation in fibrillar form. The second way is to cleave off hydrophilic peptides. We have shown by charge shift electrophoresis that the precursor is usually less hydrophobic than its amyloidogenic derivatives. So, to create amyloid one has to clip off hydrophilic peptides. The resulting less soluble peptide can aggregate to insoluble fibrils in which the polypeptides are packed very tightly and which cannot easily be broken down by enzymes of macrophages, let alone extracellular enzymes.

Greiling

Is the deposition of amyloid in osteoarthrosis the same – does it have the same composition as in the other tissues?

Linke

Nobody knows at present. It was on my list of unknown types, that I showed you on a slide.

References

Allsop D (1986) Biochemistry of cerebral amyloid in Alzheimer's disease, the unconventional slow virus diseases and Icelandic cerebrovascular amyloidosis. In: Marrink J, Van Rijwijk MH (eds) Amyloidosis. Martinus Nijhoff, Amsterdam, p 243–253

Araki S (1986) Familial amyloidotic polyneuropathies. In: Marrink J, Van Rijwijk MH (eds) Amyloidosis. Marinus Nijhoff, Amsterdam, p 195–218

Benditt EP, Eriksen N (1971) The chemical classes of amyloid substance. Am J Pathol 65: 231–249

Benditt EP, Eriksen N (1971) The major proteins of human and monkey amyloid substance: common properties including unusual N-terminal amino acid sequences. FEBS Lett 19: 169–173

Bennhold H (1922) Eine spezifische Amyloidfärbung mit Kongorot. Münch Med Wochenschr 69: 1537–1549

Buerger L, Braunstein H (1960) Senile cardiac amyloidosis. Am J Med 28: 357–367

Cohen AS (1967) Amyloidosis. N Engl J Med 277: 522–530; 574–583; 628–638

Cohen DH, Feiner H, Jensson O, Frangione B (1983) Amyloid fibril in hereditary cerebral hemorrhage with amyloidosis (HCHWA) is related to the gastroenteropancreatic neuroendocrine protein, gamma trace. J Exp Med 158: 623–628

Connors LH, Shirahama T, Skinner M, Fenves A, Cohen AS (1985) In vitro formation of amyloid fibrils from intact β_2-microglobulin. Biochem Biophys Res Commun 131: 1063–1068

Cornwell III GG, Murdoch WL, Kyle RA, Westermark P, Pitkänen P (1983) Frequency and distribution of senile cardiovascular amyloid. A clinicopathologic correlation. Am J Med 75: 618–623

Costa PP, Figueira AS, Bravo FR (1978) Amyloid fibril protein related to prealbumin in familial amyloidotic polyneuropathy. Proc Natl Acad Sci USA 75: 4499–4503

Diringer H, Gelderblom H, Hilmert H, Ozel N, Edelbluth C, Kimberlin RH (1983) Scrapie infectivity, fibrils and low molecular weight proteins Nature 406: 376–478

Dische FE, Wernstedt C, Westermark GT, Westermark P, Pepys MB, Rennie JA, Gilbey SG, Watkins PJ (1988) Insulin as an amyloid-fibril protein at sites of repeated insulin injections in a diabetic patient. Diabetologia 31: 158–161

Floege J, Brandis A, Nonnast-Daniel B, Westhoff-Bleck M, Linke RP, Koch KM (1989) Subcutaneous amyloid-tumor of β_2-microglobulin origin in a long-term hemodialysis patient. Nephron 53: 73–75

Gejyo F, Yamada T, Odani S, Nakagawa P, Arakawa M (1985) A new form of amyloid protein associated with hemodialysis was identified as β_2-microglobulin. Biochem Biophys Res Commun 129: 701–706

Gejyo F, Homma N, Maruyama H, Ohara K, Avakawa M (1988) Coexistence of β_2-microglobulin-derived amyloid deposits and extopic calcification in the heart of a chronic hemodialyzed patient. In: Isobe T, Araki S; Uchino F; Kito S, Tsubura G (eds) Amyloid and Amyloidosis. Plenum Press New York and London p 617–622

Glenner GG (1980) Amyloid deposits and amyloidosis. The β-fibrilloses. N Engl J Med 302: 1283–1292; 1333–1343

Glenner GG, Wong CW (1984) Alzheimer's disease: initial report on the purification and characterization of a novel cerebrovascular amyloid protein. Biochem Biophys Res Commun 120: 885–890

Glenner GG, Bladen HA, Linke RP, Termine JD (1974) β-Pleated sheet fibrils: a comparison of native amyloid with synthetic protein fibrils. J Histochem Cytochem 22: 1141–1158

Hodkinson HM, Pomerance A (1977) The clinical significance of senile cardiac amyloidosis. A prospective clinicopathological study. Q J Med 183: 381–387

Johannsson B, Wernstedt C, Westermark P (1987) A final natriuretic peptide deposit as atrial amyloid fibrils. Biochem Biophys Res Comm 148: 1087–1092

Kedar I, Ravid M, Sohar E (1976) In vitro synthesis of "amyloid" fibrils from insulin, calcitonin and parathormon. Isr J Med Sci 12: 1137–1143

Linke RP (1981) Amphiphilic properties of the low molecular weight component of serum amyloid A protein shown by charge shift electrophoresis. Biochem Biophys Acta 668: 388–396

Linke RP (1982) Immunohistochemical identification and cross reactions of amyloid fibril proteins in senile heart and amyloid in familial polyneuropathy. Lack of reactivity with cerebral amyloid in Alzheimer's disease. J Clin Neuropathol 4: 172–182

Linke RP (1983) Senile cardiac amyloid. Biochemical and immunohistochemical results. In: Platt D (ed) Cardiology and aging. Schattauer, Stuttgart, p 81–97

Linke RP (1985) Immunochemical typing of amyloid deposits after microextraction from biopsies. Appl Pathol 3: 18–28

Linke RP, Sipe JD, Pollock PS, Ignaczak TF, Glenner GG (1975) Isolation of a low-molecular weight serum component antigenically related to an amyloid fibril protein of unknown origin. Proc Natl Acad Sci USA 72: 1473–1476

Linke RP, Nathrath WB, Wilson PD (1983) Immuno-electron microscopic identification and classification of amyloid in tissue sections by the postembedding protein-A gold method. Ultrastruct Pathol 4: 1–7

Linke RP, Nathrath WBJ, Eulitz M (1986a) Classification of amyloid syndromes from tissue sections using antibodies against various amyloid fibril proteins: report of 142 cases. In: Glenner GG, Osserman EF, Benditt EP, Calkins E, Cohen AS, Zucker-Franklin D (eds) Amyloidosis. Plenum, New York, p 599–605

Linke RP, Bommer J, Ritz E, Waldherr R, Eulitz M (1986) Amyloid kidney stones of uremic patients consist of beta$_2$-microglobulin fragments. Biochem Biophys Res Commun 136: 665–671

Linke RP, Voigt C, Störkel FS, Eulitz M (1988a) N-terminal amino acid sequence analysis indicates that isolated atrial amyloid is derived from atrial natriuretic peptide. Virchows Arch [Cell Pathol] 55: 125–127

Linke RP, Logan C, Muckle TJ, Simon G (1988b) Immunological examination of senile amyloidosis of the temporal artery. In: Isobe T, Araki S, Uchino F, Kito S, Tsubura E (eds) Amyloid and Amyloidosis. Plenum Press New York and London p 657–659

Lubarsch O (1929) Zur Kenntnis ungewöhnlicher Amyloidablagerungen. Virchows Arch, Path Anat 271: 867–891

Masters CL, Simms G, Weinmann NA, Multhaupt G, McDonald BL, Beyreuther KC (1985) Amyloid plaque core protein in Alzheimer disease and Down syndrome. Proc Natl Acad Sci USA 82: 4245–4249

Missmahl HP, Hartwig H (1953) Polarisationsoptische Untersuchungen an der Amyloid-Substanz. Virchows Arch, Path Anat 324: 489–508

Muckle TJ (1986) Peripheral angiopathy In: Marrink J, Van Rijwijk MH (eds) Amyloidosis. Martinus Nijhoff, Amsterdam, p 271–282

Pitkänen P, Westermark P, Cornwell III GG (1984) Senile systemic amyloidosis. Am J Pathol 117: 391–399

Pomerance A (1966) The pathology of senile cardiac amyloidosis. J Pathol Bact 91: 357–367

Pras M, Schubert M, Zucker-Franklin D, Rimon A, Franklin EC (1968) The characterization of soluble amyloid prepared in water. J Clin Invest 47: 924–933

Prusiner SB (1982) Novel proteinaceous infectious particles cause scrapie. Science 216: 136–144

Puchtler H, Sweat F, Levine M (1962) On the binding of Congo red by amyloid. J Histochem Cytochem 10: 355–364

Roberts WC, Walter BF (1983) Cardiac amyloidosis causing cardiac dysfunction: analysis of 54 necropsy patients. Am J Cardiol 52: 137–146

Rokitanski KFV (1842) Handbuch der pathologischen Anatomie, Vol 3. Braunmüller and Seidel, Wien

Saraiva MJM, Linke RP, Gawinowicz MA, Goodman DS (1988) Senile cardio-vascular amyloid: lack of evidence for differences between amyloid fibril protein and normal transthyretin. In: Isobe T, Araki S, Uchino F, Kito S, Tsubura G (eds) Amyloid and Amyloidosis. Plenum Press, New York and London, p 641–645

Schwarz P (1970) Amyloidosis. Cause and manifestation of senile deterioration. Charles C. Thomas, Springfield, Ill.

Sletten K, Westermark P, Natrig JB (1976) Characterization of amyloid fibril proteins from medullary carcinoma of the thyroid. J Exp Med 143: 993–998

Sletten K, Westermark P, Natrig JB (1980) Senile cardiac amyloid is related to prealbumin. Scand J Immunol 12: 503–506

Stein K, Störkel S, Linke RP, Goebel HH (1987) Chemical heterogeneity of amyloid in the carpal tunnel syndrome. Virchows Arch [A] 412: 37–45

Störkel S, Schneider HM, Thoenes W (1983) Manifestation and ultrastructural typing of amyloid deposits in the heart. Virchows Arch [A] 401: 185–201

Virchow R (1854) Über eine im Gehirn und Rückenmark des Menschen aufgefundene Substanz mit der chemischen Reaktion der Cellulose. Virchows Arch, Path Anat 6: 135–138

Westermark P, Wilander E (1978) The influence of amyloid deposits on the islet volume in maturity onset diabetes mellitus. Diabetologia 15: 417–421

Westermark P, Johansson B, Natrig JB (1979) Senile cardiac amyloidosis: the existence of two different amyloid substances in the aging heart. Scand J Immunol 10: 303–308

Westermark P, Wernstedt C, Wilander E, Hayden DW, O'Brien TD, Johnson KH (1987) Amyloid fibril in human insulinoma and islets of Langerhans of the diabetic cart are derived from a neuropeptide-like protein also present in normal islet cells. Proc Natl Acad Sci USA 84: 3881–3885

Wright JR, Calkins E (1975) Amyloid in the aged heart. Frequency and clinical significance. J Am Geriatr Soc 23: 97–103

Wright JR, Calkins E, Humphrey RL (1977) Potassium permanganate reaction in amyloidosis. A histologic method to assist in differentiating forms of this disease. Lab Invest 36: 274–281

Metabolism and Nutrition in the Elderly

Changes in Structure and Metabolism of Proteoglycans in Aging

H. Greiling, R.N. Schöngen, K. Kleesiek, and H.W. Stuhlsatz[1]

Besides the various collagen types I–XII and the elastins, the so-called ground substance, which is composed of glycosaminoglycans and proteoclycans, is produced by specific cells in connective tissues. They are developed from a primitive mesenchymal cell. Specific cells – fibroblasts, chondrocytes, etc. – produce specific tissue types which have a characteristic composition of macromolecules, and also glycosaminoglycans and proteoglycans, which determine the biomechanical properties of the tissue.

There are age-dependent changes in proteoglycan structure which are different in various connective tissue types. The proteoglycan subunit in cartilage consists of chondroitin sulfate and keratan sulfate chains connected to a protein core. Numerous proteoglycan subunits are aggregated by means of a hyaluronate chain. Since the early report of Kaplan and Meyer (1959) which described for the first time age-dependent changes in the composition of the glycosaminoglycans in human costal cartilage, further studies have confirmed both in animal and human cartilage an age-dependent decrease in total chondroitin sulfate combined with an increase in the ratio of chondroitin 6-sulfate to chondroitin 4-sulfate (Greiling and Baumann 1973). In addition to the decrease in the total glycosaminoglycan concentration with age, the number of unsulfated disaccharide units present in chondroitin sulfate is reduced. Mathews and Glagov (1966) found a relative increase in keratan sulfate in human costal cartilage with age.

Roughley and White (1980) found that the proteoglycan content of the human articular cartilage decreases with age; the same is true for the size of the proteoglycan subunit. The results of these authors confirmed our findings concerning the ratio of chondroitin sulfate to keratan sulfate in human knee joint cartilage: an increase in keratan sulfate relative to chondroitin sulfate, and an increase in chondroitin 6-sulfate relative to chondroitin 4-sulfate. In addition, Roughley and White oserved an increase in protein relative to glycosaminoglycans and a decrease in serine and glycine in relation to an increase in arginine of the proteoglycan core protein with age. Similar results were also obtained by Inerot et al. in canine hip articular cartilage. They found that the extracted proteoglycans were smaller in the older proteoglycan monomers (Inerot et al. 1978). Aging of human cartilage is also accompanied by an increase in the hyaluronate binding region and partially fragmented link proteins (Roughley and Mort 1986).

---

[1] Institute of Clinical Chemistry and Pathobiochemistry, Medical Faculty, Aachen University of Technology, Pauwelsstr., D-5100 Aachen / FRG

Gerontology
Ed. by D. Platt
© Springer-Verlag Berlin Heidelberg 1989

In the human aorta, too, a lage aggregating chondroitin sulfate proteoglycan is found besides aortal proteoglycans with lower molecular weight and a high dermatan sulfate content with enriched iduronic acid (Heinegard and Paulsson 1984). We could detect an increase in keratan sulfate and a decrease in chondroitin sulfate with increasing age (Stuhlsatz et al. 1982).

Since the increasing deposition of calcium phosphate in each aortic segment correlates with an enhancement of the concentration and relative proportion of keratan sulfate, both topographically increasing from the aortic arch to the bifurcatio aortae, a kind of nucleating function may also be considered for keratan sulfate with age. As ion exchanging macromolecules, the glycosaminoglycans exhibit different affinities to Ca^{2+} which is high in chondroitin sulfates, especially chondroitin 6-sulfate, and lowest in keratan sulfate. A decrease in chondroitin sulfate content of the aortic proteoglycans in favor of keratan sulfate which binds Ca^{2+} to a much lesser extent would increase the portion of deimmobilized Ca^{2+} which may give rise to insoluble calcium phosphate. Such a microprecipitate could then serve as a crystallization nucleus.

Aorta proteoglycans are capable of interacting with low density lipoproteins (LDLs). The higher the anionic part of the glycosaminoglycans, the better the precipitation which means the higher the insolubility of the LDL-glycosaminoglycan complex. Another important aspect is the age-related advanced glycosylation of connective tissue components, e.g. collagen, also in atherosclerosis. LDLs are covalently bound by glycosylated collagen more than threefold as much as by normal collagen (Vlassara et al. 1986). Collagen from normal subjects shows an age-related increase in the accumulation of advanced glycosylation end products. In diabetes mellitus the thickening of basement membranes and intima are related to this phenomenon.

How can we explain the age-dependent changes of decreased chondroitin sulfate and increased keratan sulfate on a molecular level? Some studies indicate an age-associated depression in the biosynthesis of proteochondroitin sulfate in both animal and human cartilage. The enzyme activity catalyzing the covalent attachment of xylose to the seryl residues of the core protein has been suggested to be rate limiting in the biosynthesis of the glycosaminoglycan chain of proteochondroitin sulfate. Therefore we studied the activity of UDP-xylose: proteoglycan core protein xylosyltransferase in the costal cartilage of young and senescent rats.

The activity of xylosyltransferase measured in samples of old and young costal cartilage is decreased about 70% in the tissue of old rats, related to cartilage wet weight and protein. In old cartilage, there was a reduction of cell number, as checked by the decline in extractable DNA to about 30%. However, the decrease in the activity of xylosyltransferase in relation to the concentration of DNA in old cartilage was similar to that reported above (about 70%). The results suggest that the reduced xylosyltransferase activity might lead to a diminished concentration of proteochondroitin sulfate in the cartilage of old animals (Wolf et al. 1982).

When the activity of xylosyltransferase was related to galactosamine as a measure of the concentration of chondroitin sulfate, no significant differences between young and old rats were detectable. Thus, there is a coordinate decrease in both xylosyltransferase activity and chontroitin sulfate content in the cartilage of old rats in comparison to that of young animals.

Our findings point to xylosyltransferase as a possible regulator of proteochondroitin sulfate synthesis at the posttranslational level. This is in agreement with the findings of Schwartz (1977) which show the independence of proteochondroitin sulfate synthesis from the biosynthetic rate of the respective core protein. The rather short half-life of xylosyltransferase as compared to other enzymes involved in the glycosaminoglycan chain synthesis indicates the possible regulatory role of this enzyme in chondroitin sulfate proteoglycan production.

Since a reduction of xylosyltransferase activity was also found in our experiments if related to the concentration of DNA, a loss of chondrocytes as a cause of this change is excluded. The activity of another cytosolic enzyme, lactate dehydrogenase, was found to be nearly unaffected by the age of the animals, if related to DNA. Therefore it is conceivable that, due to the reduction of xylosyltransferase activity in old cartilage, the enzymatic attachment of xylose to the seryl residues of core protein becomes rate limiting under such conditions. In accordance with this assumption, Inerot et al. (1978) have shown similar chain length (molecular weight) of chondroitin sulfate in old and young cartilage, and Honda et al. (1979) have presented evidence that the glycosaminoglycan chain elongation reaction is not impaired in the cartilage of senescent rats. Thus, the age-dependent diminution of total chondroitin sulfate is due to a reduced number of initiated carbohydrate side chains along the core protein which is likely to be caused by decreased xylosyltransferase in old tissue.

Our results do not answer the question of whether there is a decrease in the specific activity of this enzyme or a diminution of enzyme protein. The nature of the primary event that causes diminished xylosyltransferase activity is not yet known and needs further investigation. Of particular importance might be the changed composition of hormones with age, since Schiller (1976) has shown that in diabetic thyroidectomized and hypophysectomized rats the reduced synthesis of proteoglycans is due to a decreased activity of xylosyltransferase. She observed that in hormone-deficient animals the enzymatic attachment of xylose to seryl residues of the core protein becomes the rate-limiting step in the synthesis of proteochondroitin sulfate. Other authors have shown that hormones which are involved in the sulfation of proteoglycans, e.g. somatomedin and thyroxine, especially affect the activity of xylosyltransferase.

With increasing age free thyroxine concentration in blood serum decreases (Wilke 1983). We found a stimulation of chondroitin sulfate synthesis by triiodothyronine (T_3) in chondrocyte cultures. In the presence of rT_3, the antagonist of T_3, the galactosamine/glucosamine ratio diminishes which means an increase in keratan sulfate synthesis. Also the incorporation of ^{14}C-serine into the core protein increases with T_3 concentration (Greiling et al. 1986). The same occurs to thyroxine (T_4) and 3',5'-diiodothyronine which means an activation of chondroitin sulfate synthesis with T_4 and an inhibition with 3',5'-diiodothyronine. Also in human blood serum there is an increase in the rT_3/T_3 ratio after 60 years.

We postulate the following regulatory mechanism. T_4 and T_3 increase the number of serine acceptors for xylose and consequently the xylosyltransferase activity. This results in a diminished UDP-xylose pool. UDP-xylose is a feedback inhibitor of UDP-glucose dehydrogenase. A decreased UDP-xylose concentration stimulates the UDP-glucose dehydrogenase and therefore the proteochondroitin sulfate synthesis. Decreased concentrations of T_4 and T_3 in blood serum found in older animals or an increase in 3',5'-diiodothyronine or rT_3 have the inverse effect and stimulate proteokeratan sulfate synthesis, as can be seen in the elderly. Thus, the characteristic changes in connective tissue with increasing age can be explained at the regulatory enzyme level (Greiling et al. 1986).

Is there also an age-dependent degradation of proteoglycans by proteinases? Elastase seems to cleave the link protein of proteoglycan aggregates and it is known to degrade the nonhelical terminal peptides of cartilage collagen molecules which leads to disruption of the main intermolecular crosslinks in collagen fibers and to deterioration in the tensile strength of articular cartilage.

Various mechanisms are described that may cause an enzymatic destruction of the cartilage. An extracellular proteolytic activity of proteinases in the synovial system is inhibited by an excess of very potent proteinase inhibitors, such as α_1-proteinase inhibitor and α_2-macroglobulin, derived from the plasma. Thus, the occurrence of a relevant free proteinase activity in the synovial fluid is presumed to be unlikely.

Quantitation of elastase complexes to α_1-proteinase inhibitor was carried out by an enzyme-linked immunoassay. The mean concentration of elastase in the inflammatory synovial fluid was approximately 10000 μg/l, compared to 41 μg/l in noninflammatory synovial fluids (Kleesiek et al. 1986). The concentration of elastase-α_1-proteinase inhibitor complex is also elevated in synovial fluids of "activated" degenerative joint diseases which occur particularly in the elderly. But systematic studies are necessary to investigate a possible age dependency of the concentration of elastase in plasma or tissue.

Oberley and Oberley (1986) have postulated that aging occurs by damage of differentiated postmitotic cells which means aging in dividing cells is much slower than in nondividing cells in humans. The best evidence for this is that the major manifestations of human aging are heart diseases, brain dysfunction, and vessel

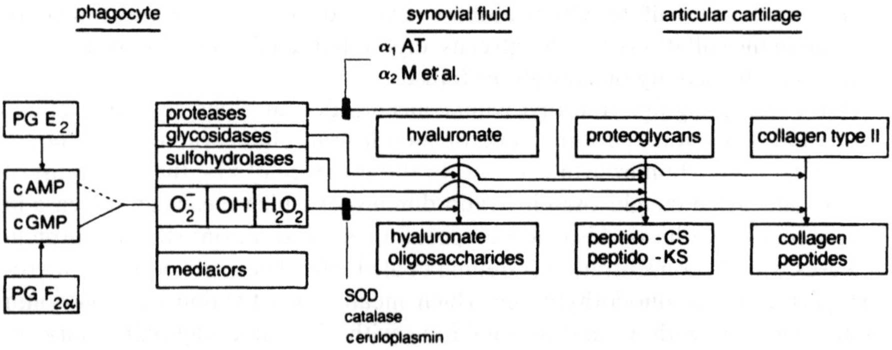

Fig. 1. Destruction of extracellular matrix components in inflammatory joint diseases and in age-dependent pathobiochemical processes. α_1AT, α_1-proteinase inhibitor; α_2M, α_2-macroglobulin; *CS*, chondroitin sulfate; *KS*, keratan sulfate; *SOD*, superoxide dismutase

diseases all of which are mainly postmitotic cell diseases involving organs with very little growth potential in the adult. Oberley and Oberley believe that the initial site of aging is mitochondrial DNA, not the nucelar DNA. They postulate that the damage to aging cells is caused by oxygen radicals which are produced about five- to tenfold in mitochondrial membranes compared with nuclear membranes (Patton et al. 1980). Cutler (1984) postulates so-called longevity genes. He has hypothesized that a number of systems may be involved in longevity including detoxification processes, antioxidants, cellular renewal processes, redundancy mechanisms, specific metabolic rate control, gene control systems, relative enzyme levels, and structural components of cells. In his opinion antioxidants determine human longevity. These are: superoxide dismutase, catalase, urate, α-tocopherol, and carotinoids. Further important antioxidants are ascorbate, ceruloplasmin, and glucose. Cutler has evaluated that afore mentioned antioxidants which also determine cartilage stabilization in aging.

We have shown that cartilage destruction by granulocytes can be inhibited "in vitro" by addition of superoxide dismutase. We developed a model for frustrated phagocytosis in which FMLP-activated granulocytes react on cartilage slices. We have shown an inhibition of the cartilage destruction by granulocytes in the presence of glycosaminoglycan polysulfates (chondroitin polysulfate, dermatan polysulfate), potent proteinase inhibitors. A diminished activity of superoxide dismutase or glutathione peroxidase in aged cartilage tissues may be responsible for the increased degradation of joint cartilage in the elderly.

We postulate that various proteinases and other lysosomal enzymes combined with superoxide radicals are responsible for the destruction of the proteoglycans and collagens of cartilage, especially I, II, and III. This process can be inhibited by α_1-proteinase inhibitor and α_2-macroglobulin, but it is also important to diminish the concentrations of superoxide and hydroxyl radicals by superoxide dismutase and of H_2O_2 by catalase (Fig. 1).

We know the role of immunochemical reactions in proteoglycan and collagen degradation. The degradation of proteoglycans and collagens by proteinases and the regulatory role of interleukin 1 are shown in Fig. 2. In the aging process there is an accumulation of proteoglycan and collagen degradation products which can also react directly on macrophages leading to an age-dependent interleukin production which increases the degradation of proteoglycans and collagen in the cartilage. The decrease in T-helper cells with increasing age has an additional effect on the degradation of cartilage.

There are many unsolved problems in the connective tissue metabolism. There is a requirement for more basic research in clinical biochemistry which is necessary for causal therapy in gerontology.

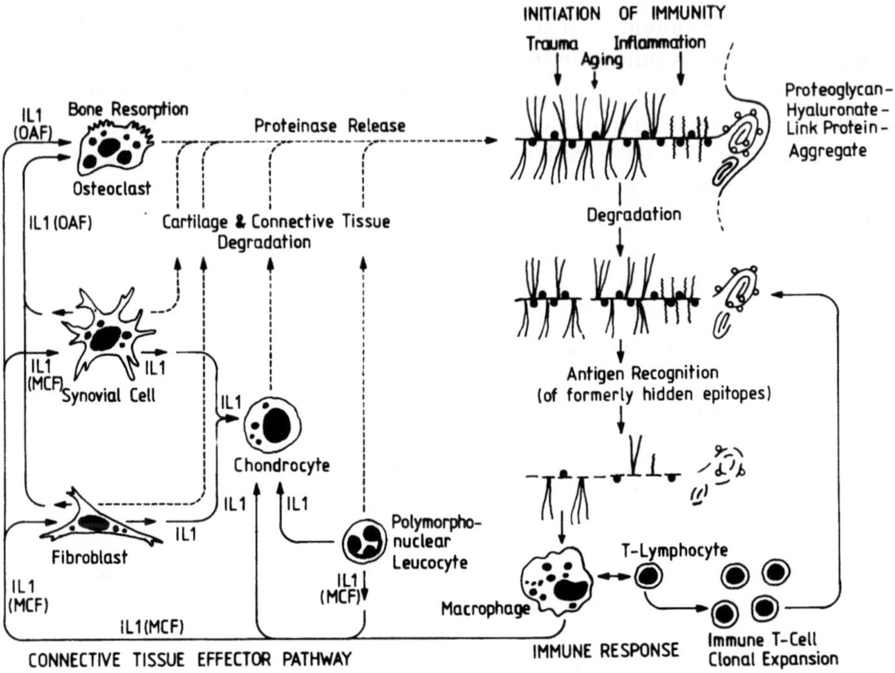

Fig. 2. Immunochemical age-dependent processes which initiate immune T cell involved interleukin 1 production. Interleukin 1 stimulated the release of proteinases from osteoclasts, chondrocytes, synovial cells, and fibroblasts. (Modified from Poole 1986)

Discussion

Platt

As you know, we looked for the degradation processes in former times. My question is: Have you looked or is there any information on glycosidases which are working in this scheme as trauma and inflammation referring to keratan sulfate?

Greiling

Yes, there are many studies about the degradation of the keratan sulfates and especially keratan sulfate proteoglycans, and these degradation processes are catalyzed by lysosomal enzymes. We know also that the keratan sulfate peptides are eliminated and excreted in the urine; therefore, I think, the first step must be the splitting of the protein core and then, as can be shown in kidney lysosomes, the other enzymes may split the carbohydrate chain, e.g. a xylosidase for chondroitin sulfate or mannosidases for keratan sulfate. And then you need *N*-acteylglucosaminidase and β-galactosidase which also can be shown in kidney lysosomes for the degradation of the disaccaride chain. In addition lysosomal enzymes from liver have been shown to split the chain. But I would say that the excretion of keratan sulfate peptides normally needs only the proteinase action to degrade the protein core. However, in the cell, especially in mucopolysaccharidosis, we have an accumulation process. One can show that the lysosomal enzymes are capable of splitting the chain, since sulfatases have also been shown in kidney and liver lysosomes.

Hofecker

Fleckenstein has shown that there is a progressive increase in calcium in the aorta and we've found the same to a much lesser extent in the aorta of the rat. My question is: Is this exclusively a function of the balance of glycosaminoglycans or are other mechanisms involved?

Greiling

This is one mechanism. I think that the LDL increasing factor is the other important mechanism. But in my opinion the atherosclerotic process is not only dependent on the lipoproteins. First the endothelium must be damaged, for instance by inflammatory processes, and all internists can show you cases with high LDL levels and no atherosclerotic lesions. First in the intima of the aorta the connective tissue must be damaged; this is necessary for the accumulation of the LDL, and in the third phase the calcium phosphate precipitation occurs. But I think the lipoprotein purists are wrong when they say that only the LDL concentration is an important factor. Additional factors are necessary for the precipitation of calcium phosphate and also LDL accumulation.

Rauterberg

Regarding the last remark: Currently, more and more extracellular matrix proteins are emerging which actively bind calcium; laminin, for instance, has a specific binding capacity for calcium. Thrombospondin which belongs to the extracellular matrix in the vessel wall has calcium-binding properties too. There may be other proteins with similar properties. But I have another question: Do you think that there is active degradation in cartilage without granulocytes? For instance, fibroblasts or synoviocytes have a complete pattern of extracellular proteases. One of these enzymes, called stromelysin, has recently been described to degrade proteoglycans. Are there indications that there are some changes in nongranulocyte enzymes with age?

Greiling

Yes, I think especially in osteoarthritic processes the inflammation process isn't needed for degradation. The proteinases from damaged chondrocytes perhaps can destroy the cartilage from the inner site. So I think two processes can come together in the special case of osteoarthritis, where in the active phase there is damage from the granulocytes while in the inactive phase the cartilage is damaged by proteinases from the chondrocytes and from the synovial cells which are also stimulated to release proteinases.

Linke

I would like to extend the idea of Dr. Rauterberg but with a different twist. Polymorph granulocytes, macrophages, fibroblasts, and many other cells secrete enzymes. Usually these enzymes stay locally and there is no problem in younger individuals, due to the presence of antiproteinases in excess. In the lung for instance, we have huge amounts of macrophages. Their secreted enzymes are neutralized by antiproteinases. In smoking, however, these antiproteinases are damaged by oxidation, so elastin is broken down with detrimental effects. What is the damage to antiproteinases here, so that enzymes become active? Did you look at the antiproteinases, which are usually protective?

Greiling

Yes, your example with antiproteinase disruption in smoking is very good. You know that in this case the mothionine is perhaps oxidized to methionine sulfoxide. A similar case might be septic arthritis in which there are so many proteinases that the capacity of antiproteases is insufficient for complex binding. In the synovial fluid in rheumatoid arthritis we have found a lower concentration of superoxide dismutase and catalase, so there is a greater probability that methionine will be oxidized to methionine sulfoxide. This could be one reason why antiproteases are insufficient in such cases, but this is a problem for future research.

References

Cutler RG (1984) Evolutionary biology of aging and longevity in mammalian species. In: Johnson JE (ed) Aging and Cell Function. Plenum Press, New York London, pp 1–147

Greiling H, Baumann G (1973) Age-dependent changes of nonsulfated disaccharide groups in the proteoglycans of knee joint cartilage. In: Vogel HG (ed) Connective tissue and ageing. Excerpta Medica, Amsterdam, pp 160–162

Greiling H, Kleesiek K, Reinards R (1986) Interaction of synovial cells and synovial fluid with cartilage. In: Kuettner K, Schleyerbach R, Hascall VC (eds) Articular cartilage biochemistry. Raven Press, New York, pp 195–210

Heinegard D, Paulsson M (1984) Structure and metabolism of proteoglycans. In: Piez KA, Reddi A H (eds) Exracellular matrix biochemistry. Elsevier, New York Amsterdam Oxford, pp 277–328

Honda A, Abe M, Nurata S, Mori Y (1979) The effect of ageing on the synthesis of hexosamine-containing substances from rat costal cartilage. J Biochem 85: 519–528

Inerot SI, Heinegard D, Audell L, Olsson S E (1978) Articular cartilage proteoglycans in aging and osteoarthritis. Biochem J 169: 143–156

Kaplan D, Meyer K (1959) Ageing of human cartilage. Nature 183: 1267–1268

Kleesiek K, Reinards R, Brackertz D, Neumann S, Lang H, Greiling H (1986) Granulocyte elastase as a new biochemical marker in the diagnosis of chronic joint diseases. Rheumatol Int 6: 161–169

Mathews MB, Glagov S (1966) Acid mucopolysaccaride patterns in ageing human cartilage. J Clin Invest 45: 1103–1111

Oberley LW, Oberley TD (1986) Free radicals, cancer, and aging. In: Johnson JE, Walford R, Harman D, Miquel J (eds) Free radicals, aging, and degenerative diseases. Liss, New York, pp 325–371

Patton SE, Rosen GM, Rackman E (1980) Superoxide production by purified hamster hepatic nuclei. Mol Pharmacol 18: 588–593

Poole AR (1986) Changes in the collagen and proteoglycan of articular cartilage in arthritis. Rheumatology 10: 316–371

Roughley PJ, White RJ (1980) Age-related changes in the structure of the proteoglycan subunits from human articular cartilage. J Biol Chem 255: 217–224

Roughley PJ, Mort JS (1986) Ageing and the aggregating proteoglycans of human articular cartilage. Clin Sci 71: 337–344

Schiller S (1976) The effect of hormones on synthesis of the region linking chondroitin sulfate to protein. Biochim Biophys Acta 451: 457–464

Schwartz NB (1977) Regulation of chondroitin sulfate synthesis. J Biol Chem 252: 6316–6321

Stuhlsatz HW, Löffler H, Mohanaradhakrishnan V, Cosma S, Greiling H (1982) Topographic and age-dependent distribution of the glycosaminoglycans in human aorta. J Clin Chem Clin Biochem 20: 713–721

Vlassara H, Brownlee M, Cerami A (1986) Nonenzymatic glycosylation: Role in the pathogenesis of diabetic complications. Clin Chem 32: B 37–B 41

Wilke TJ (1983) Influence of age and sex on the concentration of free thyroxin in serum and on the free thyroxin: total thyroxin ratio. Clin Chem 29: 1428–1430

Wolf B, Gressner AM, Nevo Z, Greiling H (1982) Age-related decrease in the activity of UDP-xylose: core protein xylosyltransferase in rat costal cartilage. Mechanisms of Ageing and Development 19: 181–190

The Effect of Dietary Restriction on Life Span

C.H. Barrows[1]

The increased life span associated with dietary restriction has been demonstrated in animals ranging in complexity from protozoans such as Tokophrya up through rotifers, campanularia, drosphila, and fish to the rodents mice and rats. Among the invertebrates the life span has been increased as much as two- or threefold, whereas among the rodents the increases have ranged from 25% to 50%. Dietary restriction has been brought about by feeding a nutritionally adequate diet, one which supports maximal growth, at reduced levels of intake on a daily basis, or intermittently such as starving every other day. Dietary restriction has also been brought about by feeding ad libitum a diet low in protein, i.e., reducing the level from 20% to 8% or 4% (Barrows and Kokkonen 1982).

It was generally believed that dietary restriction had to be initiated in young growing animals to increase the life span. However, in 1965 it was demonstrated that the life span of middle-aged rotifers could be increased by dietary restriction (Fanestil and Barrows 1965). In Table 1 it may be seen that adequately fed rotifers (I) lived 33 days, whereas those dietary restricted (II) at the end of egg production (12–13 days) lived 42 days. However, this is not as long as the 53 days lived by animals dietary restricted throughout their life span. Similar data (Table 2) have been reported in the rat by Beauchene et al. (1979). It has also been reported that reducing the level of protein from 24% to 12% increases the life span of 16-month-old female rats (Barrows and Kokkonen 1975). Since the distress of hunger deters most people from successfully carrying out a dietary-restricted program,

Table 1. The effect of dietary restriction following cessation of egg production on the life span of rotifers (Fanestil and Barrows 1965)

No.	Interval A–C[a]	Interval C–E[a]	Life span (days)
30	I[b]	I	33.4 ± 1.3
28	I	II	41.8 ± 2.6
22	II	II	53.4 ± 3.6

[a] A, day hatched; C, end of egg production; E, death.
[b] I, normal diet; II, restricted diet.

[1] Gerontology Research Center, NIA, Francis Scott Key Medical Center, Baltimore, MD 21224, USA

Gerontology
Ed. by D. Platt
© Springer-Verlag Berlin Heidelberg 1989

the life span of 16-month-old mice fed diets which contain a nonnutritive additive, cellulose, was investigated (Kokkonen and Barrows 1988). The data seen in Table 3 show a 30% increase in the life span of animals whose diet contained 50% cellulose. However, dietary restriction has been ineffective in mice which have reached their mean life span, i.e., 25 months (Kokkonen and Barrows 1985).

In 1969 Ross reported the effect of age and dietary restriction on the enzymatic activities of liver based on hepatocytic numbers and size, determined in fixed sections. The data are more understandable when the slower rates of age regression in dietary-restricted as compared to normal animals (Table 4) are known (Barrows and Kokkonen 1985). For example, there is a decrease in cell size with age and dietary restriction (Table 5). However, the decrease in cell size observed at 121 and 385 days due to dietary restriction is more obvious than at 795 days. This is due to the slower rate of age-related decrease in cell size in animals fed the restricted as compared to the commercial diet. In Table 6 a reduced hepatocytic nitrogen content is observed with age and dietary restriction. Presumably this represents changes in protein content. Table 7 shows similar changes in hepatocytic catalase activity. Ross also showed a direct and straight line relationship between cell size and either nitrogen content or enzymatic activities among all dietary groups. However, values, for the same size cells, obtained from animals fed the low protein diet were lower than those from the other groups. Furthermore, when Ross attempted to relate life expectancy to hepatocytic enzymatic activities, values obtained from the animals fed the low protein diet were always displaced from the curves.

Table 2. The effect of intermittent feeding on the life span of male Wistar rats (Beauchene et al 1979)

No.	Diet	50% Survivorship (weeks)
25	Ad libitum	135
30	A libitum–restricted[a]	156
30	Retricted[b]	172

[a] Fed every other day at 1 year.
[b] Fed every other day throughout life span.

Table 3. The effect of feeding cellulose on the remaining life span of 16-month-old male mice (Kokkonen and Barrows 1988)

	Life span (days)	
Diets	Experiment I	Experiment II
24% caseine	273 ± 14	294 ± 15
33% cellulose	311 ± 18	322 ± 15
50% cellulose	334 ± 16	383 ± 28

Table 4. The effect of dietary restriction on age regressions in livers of male mice (Barrows and Kokkonen 1985)

	24% casein	4% casein	Intermittently fed	Intermittently fasted
DNA[a]	8.9 ± 0.1	0.8 ± 0.1	3.5 ± 0.1	3.7 ± 0.1
Protein[b]	−1.8 ± 0.2	0.1 ± 0.1	−0.4 ± 0.2	−1.3 ± 0.2
Malic dehydrogenase[c]	−2.1 ± 0.3	0.2 ± 0.2	0.58 ± 0.3	−1.3 ± 0.4
Succinic dehydrogenase[d]	−5.6 ± 0.4	0.1 ± 0.1	0.4 ± 0.1	−2.5 ± 0.7

[a] (γ/mg tissue) (10^{-2}) per month.
[b] (mg/γ DNA) (10^{-3}) per month.
[c] (mmol DPNH/bn/γ DNA) (10^{-4}) per month.
[d] (μmol succ/min/mg DNA) (10^{-2}) per month.

Table 5. The effect of age and diet on the size of hepatocytes (Ross 1969)

	Diet		
Age (days)	Commercial	A	C
121	5819[a]	4196	4198
385	5831	4754	4701
795	4558	4075	4677
995		3925	4233

[a] Expressed as μ^3.

Table 6. The effect of age and diet on the nitrogen content of hepatocytes (Ross 1969)

	Diet		
Age (days)	Commercial	A	C
121	26.1[a]	18.1	14.8
385	27.1	20.6	18.2
795	20.6	17.6	17.8
995		18.1	15.1

[a] mg of nitrogen × 10^8 per hepatocyte.

Therefore, it became important to establish whether different methods of dietary restriction altered the enzymatic activities of cells of the same size from those of normal animals and what, if any, was the significance of such alterations. The studies (Barrows and Kokkonen 1985; Leto et al. 1976) showed that not all but most enzymatic activities were lower per mg DNA in dietary-restricted and old animals. In addition, the greatest differences were found in liver, less in kidney, only a small change in heart, and no differences in brain or spleen. In Table 8 the effect of dietary restriction and age on the DNA and protein content of liver is presented. The use of DNA as a basis for expressing biochemical measurements in aging and nutritional studies has been justified previously (Barrows and Kokkonen 1985). The increased concentration of DNA in liver with age and dietary restriction seen in Table 8 may represent an increased concentration of nuclei, which is in agreement with the data of Schmucker (1978). An increased concentration of nuclei suggests that aging and dietary restriction result in small cells and is in agreement with the data of Ross based on actual counts and size measurements in fixed sections. The decreased protein per mg DNA presumably per cell with age and dietary restriction agrees with the data of Ross based on hepatocytic counts in fixed sections.

Figure 1 shows a straight line relationship between the malic dehydrogenase activity per mg DNA and the γ DNA per mg liver tissue among all diets. The data are compatible with the concept that small cells contain low enzymatic activities. As the control animals (Fig. 1A) age, the cells become small and contain low enzymatic activities. The effect of age is not as obvious in the dietary-restricted animals. A comparison of the enzymatic activities of cells of the same size (same γ DNA per mg tissue) indicates low levels in low protein fed animals (Fig. 1B), high levels in animals following a 24-h fast (Fig. 1D), and the same levels as controls following a 24-h refeeding period (Fig. 1C). However, it seems unlikely that these findings are of significance in terms of life span since animals fed diets

Table 7. The effect of age and diet on the catalase activity of hepatocytes (Ross 1969)

Age (days)	Diet Commercial	A	C
121	62.3[a]	31.3	22.0
385	64.0	36.5	30.8
795	42.6	25.5	30.1
995		21.4	19.6

[a] Units of activity $\times 10^8$ per hepatocyte.

Table 8. The effect of age and dietary restriction on DNA and protein in the livers of male mice (Barrows and Kokkonen 1985)

Age (mo)	28% casein	4% casein	Intermittently fed	Intermittently fasted
DNA (γ/mg tissue)				
13.5	2.7 ± .1	3.5 ± .1	3.4 ± .1	4.5 ± .1
32.5	4.3 ± .2	3.3 ± .2	3.9 ± .1	4.9 ± .2
Protein (mg/γ DNA)				
13.5	68.3 ± 3	43.6 ± 2	50.6 ± 2	62.0 ± 3
32.5	39.1 ± 2	45.6 ± 2	43.8 ± 2	43.0 ± 2

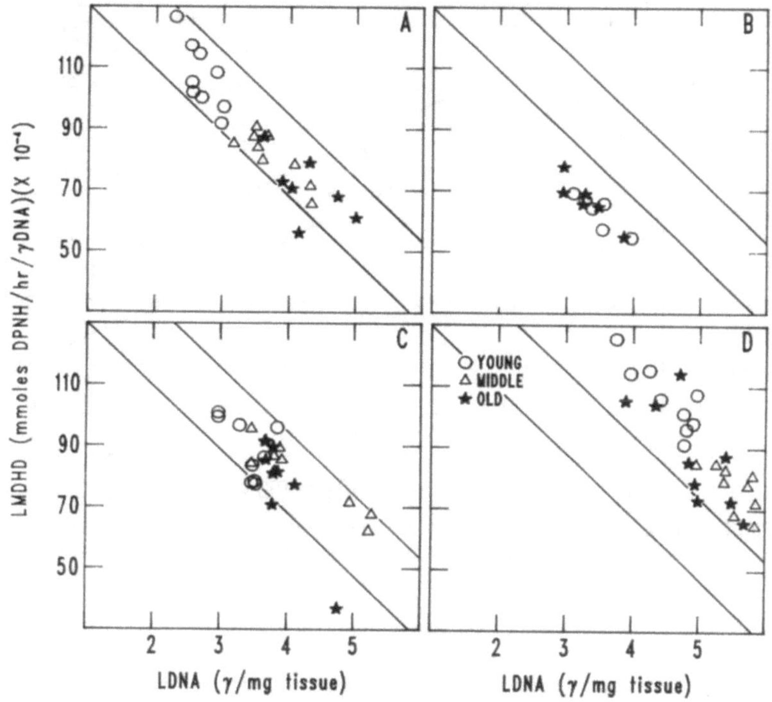

Fig. 1 A–D. The relationship between cellular malic dehydrogenase (*LMDHD*) and DNA (*LDNA*) in the livers of $B_6D_2F_1$ male mice fed different dietary regimes: **A** 24% protein ad libitum; **B** 4% protein ad libitum; **C** intermittently fed; **D** intermittently fasted

which contain cellulose live longer than controls, but their enzymatic acitivies based on cell size are the same as those of controls (Fig. 2).

All types of dietary restriction result in small cells which contain low protein levels and enzymatic activities. This suggests that dietary restriction is associated with reduced protein synthesis. The rates of disappearance of radioactivity (k) from the proteins of liver of normal mice and those fed dietary cellulose were the same (Table 9) (Kokkonen and Barrows 1988). Therefore, the time to turnover of 50% of the liver proteins, i.e., the half-life, was the same. However, the cellular protein synthesized per day (50% cellular protein ÷ half life) was reduced in the dietary-restricted mice. This was also observed in the animals fed low protein diets or intermittently (Table 10) (Barrows and Kokkonen 1987). Since aging results in small cells, reduced protein synthesis with age was an expected finding (Table 11) (Barrows and Kokkonen 1987).

The common characteristic of all dietary-restricted animals is a reduced protein synthesis. Reduced protein synthesis may limit the synthesis of regulatory proteins and perhaps RNA necessary for genetic code read out and thereby lengthen the time of maturation. This proposal was tested by introducing cycloheximide, an inhibitor of protein synthesis, into chick embryos (Barrows and Kokkonen 1975). The results (Table 12) show a markedly slower rate of develop-

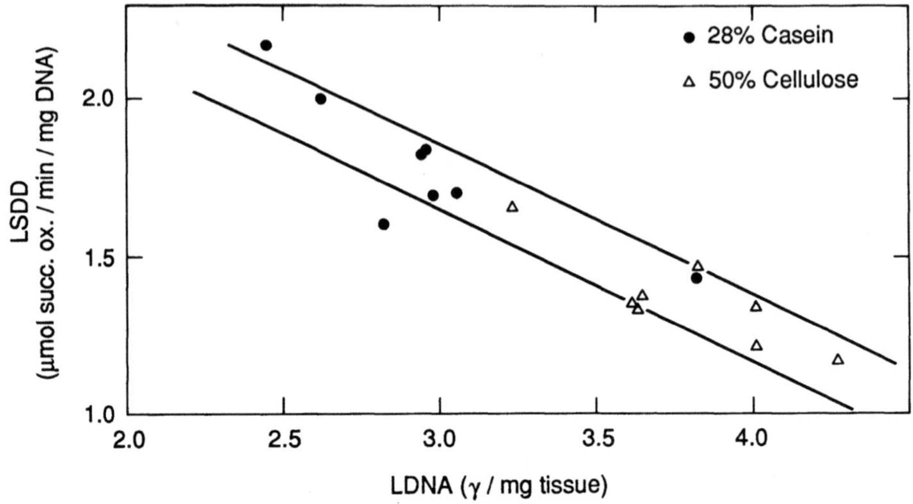

Fig. 2. The relationship between cellular succinic dehydrogenose (*LSDD*) and DNA (*LDNA*) in the livers of C57BL/6J male mice fed different diets

Table 9. The effect of diets on cellular protein synthesis in livers of male mice (Kokkonen and Barrows 1988)

	24% casein	33% cellulose	50% cellulose
k	0.23 ± 0.02	0.19 ± 0.02	0.19 ± 0.02
Half-life (days)	3.1	3.7	3.7
Cellular protein (mg/γ DNA)	63.8 ± 1.6	53.2 ± 1.6	54.8 ± 1.4
50% cellular protein (mg)	31.9	26.6	27.4
Cellular protein synthesized (mg/day)	10.5	7.2	7.5

Table 10. The effect of diets on cellular protein synthesis in livers of male mice (Barrows and Kokkonen 1987)

	24% casein	4% casein	Intermittently fasted	Intermittently fed
k	0.21 ± 0.02	0.21 ± 0.02	0.18 ± 0.02	0.21 ± 0.02
Half-life (days)	3.3	3.3	3.8	3.3
Cellular protein (mg/γ DNA)	58.0 ± 1.5	41.4 ± 0.9	49.3 ± 1.1	57.9 ± 1.7
50% cellulose protein (mg)	29.0	20.7	24.6	28.9
Cellular protein synthesized (mg/day)	8.8	6.2	6.4	8.8

Table 11. The effect of age on cellular protein synthesis in livers of male mice (Barrows and Kokkonen 1987)

	Age (months)			
	12	18	24	33
k	0.19 ± 0.01	0.20 ± 0.01	0.19 ± 0.02	0.22 ± 0.02
Half-life (days)	3.6	3.3	3.6	3.1
Cellular protein (mg/γ DNA)	63.1 ± 1.6	55.6 ± 2.1	52.7 ± 1.5	39.6 ± 2.4
50% cellular protein (mg)	31.5	27.8	26.3	19.8
Cellular protein synthesized (mg/day)	8.7	8.4	7.3	6.3

Table 12. The effect of cycloheximide[a] on the development of chick embryos (Barrow and Kokkonen 1975)

Days	Length (mm)	Number of somites	Shape of development	Heart rate (beats/Min)
2 C	4.3 ± 0.1	16.5 ± 0.7	12.6 ± 0.2	15.0 ± 2
E	3.5 ± 0.2	12.7 ± 0.9	10.8 ± 0.5	7.0 ± 1
3 C	5.8 ± 0.1		16.2 ± 0.2	40.0 ± 8
E	5.3 ± 0.1		15.2 ± 0.2	29.0 ± 4

[a] 1 γ/egg.

ment. The fact that dietary restriction is effective in adult animals demands another proposal if no new genetic information is expressed in adult life. It was proposed by Orgel (1963) that aging results from errors which occur during transcription and translation of genetic information. If it may be assumed that such age-related errors occur because of the use of the genetic code, limiting protein synthesis would minimize the code's use and be beneficial. Imperfections in the genetic code, if they occur with age, could result in incomplete synthesis of a given protein such as an enzyme and may be extensive enough to impair total tissue protein synthesis. These age-related changes have been reported. If the synthesis of the protein is completed, errors may be expected to be present. Our attempts to show a delay in the occurrence of error-laden proteins were unsuccessful due to inconsistencies in the presence of age-related errors in aldolase (Barrows and Kokkonen 1981). One other attempt was made to "protect the genetic code from use" by inhibiting RNA and protein synthesis in adult rotifers. Both inhibitors were effective in increasing the life span (Table 13).

Finally, I would like to discuss briefly the effect of dietary restriction on disease. This was first reported in 1945 by Saxton. He showed that the onset of a large variety of diseases found in rats was delayed by dietary restriction. This finding has been repeatedly confirmed (Barrows and Kokkonen 1982). However, because of the lack of information regarding the etiology and progression of diseases in rodents, these data contributed little information in terms of the mechanism of dietary restriction. A few years ago a genetically defined mouse that became diabetic was made available (Hummel et al. 1966). The progress of the disease was well defined until death. Dietary restriction increased the life span of these animals (Tables 14, 15) (Kokkonen and Barrows, unpublished data). Although quantitative data are not available, at 21 days of age many of the animals expressed the disease by polyuria and glycosuria. Following 3–4 days of feeding the restricted diets, these symptoms disappeared. The control animals gained weight to about 30–35 g. At this time they lost weight, showed extreme polyuria and glycosuria, and died. On the other hand the dietary-restricted animals continued to gain weight to 50–60 g. These animals are also genetically obese. The animals maintained this body weight until shortly prior to death, at which time there was a loss of body weight (to approximately 20 g), which was associated with extreme polyuria and glycosuria. These data suggest that dietary restriction

Table 13. The effect of the inhibition of protein and RNA synthesis on the life span of rotifers

Treatment	No.	Mean life span ± SEM (days)
Controls	24	25.2 ± 1
1×10^{-4} M cycloheximide	30	32.0 ± 1
1γgml actiomycin	24	35.8 ± 1

γgml = microgram/ml.

Table 14. The effect of diet on the life span of diabetic mice (C57BL/KsJ-db/db)

Diet	No.	Life span (days)
20% casein	20	157 ± 16
50% cellulose	22	101 ± 6
4% casein	20	273 ± 28
Intermittent	17	356 ± 45

Table 15. The effect of diet on the life span of diabetic mice (C57BL/KsJ-db/db)

Diet	No.	Life Span (days)	Survivors (%)[a]
20% casein	53	205 ± 17	0
50% cellulose	34	251 ± 19	0
4% casein	49	319 ± 23	4
Intermittent	37	338 ± 26	33
33% cellulose	35	523 ± 21	46

[a] On the 640th day of feeding.

more than delays the onset of diseases; it can cause a remission of an active genetically programmed disease for a prolonged period of time, i.e., 2 or 3 times the life expectancy of fully fed animals.

At present no experiments have been carried out to test the effect of dietary restriction on the life span of man. The interpretation of retrospective studies is at best tenuous. Most of these involve nutritional deprivation during war or famine, which produces marked nutritional imbalances rather than low intakes of a nutritionally adequate diet. On the basis of current knowledge I know of no reasons that would exclude man from responding positively to dietary restriction.

Discussion

Medvedev

Your usually keep male and female rats and mice separate. But what happens if you give them the chance to live together, to reproduce normally, etc. Would they live longer?

Barrows

Studies which have housed male and female rats together have not been carried out. However, such studies could be conducted by dietarily restricting the animals by intermittent feeding.

Hayflick

I think it's important for the group to have your thoughts on this suggestion: If feral animals live under circumstances in which dietary restriction is a natural circumstance in their lives, then what you and your colleagues have discovered is not that underfed animals live longer but that ad libitum fed animals have a reduced life span.

Barrows

I am not convinced that animals living in the wild are necessarily underfed. It seems to me that under ad lib feeding animals and probably men will eat until they are satisfied. Whether this represents adequate or overnutrition is the question. Animals which are not fed ad lib but fed restricted intakes live longer.

Rauterberg

I would be very interested to hear about the influence of physical training on the aging process. This would be another way to enhance protein synthesis without overnutrition.

Barrows

Dr. Charles Coodrick has reported that voluntary wheel running did not increase the life span of 10.5- and 18-month-old ras although the former group experienced a reduction in body weight.

Greiling

With respect to the radical theory of aging, the superoxide dismutase activity is in my opinion very important. Have you looked to the superoxide dismutase activity in the protein-rich and the carbohydrate-rich animals?

Barrows

No, I haven't.

Brocklehurst

If diabetic monkeys are obese animals, are they analogous to humans with maturity-onset diabetes? And if so then by restricting diet, aren't you curing the diabetes in the same way as we do in maturity-onset diabetics.

Barrows

I don't believe so, since diabetes was evident in the very young growing animals.

References

Barrows CH, Kokkonen GC (1975) Protein synthesis development, growth and lifespan. Growth 39: 523–533

Barrows CH, Kokkonen GC (1981) Inconsistencies in the presence of age-associated altered aldolase in the livers of mice. Age 4: 123–125

Barrows CH, Kokkonen GC (1982) Dietary restriction and life extension – biological mechanisms. In Moment GB (ed): Nutritional Approaches to Aging Research. CRC Press, Boca Raton, FL pp 219–243

Barrows CH, Kokkonen GC (1985) The effect of age and diet on biochemical characteristics of the tissues of mice. Age 8: 101–112

Barrows CH, Kokkonen GS (1987) The effect of age and diet on the cellular protein synthesis of livers of male mice. Age 10: 54–57

Beauchene RE, Bales CW, Smith CA, Tucker SM, Mason RL (1979) The effect of food restriction on body composition and longevity of rats. Physiologist, 22:4

Fanestil DD and Barrows CH (1965) Aging in the rotifer. J Gerontol, 20: 462–469

Hummel KP, Dichie MM, Coleman DL (1966) Diabetes, a new mutation in the mouse. Science 153: 1127–1128

Kokkonen GC, Barrows CH (1985) The effect of dietary vitamin, protein, and intake levels on the life span of mice of different ages. Age 8: 13–17

Kokkonen GC, Barrows CH (1988) The effect of dietary cellulose on life span and biochemical variables of male mice. Age 11: 7–9

Leto S, Kokkonen GC, Barrows CH (1976) Dietary protein, life span, and biochemical variables in female mice. H Geront 31: 144–148

Orgel LE (1963) The maintenance of the accuracy of protein synthesis and its relevance to ageing. Proc Nat Acad Sci (USA) 49: 517–521

Ross MH (1969) Aging, nutrition and hepatic enzyme activity patterns in the rat. J Nutr 97: 565–602

Saxton JA (1945) Nutrition and Growth and their influence on longevity in rats. Biological Symposia 11: 177–195

Schmucker DL (1978) A quantitative morphological evaluation of hepatocytes in young, mature, and senescent Fischer 344 male rats. In Kitani K (ed): Liver and Aging, Amsterdam, Elsevier/North Holland Biomedical Press, pp 21–34

Nutritional Problems in Geriatric Patients

G. Schlierf[1], D. Volkert[1], C. Frauenrath[1], R. Hüppe[2], W. Kruse[1], and P. Oster[1]

As long as we do not have a "Fountain of Youth" (Jungbrunnen) as quite vividly depicted by Lucas Cranach Jr., we have to make every effort to prolong health. Without doubt, one most important prerequisite is proper nutrition.

If one looks at dietary data from the Federal Republic of Germany (Ernährungsbericht 1984) in young adults and in the elderly, one can see that overnutrition appears to prevail into old age. Over 65 year olds, according to this source, consume more calories than recommended and even more than the young; there is a high protein intake with potential problems, there is too much fat, etc. This picture may be different in the very old and particularly in geriatric patients, who even in an affluent society may suffer from poor nutrition (Gofferje et al. 1979), which will be the main topic of this presentation.

There are many causes of malnutrition in the elderly and particularly in very old patients, as summarized by Bowman and Rosenberg (1982). They range from social isolation and ignorance about proper food to problems with appetite and chewing and to interactions with drugs.

This chapter presents preliminary data from a study which we call BEST – Bethanien-Ernährungs-Studie (supported by the Bundesminister für Forschung und Technologie, Bonn). It is a nutrition and health survey in a geriatric hospital. The study involves 300 patients at or above age 75. The mean age of the patients is 82 years. Main diagnoses are cardiovascular disease, pulmonary disease, neoplasms, and psychiatric disorders. The aims of this study are fourfold. First, we want to define malnutrition according to kind and frequency; second, we want to find causes; third, in observing these people longitudinally we want to relate malnutrition and mortality; and finally in an interventional step in half of the 300 subjects over 18 months, we wish to establish whether it is possible even in these very old patients to improve poor nutrition. The data shown here will be devoted to the first question, namely the definition of malnutrition, and we will focus further on vitamin malnutrition in the first 100 patients. Space does not permit citation or discussion of the numerous previous studies of this problem in West Germany and in other countries, as, for example, summarized by Durnin (1978). In acknowledging valuable contributions by others we shall restrict this paper to the nutritional situation of geriatric patients now and in the city of Heidelberg.

[1] Bethanien-Krankenhaus Heidelberg, Abt. Innere Medizin/Geriatrie, Rohrbacher Str. 149, D-6900 Heidelberg / FRG

[2] Institut für Ernährungswissenschaft an der Justus-Liebig-Universität, D-6300 Giessen / FRG

Gerontology
Ed. by D. Platt
© Springer-Verlag Berlin Heidelberg 1989

Table 1. BEST: Patients' characteristics (n = 100)

Living situation	alone	26%	
	with someone	57%	
	o.p. home	17%	
Dependence	none	48%	
	bathing etc.	11%	
	dressing	8%	
	eating	19%	
Nutritional status	underweight	23%	
	overweight	27%	
Dementia	none	33%	
	mild	16%	
	severe	36%	
Able to walk	unrestricted	25%	
	with help	26%	
Unable to walk	housebound	40%	
	bound to room	2%	49%!
	bedridden	7%	
Able to cut meat/fruit		58%	
Able to cut meat/fruit with difficulties		15%	
Unable to cut meat/fruit		27%	
Dentures		87%	
Poor appetite		26%	
Difficulty in swallowing		18%	
Difficulty in chewing		50%	
On diet, mostly diabetics		29%	

Table 1 characterizes the patients under study. Eighty-three live at home, eight in old peoples' residences, and nine in nursing homes. The table also shows activities of daily life and the abilities of these people. Twenty-five are able to walk without problems, an additional quarter can walk with help, and the others are housebound or even bedridden. So 50% of the patients are actually in a very poor state of health as defined by criteria of mobility. Only half of the patients are able to cut meat or fruit without any difficulty; 15% can do so but with difficulty and more than one-quarter cannot perform this function themselves. Almost all have dentures. One-quarter complain about poor appetite, one-fifth have difficulty in swallowing, one half have difficulty in chewing, even with dentures, and almost one-third are diabetics.

Table 2 shows nutrient intakes for women and for men, which we tried to estimate by 24-h recalls. I will not go into the problems of this method in the very old except to state that there are big problems. Thus, the figures have to be interpreted with reservation.

In the very old female patients there is a low energy intake as compared to the recommendations (Empfehlungen für die Nährstoffzufuhr 1985). With regard to these recommendations of the German Nutrition Society, one must keep in mind that they are defined for persons 65 years and older and we do not have recommendations for specific age groups above 65. Thus, not only the calculated

Table 2. BEST: Median nutrient intake (24-h recall in women (n = 69) and men (n = 25)

	Women		Men	
	Intake	DGE recom.	Intake	DGE recom.
Energy (kcal)	1533	1700	1678	1900
Protein (g)	55	45	62	55
Fat (g)	66	<55	73	<61
Carbohydrate (g)	158		172	
Alcohol (g)	0.02		5	
Fiber (g)	13		15	
Purine (mg)	310		448	
Cholesterol (mg)	220		300	
Na (mg)	1504		2174	
K (mg)	2208	3500	2095	3500
Mg (mg)	184	300	196	350
Ca (mg)	445	800	454	800
Fe (mg)	10	12	12	12
P (mg)	873	800	969	800
Retinol (mg)	0.51	0.8	0.66	1.0
Vit. D (μg)	1.29	5	1.32	5
Vit. E (mg)	7.64	12	7.76	12
Folate (μg)	143.96	160	136.10	160
Vit. B_1 (mg)	0.97	1.1	0.98	1.3
Vit. B_2 (mg)	1.02	1.5	0.99	1.7
Vit. B_6 (mg)	1.21	1.6	1.35	1.8
Vit C (mg)	102.02	75	57.84	75

intakes but also the reference values are rather weak. There appears to be no problem with protein intake or with fat intake. It follows that particularly carbohydrate-containing foods are not consumed in sufficient amounts. Dietary fiber is at 13 g per day instead of about 30 g.

If one looks at intakes of cholesterol, purine, and sodium, our female patients perform excellently. There appear, however, to be problems with calcium intake, and this of course is to be discussed in connection with the osteoporosis problem. Magnesium intake is low, presenting a problem for people taking diuretics.

Let us now consider vitamin intakes, again in comparison to recommendations. Retinol is 0.5 mg as compared to 0.8. Vitamin D, which of course has a significant endogenous synthesis if people are able to go out and be exposed to sunlight, is low. Vitamins B_1, B_2, and B_6 are rather low, usually only about 60% of the recommended levels. In summary, our group appears to have energy-vitamin malnutrition relating to many vitamins. Men show a similar picture: there may be a vitamin E problem, there is a similar vitamin D problem, and there are low intakes of vitamins B_1, B_2, B_6, and also C.

We have measured food consumption by two methods. One was the 24-h recall, the other was the food frequency, which indicates whether different food groups, e.g., dairy products, are consumed daily, often, sometimes, or never. As

Table 3. Vitamin status of elderly people: frequency of values outside conventional limits

	Healthy elderly (>65 years)	Geriatric patients (>75 years)
Vit. A	7%	43%
Vit. C	8%	26%
Vit. B_1 – αETK	3%	15%
Vit. B_2 – αEGR	4%	20%
Vit. B_6 – αEGOT	8%	14%

Table 4. BEST: vitamin status

Satisfactory	33%
One vitamin "deficient"	36%
Two vitamins "deficient"	15%
Three vitamins "deficient"	9%
Four vitamins "deficient"	6%

an example, dairy products are consumed daily or often by only 40% or the patients and this is certainly one of the causes of the very low calcium intake in this group.

Wholemeal products such as muesli, which is of course not a common food in the very old because they have not been used to it in their youth, or wholemeal bread, which is not very easy to chew, are not liked very much by old patients.

Vegetable consumption appears to be good; cooked vegetables are eaten daily or often by more than 80% of these patients. Finally, to our surprise, 80% eat fresh fruit daily or often.

One additional note of caution is necessary with such questions: Everyone who does dietary surveys knows that people tend to report what they should eat, not what they really eat. Since fresh fruit has a healthy image, it is easy to answer "of course, I do eat fresh fruit," although this has nothing to do with reality. For this and other reasons harder data are desirable. We therefore measured vitamins or vitamin-dependent parameters in these patients in conjunction with the Institute for Nutritional Science in Giessen (Table 3). If we take as cut-offs conventional limits, in these patients vitamin A is below them in more than one-third of these very old patients, vitamin C in about 20%, and vitamins B_1, B_2, and B_6 in one-sixth. In interpreting these values, one has to keep in mind that again the conventional limits are set for those aged 65 years and older, and we actually have no hard data on whether 80 year olds really do require the same amounts of vitamins as 65 years olds. Since we previously had a chance to study 65- to 74-year-old "free-living" elderly (Ernährung und Alter 1986), we can compare the data and it appears that among this group the vitamin situation is much better. Therefore, either the difference in age or the difference between health and disease or both explain the differences in the frequency of low vitamin levels.

Many patients have multiple vitamin deficiencies (Table 4). Thirty-three percent of our old patients had a satisfactory vitamin status; 36 had one vitamin deficient, two vitamins were deficient in one-sixth, and three or four vitamins were deficient in a sizeable percentage of patients. None of these patients showed overt clinical signs of vitamin deficiencies, in accordance with other studies. It is another question whether unspecific "symptoms" of vitamin deficiency such as loss of memory, lack of concentration, or depression are more common in such patients (Heseker and Kübler 1983; Wenger 1982). Neither age nor living situation nor severity of disease nor presence or absence of dementia was indicative of a poor or a better vitamin status. There were, however, different vitamin deficiencies according to the nutritional status (normal, under- or overweight) and we found differences in males and females. Males in general had a vitamin status which was less satisfactory than women, and this concerned all vitamins except vitamin B_6. Men, if they get very old, may have more problems in getting proper food than women.

It remains to be seen which causes and conditions are, in addition, associated with biochemical vitamin deficiencies and, more importantly, whether these relate to prognosis. We will also learn whether malnutrition can be improved in the very old. Most probably, as with other conditions, preventive measures should be implemented as early as possible. Learning in childhood about proper nutrition may still be the best guarantee of being well nourished in the last decades of life.

Discussion

Medvedev

I know that in the United States and in Britain nearly everybody now takes multivitamins. How is it in Germany? Do people easily take multivitamins and compensate the deficiency?

Schlierf

It's of course possible to buy multivitamins in Germany, just as it is in the United States. Of our patients only 6% used to take vitamins. If, instead of tedious dietary counseling, we were just to prescribe some vitamins we might have a new problem related to compliance for other drugs. Sixty percent of patients do not take the prescribed drugs, and if we prescribe vitamins we are not sure they take them. So it's not as easy as it appears. Secondly, I did not show it, but we have a rather high frequency of low albumin levels and low protein levels. When we measure retinol-binding proteins or other acute proteins, they are also low and this cannot be corrected by the vitamin pill. We have to improve general nutrition. And probably we have to improve general nutrition *before* people are very old and *before* they are very sick.

Beischer

Which food was offered to the patients? Was it just normal food or was tube feeding also involved?

Schlierf

Well, the food we measured was the food consumed at home, before they entered the hospital. There were no patients on tube feeding when they came to our hospital, if the diagnosis was stroke for instance. There is a report in the literature that if you look at what people eat in a geriatric hospital, people who get fed are better nourished than people who are considered by doctors or nurses to be able to feed themselves. A lot of unused food items are returned with the trays, and if you feed the patient you know what he's eaten.

Greiling

A question regarding the so-called vitamin status. We have looked for reference values in plasma and serum for various vitamins and found no precise values regarding the age dependency. For the past 10 years HPLC methods have been available for the determination of vitamins in blood serum. My question is: Is your vitamin status in relation to the vitamin concentration in the foods or do you also have results about the concentration of water- or fat-soluble vitamins in blood plasma? In my opinion this is necessary for the future. For instance, what about vitamin B_1? In the cells there is thiamin pyrophosphate, thiamin triphosphate, and thiamin monophosphate, but only a low concentration of the free thiamin monophosphate, but only a low concentration of the free thiamin vitamin B_1. In my opinion many problems remain in the definition of a so-called vitamin status. To repeat the question: Have you measured all these vitamins in blood plasma or is the vitamin status related to the vitamin concentration in the food?

Schlierf

I showed two sets of data. I showed you what people ate and I showed blood levels. The slide showing that about 40 % of patients were low in vitamin A meant they had low blood levels, and of the 100 patients there were actually three who had less than 10 μg/100 ml vitamin A. The deficiency cut-off point is 35, and if you read the general literature they should be blind and deaf and everything with levels at 10, which they were not at all. This makes me question the recommendations or the established normal values for these variables.

Greiling

Have you evaluated the concentrations of free vitamin or the metabolites?

Schlierf

This analysis has been done in Giessen by Professor Kübler.

Greiling

But there are many conflicting datas in the literature about the concentration and the blood levels of vitamin A and the metabolites.

Schlierf

The blood vitamin status of the vitamins A, B_1, B_2, B_6, and C was assessed: The plasma concentration of retinol was determined by HPLC. The ascorbic acid concentration in plasma was measured photometrically after the coupling reaction with 2,4-dinitrophenylhydrazine. The status of the B vitamins was evaluated using the acitivty coefficients of the erythrocyte enzymes trandsketolase (α-ETK), glutathione reductase (α-EGR), and glutamic oxalate aminotransferase (α-EGOT).

Brocklehurst

We also looked at the water-soluble vitamins in the 1960s in a group of geriatric patients and we found that a large number of old people admitted to hospital had levels of leukocyte ascorbic acid and thiamin on transketolase testing that were low and that could be brought up to normal values by supplementation. We then wanted to see whether there were any clinical signs that were particularly associated with these low levels and so for a year we studied a group of old people in long-stay geriatric wards. Fifty percent of them were given vitamin C and vitamin B and the other 50% were given placebos. They were examined once every 3 months by an independent observer who looked at them generally, and particularly at the tongue, the skin, the lips, and so on. At the end of the year he was able to identify almost 100% of the supplemented group on overall impression. There were also rather fewer pressure sores in the supplemented group. So the question really does arise as to whether these are subclinical signs of vitamin deficiency. The tongue changes, angular stomatitis, and so on have many causes and therefore one can't say that people with these changes are clearly vitamin deficient. But the question does arise as to whether we should not be supplementing these patients with water-soluble vitamins and probably, as you indicate, with multivitamins.

Schlierf

I think this will of course be the conclusion if general dietary measures are not successful. Presently we go into the patient's house or into the nursing home every 3 months, accompanied by the dietitian. We talk about our findings, we talk about nutrition, we see whether some change has been made. If we find after our controlled study that this did no good at all then we would say: it would be better to give vitamins than to do nothing. I know your study and there were others on this problem, but presently measuring vitamins is not a clinical procedure. So unless one has a scientific interest in this, and even if two-thirds of patients are afflicted by a low vitamin status, vitamins are not measured in usual hospital circumstances and one cannot treat these patients if one does not have a diagnosis.

Heckers

Do you have any idea why these old people have such a low intake of milk and dairy products? Is it a question of intolerance?

Schlierf

No, intolerance for milk could be at most in 10%. They just don't like to drink milk. That is what we usually get as an answer. They don't like to drink milk.

Kennedy

Feeding difficulties in this age group are a major problem. You indicated many of your patients could have fallen into this group. Did you look at them as a separate group and did they have a higher incidence of poor dietary intake of the vitamins you studied?

Schlierf

In these first 100: no. We had thought the demented patients would have particularly poor nutritional status. This was not the case. They were cared for by someone who paid at least as much attention to the diet as many who fed themselves.

Barrows

We were concerned as to whether the decreased food intake in senescent humans and animals resulted in an increased mortality due to reduced intake of vitamins. We fed diets which contained 50% less vitamins to mice of different ages and found a marked increase in mortality of the animals, including the old ones. Therefore, we suggest that older people supplement their diet with one RDA vitamin supplement. In addition, we failed to observe any age-related impairment in the absorption of either water- or fat-soluble vitamins in studies employing radioactive vitamins administered at physiological levels.

Schlierf

I'd agree. I don't think it's a matter of absorption, at least not in the majority of patients; it's a matter of poor nutrition and maybe of interactions.

References

Bowman BB, Rosenberg IH (1982) Assessment of the nutritional status of the elderly. Am J Clin Nutr 35: 1142–1151

Durnin JVGA (1978) In: Brocklehurst JC (ed) Textbook of geriatric medicine and gerontology. The gastrointestinal system: Nutrition Part II, chap 10 pp 417–432 Churchill Livingstone, Edinburgh

Empfehlungen für die Nährstoffzufuhr, 4th extended revision (1985) Deutsche Gesellschaft für Ernährung (ed). Umschau, Frankfurt am Main

Ernährung und Alter (1986) Wissenschaftliche Verlagsgesellschaft, Stuttgart

Ernährungsbericht (1984) Deutsche Gesellschaft für Ernährung (ed) Im Auftrag des Bundesministers für Jugend, Familie, Frauen und Gesundheit

Gofferje H, Fekl W, Brand O, Rupprecht M (1979) Untersuchungen zur Mangelernährung in einer medizinischen Klink. Z Ernähr Wiss 18: 62–70

Heseker H, Kübler W (1983) Die Bedarfsdeckung älterer Menschen mit Vitaminen. Ernährungs-Umschau 30: 366–369

Wenger R (1982) Mangelernährung im Alter. In: Mangelernährung in Mitteleuropa. Wissenschaftliche Verlagsgesellschaft, Stuttgart, pp 161–169

Results from a Longitudinal Study of Initially 70-Year-Old Subjects in Giessen Followed Up for 10 Years

H. Heckers[1] and D. Platt[2]

Introduction

Diseases of the heart and blood vessels are the most important causes of death in old age. The National Center of Health Statistics has estimated that life expectancy at birth would gain 18 years in the United States if it were possible to eliminate deaths from cardiovascular-renal diseases, heart diseases, and vascular diseases affecting the central nervous system, which all are predominantly of atherosclerotic origin.

Even at age 65, the elimination of these diseases should yield a 16-year gain in life span (Table 1). These data emphasize the importance of atherosclerosis, which is a multifactorial, time-related process. Though aging makes atherosclerosis universal given adequate longevity, the influence of secondary factors is more prominent at least in young and middle-aged people. In old age, however, the predictive contribution of risk factors is controversial, especially because direct evidence for the effectiveness of preventive measures is limited and, in respect of lipid disorders, completely absent. For this reason we started a number of studies on the prevalence, incidence, and clinical impact of lipid disorders on atherosclerosis in randomly selected subjects beyond the age of 70 years.

Are Hyperalphalipoproteinemia and Hypobetaliproteinemia Longevity Syndromes?

In 1982 we reported on 103 randomly selected nonagenarians studied in 1977/78 (Heckers et al. 1982). In contrast to former studies by Glueck et al. (1975a, b, 1976), our results did not confirm that primary familial hyperalphalipoproteinemia (HAL) and hypobetalipoproteinemia (HBL) are markers for high life expectancy. Compared with the results in a control group exactly 70 years old when sampled and likewise randomly selected, the relative occurrence of HAL was smaller in the female subgroup and in the whole group of nonagenarians, but the difference

[1] Center of Internal Medicine, Justus-Liebig-University, D-6300 Giessen / FRG
[2] Lehrstuhl für Innere Medizin – Gerontologie der Universität Erlangen-Nürnberg
Heimerichstr. 58, D-8500 Nürnberg / FRG

Gerontology
Ed. by D. Platt
© Springer-Verlag Berlin Heidelberg 1989

Table 1. Gain in expectation of life at birth and at the age of 65 due to elimination of various causes of death (Source: Life tables published by National Center of Health Statistics, US Public Health Service & US Bureau of Census, »Some demographic aspects of aging in the United States«, February 1973)

Cause of Death	Gain (yr) in expectation of life if cause was eliminated	
	At birth	At age of 65
Major cardiovascular-renal diseases	10.9	10,0
Heart diseases	5.9	4.9
Vascular diseases affecting central nervous system	1.3	1.2
Malignant neoplasms	2.3	1.2
Accidents, excluding those caused by motor vehicles	0.6	0.1
Motorvehicle accidents	0.6	0.1
Influenza and pneumonia	0.5	0.2
Infectious diseases (excluding tubertculosis)	0.2	0.1
Diabetes mellitus	0.2	0.2
Tuberculosis	0.1	0.0

between the two age groups was not significant (Table 2). In another study of 180 unselected octo- and nonagenarians, 13 women and 10 men out of the total number of 77 female and 103 male subjects exhibited HAL (Schneider 1980). When comparisons were made with our two studies, no significant differences in the occurrence of HAL could be calculated for women and for men. In a later study, Glueck and associates also did not report an aggregation of HAL and HBL when they focused on the lipid and lipoprotein distribution in a cross-sectional unrepresentative sample of 124 octogenarians and 13 nonagenarians (Nickolson et al. 1979). All these data give evidence that Glueck et al. (1975a, b, 1976) misinterpreted their results. They studied octogenarian kindreds who were not randomly selected but self-referred by either two siblings or a parent and a child living to an age of 80 years or more. Since the kindreds studied were selected because of their distinctive familial longevity, it is no wonder that these families had an average higher life expectancy than the general US population. Comparisons, if at all, can be made only with equally selected kindreds in whom metabolic syndromes such as HAL and HBL are missing. Moreover, if the individual mean life expectancy is indeed influenced by HAL and HBL, it is necessary, for statistical purposes, to distinguish between family members who are carriers of these metabolic syndromes and those who are not. For the same reason it is not understandable why all first-degree relatives (108 persons in 14 kindreds) were included in the statistical analysis of morbidity and mortality for myocardial infarction instead of the 18 persons in 14 kindreds carrying these metabolic markers.

Table 2. Occurrence of primary HAL and HBL in randomly selected groups of 103 nonagenarians and 109 70-year-old subjects (Hekkers et al. 1982) and in 180 unselected octogenarians (Schneider 1980)

	Study population		HAL[a]		HBL[b]
	Years	No.	No.	(%)	No.
All	70	109	23	(21)	–
	80+	180	23	(13)	
	90+	103	17	(17)	1
Females	70	61	20	(33)	–
	80+	77	13	(17)	
	90+	70	13	(19)	1
Males	70	48	3	(6)	–
	80+	103	10	(10)	
	90+	33	4	(12)	–

[a] HDL-C $\geqq$70 mg/dl serum; [b] LDL-C $\leqq$70 mg/dl serum.

Table 3. Prevalence (%) of Dyslipoproteinemia in old and very old randomly selected subjects

Dyslipoproteinemia	No.	IIa	IIb	IV	IIa+HA	IIb+HA	IV+HA	HA	All
Males									
70 yrs	48	14.6	8.3	22.9	–	–	10.4	18.8	54.2
75 yrs	36	22.2	2.8	16.7	–	–	8.3	22.2	55.6
90+ yrs	33	12.1	–	–	3.0	–	–	9.1	18.1
Females									
70 yrs	61	29.2	9.8	11.5	4.9	9.8	4.9	24.6	55.5
75 yrs	49	30.6	10.2	18.4[a]	4.1	10.2	18.4	46.9	73.5
90+ yrs	70	10.0	1.4	14.3	5.7	1.4	8.6	34.3	44.3

Definitions: IIa = 190 mg/dl LDL-C; IV = 200 mg/dl triglycerides; hypoalphalipoproteinemia (HA) = $\leqq$45 mg/dl (females) and $\leqq$35 mg/dl (males) HDL-C.
[a] Additionally one woman showed type V hyperlipoproteinemia.

Even if the great abundance of human genetic variants gives rise to the possibility that certain mutations will effect genes involved in longevity, a well-defined syndrome which appears to prolong human life expectancy to a fixed life span remains to be detected.

Prevalence of Dyslipoproteinemia and Aging

The control group of 109 70-year-old subjects (61 women and 48 men) was followed up and rexamined 5 years later in 1982/83, and again 10 years later in 1987/88.

Table 3 summarizes the prevalences of different types of lipid disorder in our studies. It is demonstrated that dyslipoproteinemia in old age is very frequent. More than 50% of the 70-year-old subjects of both sexes exhibited pathological lipoprotein values. Five years later the prevalence of dyslipoproteinemic survivors of this group remained unchanged in males, whereas in women a considerable increase developed to nearly 75%, characterized by increasing VLDL and decreasing HDL fractions.

The data obtained at the third examination, when the 68 survivors were 80 years old, are still incomplete; based on a preliminary evaluation the prevalence of dyslipoproteinemia in men remained constant in the whole eighth decade, whereas in women the rate declined after the second examination to the initial level of 50%.

LDL and HDL Levels and Risk Factor Accumulation in the Eighth Decade, as Revealed by Longitudinal Surveillance

Figures 1 and 2 give the LDL-C and HDL-C concentrations and Fig. 3 the ratios of LDL-C and HDL-C at age 70 in relation to the same parameters at ages 75 and 80. The linear regression lines demonstrate that within the eighth decade of life there is a progressive tendency for HDL-C to fall, and for LDL-C and the LDL-C to HDL-C ratio to rise.

These trends revealed by longitudinal surveillance diverge from findings in cross-sectional studies. One main factor responsible for the progressive increase in LDL-C with age is a decline in the activity of LDL receptors, leading to a reduced fractional rate of catabolism of LDL that most likely results from such exogenous factors as Western nutrition and lifestyle, and not as an inevitable consequence of the aging process (Miller 1984).

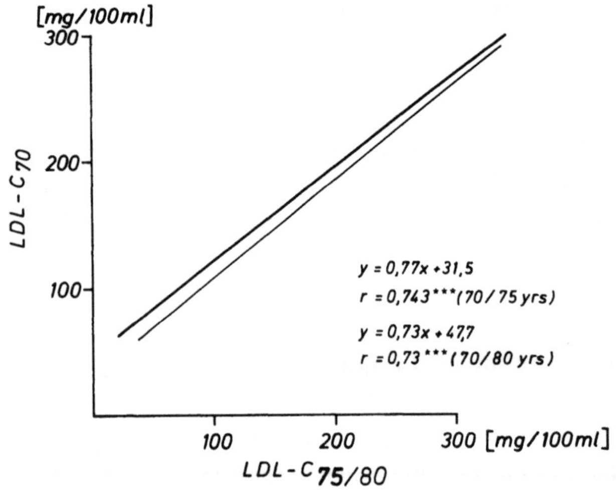

Fig. 1. LDL-C concentration at age 70 in relation to that at ages 75 and 80

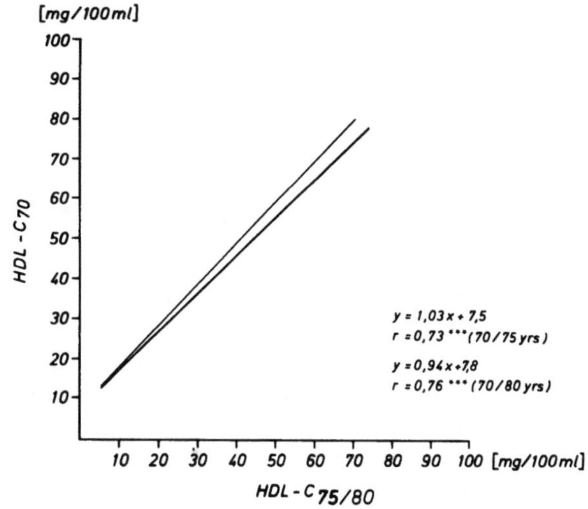

Fig. 2. HDL-C concentration at age 70 in relation to that at ages 75 and 80

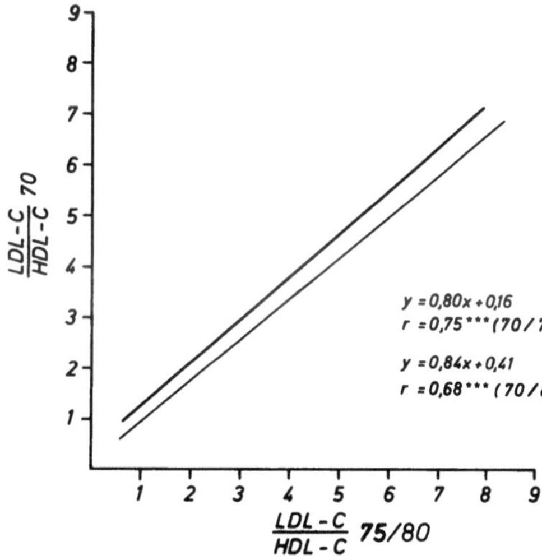

Fig. 3. LDL-C to HDL-C ratio at age 70 in relation to that at ages 75 and 80

Table 4. Accumulation of cardiovascular risk factors among 85 subjects aged 70 and 75 years

No. of risk factors	At age 70 ($n = 85$)	At age 75 ($n = 85$)
0	27	9
1	29	27
2	15	25
3	10	12
4	3	10
5	0	2

Within the 5-year period from age 70 to 75, the individual frequency of risk factors (Table 4) shifts from lower to higher prevalences which – as shown in Table 5 – is related to all factors except hypertriglyceridemia. The shift is more pronounced in women than in men.

Mortality and Cardiovascular Risk Factors in Old Age

Nearly two-thirds of the participants in our study are still alive at the end of 10 years. Forty-one septuagenarians, 24 men and 17 women, died within the eighth decade. Based on a more differentiating evaluation of risk factors according to a score, the accumulated individual risk was defined in all probands. Figure 4 shows the distribution of individual risk among the whole study group at entry and the associated deaths within the following 10 years, based on a preliminary and incomplete appraisal. To study whether any association exists between LDL-C,

Table 5. Prevalence of cardiovascular risk factors among 85 subjects aged 70 and 75 years

	At age 70 (n = 85)	At age 75 (n = 85)
Hyperbetalipoproteinemia	23	29
Hypertriglyceridemia	24	22
Hypoalphalipoproteinemia	16	31
Adiposity	8	11
Diabetes mellitus	9	20
Hypertension	20	50

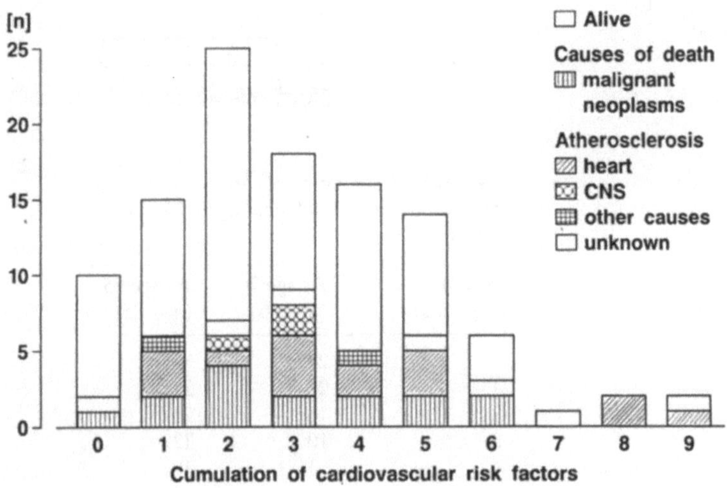

Fig. 4. Ten-year mortality according to cardiovascular risk factors at age 70

HDL-C, LDL-C/HDL-C, and triglycerides and the risk of death, the probands were grouped according to concentration quartiles, and the risk ratios were calculated in relation to the lowest quartile. The risk ratios obtained indicated that there is no association between any of the lipid/lipoprotein parameters and total, cardiovascular, or cancer-related mortality. These results may have been influenced by the unexpectedly high number of 15 deaths caused by malignant neoplasms and by the small number of probands. Only subjects with 6 or more points of risk have a slightly greater likelihood of dying within the eighth decade when compared with the group with no or one point of risk.

Discussion of Results

Not all risk factors predictive for coronary heart disease at younger ages are equally predictive at older ages. A number of studies (but not all) like the Framingham Study (Gordon et al. 1977), the Pooling Project (The Pooling Project Research Group 1978), the Los Angeles Heart Study (Chapman and Massey 1964), and the study performed in Busselton, Australia, by Welborn and Wearne (1979) have found that the predicitive value of total cholesterol diminishes with advancing age. By age 65, cholesterol is apparently no longer a cardiovascular risk factor while LDL-C and HDL-C appear to be as predictive in middle-aged and old people (up to 82 years) as in young men and women (Castelli et al. 1986; Gordon et al. 1977). A similar effect has been reported in the Framingham and the Pooling Project studies for cigarette smoking, while blood pressure remained a significant contributor to coronary heart disease prediction in the Framingham and the Pooling Project studies but not in the Busselton study.

The number of prospective studies in old age relating clinical findings to death rates and causes of death is even more limited. Barrett-Connor et al. (1984) have followed a cohort of 3187 men and women aged 50–79 years in Southern California for almost 10 years. Comparing subjects aged 50–64 years with those aged 65–79 years, they found that cholesterol remained a significant independent predictor of ischemic heart disease mortality at older ages for both sexes, while cigarette smoking and hypertension were significatly related to all-cause mortality but not to ischemic heart disease mortality. In another 10-year prospective study performed in Glostrup, Denmark (Agner and Hansen 1983), which included 230 men and 210 women aged exactly 70 years at entry, high cholesterol values were associated with excess cardiovascular disease mortality, and heavy smoking even in the eighth decade with excess total mortality, but not with excess cardiovascular mortality. Data from a longitudinal study of 2674 persons in Illinois aged 65–74 years and followed up for 5 years ascertained that cigarette smoking retained its adverse effect on survival while cholesterol did not. The excess risk of mortality declined within 1–5 years after smoking was stopped (Jajich et al. 1984). Last but not least, the data of Deutscher et al. (1986) should be mentioned; they found that mortality over a 6-month period in a group of 94 men after age 80 was directly related to the LDL level and possibly inversely related to the HDL_2 level.

All these data suggest that it is premature to dismiss the importance of the classical risk factors in old age, which, as demonstrated in our representative study, are very common in the eighth decade. For the present it seems prudent to counsel elderly adults with such risk factors along the same lines as are recommended for younger persons. In the future, risk factor intervention studies with respect to LDL and HDL also at older ages will be necessary but only in persons who are in good health because conclusions based on studies of younger adults are not necessarily applicable to older persons for many reasons. If the control of risk factors is of value even in the elderly population, such interventions may be expected to have a greater absolute short-term effect than among younger people. A 10% reduction saves more lives in 1 year than does a 50% reduction in the same number of younger people.

Discussion

Schlierf

Dr. Heckers, you mention that several other studies on risk factors in the very old indicate that lipids lose their prognostic significance, and at least in some studies, body weight and blood pressure do too. One explanation could be as follows. Dr. Greiling has pointed out that atherosclerosis is multifactorial. We do not have measures to weigh the importance of the risk factors cholersterol, blood pressure, or smoking in the individual. We only know their importance for groups. So it's possible that in 70 year olds cholesterol is not a very potent risk factor because otherwise they wouldn't have reached that age. We also have few data on protective factors. Since there are many people with risk factors and no atherosclerosis, there must be protective factors. As we have little information on these, we cannot measure them. The other possibility is that there are new hypercholesterinemias, for example induced by diuretics or β-blockers, which just don't last long enough to cause many problems. This would be the second explanation. Now the conclusion you draw, that presently it's prudent to deal with the risk factors in the old and in the very old in a way similar to that which we employ in the young, is to my mind problematic because in the young one says "eat less" while in the very old many data suggest we should say "eat more". And if we make them eat even less, they may experience ill-effects.

Heckers

Though the concept of cardiovascular risk factors is based on data measured in groups, it is also valid – though less important – in individuals. Taking into account much more individual information derived from the family history and from detailed analyses of lipoproteins and apolipoproteins including, for instance, apo E isoforms, Lp(a) concentrations, and genetic variants of apo B and apo AI, we can predict the individual cardiovascular risk with relatively high validity. Nevertheless, the most important risk factor for atherosclerosis is old age. To be free of clinically apparent atherosclerosis at age 70 does not necessarily mean that the old subject will remain free from atherosclerosis in the future, because most of the deaths caused by the atherosclerotic process occur at age 75+.

Protective factors against atherosclerosis are unknown and a matter of speculation. Indeed, it seems reasonable to suppose that most of the relevant serum lipid disorders in old age are not of primary origin but are induced by drugs like diuretics or β-blockers or a number of other pathological conditions. However, our own studies do not support this hypothesis. Our recommendation for adequate treatment of lipid disorders in old age as a preventive measure is related to patients who are younger biologically than chronologically and not to multimorbid individuals. This group does not suffer from poor nutrition.

Hofecker

I would like to try and formulate a problem concerning the evaluation of survival or mortality data in very old age. If we look at mortality data in young people, death is an unnatural event. If we look at mortality data in very old people, we have a quite different situation because if we approach our maximum life span, we must die from one or other cause. So if we prevent an individual from dying from heart attack, he or she will die from another cause. The question is, what should the individual die from and what does it tell us about the success of treatment if we reduce mortality from heart attacks and the individual dies from renal failure or some other cause? So, how should we evaluate these data? Would it be sensible to put them into relation to the age-specific mortality?

Greiling

Very difficult to answer.

Heckers

As you all know, the mean life expectancy in men and women amounts to 70 and 77 years, respectively. However, the average natural limit – independent of disease – is about 85 years or even more. The addition of years to the lives of people by elimination of negative environmental factors would not necessarily be detrimental but should be oriented toward extension of the period of health and vigor. The development of segmental interventions will certainly be related to the state of the art of gerontological research.

Blaschke

I agree with your statement about the need for interventional studies in the older population. I want to raise a point of concern, however. Epidemiologists use a number called the »number needed to be treated«; that is, the number of patients who must be treated in order to prevent one heart attack, stroke, or whatever adverse outcome is to be avoided. My concern is that, with the relatively crude risk factors that you're using, there is no way of narrowing down that overall population which must be treated. I wonder if you have any comments about whether some of the more recent noninvasive techniques might be useful in trying to narrow down that treated population, so that, for example, only those patients with abnormal lipids are treated who are more likely to benefit from treatment. This also helps overcome the concern that I think was appropriately expressed about generally recommending changes in diet or changes in lifestyle. Could we do better if we had some improved way of identifying the subpopulation form your population that is at greatest risk for cardiac disease and then treated only that subpopulation?

Greiling

There are many controversial results about the concentration of HDL and also cholesterol in olders people. The Würzburg Study Group of Franke examined the cholesterol concentration in a 100-year-old group and found normal levels. In the literature the opinion has been expressed that there is a genetically programmed messenger RNS for the apolipoproteins of HDL. Therefore my question is, are there any new results about the HDL concentations in older people?

Heckers

I agree with Dr. Blaschke that we need better noninvasive imaging methods to diagnose early atherosclerotic changes. Preliminary results demonstrate that high resolution Duplex sonography and computed tomography of the enhanced abdominal aorta may be useful approaches, but neither method is useful for the coronaries.

High HDL-C and low LDL-C concentrations, called familial hyperalphalipoproteinemia and familial hypobetalipoproteinemia, are – though it would fit best – not markers of a high life expectancy. This thesis, first described by Charles Glueck and co-workers in 1975, could not be confirmed by reinvestigations by our group and others. Glueck had studied octogenarian kindreds, not randomly selected but self-referred by either two siblings or a parent and a child living to age 80 years or more. As the kindreds were selected because of their distinctive familial longevity – longevity is chiefly influenced by genetic predisposition – it is no wonder that these families had a higher average life expectancy than the general US population.

Hans Franke never studied lipoproteins in centenarians.

Schlierf

Dr. Heckers, you showed two sets of data. One indicated that high LDL and low HDL are not predictors of longevity in very old people, and the second, that mortality and cardiovascular mortality are not related to the lipids. These are the findings. How you say we should study these points in intervention studies, and I agree. But I do not think it prudent to conclude, as you do, that presently older patients should be treated like younger patients in respect of dietary advice.

Heckers

The second conclusion refers to findings by other investigators.

Schlierf

But your recommendations conflict with your data.

Heckers

Our own data on total and selective mortality are incomplete and preliminary and may be inconclusive because of the high number of malignancies. Our recommendation for adequate treatment of the lipid/lipoprotein-associated risk factors in the eighth and ninth decades of so far healthy persons is based on the reported data of the literature which show significant associations even in the aged population. What we need are controlled intervention studies in old people too, for instance with one of the recently registered highly effective HMGCoA-reductase inhibitors, performed for 2 or 3 years only in study groups of no more than 500 subjects each.

Schlierf

We should not treat, we should study.

Frenzel

Alcohol consumption is increasing. Would you please comment on alcohol consumption as a risk factor for cardiovascular disease. Both protection and aggravation have been reported in the literature.

Heckers

There is now substantial evidence that moderate alcohol consumption provides some protection against coronary heart disease and this is apparently explained by elevations in the level of HDL. Based on dietary and alcohol consumption data from 18 countries, Hegsted and Ausman (J Nutr 118: 1184, 1988) found simple correlations with coronary heart disease for saturated fat (r = 0.71), for polyunsaturated fat (r = – 0.34), and for total alcohol consumption (r = – 0.58). A multiple regression equation incorporating the dietary and alcohol data yielded an r of 0.92.

Linke

I would like to expand on the diet. I will give a short answer to Dr. Frenzel. Maybe individuals who drink alcohol don't eat so much fat und other food and thus "fast" more than others. I have another point pertaining to diet, because diet is most important in this respect. There are certain religious groups who eat a very restricted diet. Perhaps you can comment on how they feel in old age and on what changes occur in their blood chemistry.

Heckers

Vegetarians like the most often studied Seventh-Day Adventist vegetarians exhibit better health and nutritional status than nonvegetarians. They have lower body weight, lower blood pressure, and better lipid and lipoprotein values. They are nearly exclusively nonsmokers, have a high level of physical activity, and do not drink alcohol. Consequently many studies have shown that vegetarians have a 30%–70% lower rate of coronary heart disease when compared to controls. Furthermore diverticulosis, gallstones, and colorectal and breast cancer are negatively correlated to a vegetarian lifestyle. All these positive effects cause a significantly higher mean life expectancy.

References

Agner E, Hansen PF (1983) Fasting serum cholesterol and triglycerides in a ten-year prospective study in old age. Acta Med Scand 214: 33–41

Barrett-Connor E, Suarez L, Khaw KT, Criqui H, Wingard DL (1984) Ischemic heart disease risk factors after age 50. J Chron Dis 37: 903–908

Castelli WP, Garrison RJ, Wilson PWF, Abbott RD, Kalonsdian S, Kannel WB (1986) Incidence of coronary heart disease and lipoprotein cholesterol levels. The Framingham study. JAMA 256: 2835–2838

Chapman JM, Massey FJ (1964) The interrelationship of serum cholesterol, hypertension, body weight, and risk of coronary disease. Results of the first ten years follow-up in the Los Angeles Heart Study. J Chron Dis 17: 933–949

Deutscher S, Bates MW, Caines MJ, LaPorte RE, Puntereri A, Taylor FH (1986) Determinants of lipid and lipoprotein level in elderly men. Atherosclerosis 60: 221–229

Glueck CJ, Fallat RW, Millett F, Gartside P, Elston RC, Go RCP (1975a) Familial hyper-alpha-lipoproteinemia: studies in eighteen kindreds. Metabolism 24: 1243–1265

Glueck CJ, Fallat RW, Millett F, Steiner PM (1975b) Familial hyperalphalipoproteinemia. Arch Intern Med 135: 1025–1031

Glueck CJ, Gartside P, Fallat RW, Sielski J, Steiner PM (1976) Longevity syndromes: familial hypobeta- and familial hyperalphalipoproteinemia. J Lab Clin Med 88: 941–957

Gordon T, Castelli WP, Hjortland MC, Kannel WB, Dawber TR (1977) Predicting coronary heart disease in middle-aged and older persons. The Framingham study. JAMA 238: 497–499

Heckers H, Burkard W, Schmahl FW, Fuhrmann W, Platt D (1982) Hyper-alpha-lipoproteinemia and hypo-beta-lipoproteinemia are not markers for a high life expectany. Gerontology 28: 176–202

Jajich CL, Ostfeld AM, Freeman DH (1984) Smoking and coronary heart disease mortality in the elderly. JAMA 252: 2831–2834

Miller NE (1984) Why does plasma low density lipoprotein concentration in adults increase with age? Lancet I: 263–267

Nicholson J, Gartside PS, Siegel M, Spencer W, Steiner PM, Glueck CJ (1979) Lipid and lipoprotein distribution in octo-/and nonagenarians. Metabolism 28: 51–55

Schneider J (1980) High-density lipoproteins and peripheral vascular disease in octo- and nonagenarians. J Am Geriatr Soc 28: 215–219

The Pooling Project Research Group (1978) Relationship of blood pressure, serum cholesterol, smoking habit, relative weight and ECG abnormalities to incidence of major coronary events: final report of the Pooling Project. AHA Monograph No 60

Welborn TA, Wearne K (1979) Coronary heart disease incidence and cardiovascular mortality in Busselton with reference to glucose and insulin concentrations. Diabetes Care 2: 154–160

Neuropathic, Microangiopathic, and Macroangiopathic Complications in Hospitalized Diabetic Patients of Old Age

W. BEISCHER, R. BRACHMANN, and K.-H. NEDDER[1]

"Diabetes in the Elderly – a Neglected Area?" was the subject of a review article by Tattersal from the UK in 1984, published in *Diabetologia,* the official organ of the European Diabetes Association. There is no question that it was a neglected area, and this is still true. Neglected because of rarity? By no means: diabetes is a very common disease in the elderly. According to the Health and Nutrition Examination Survey 1976–1980, the prevalence of diabetes in the US population was 73/1000 males and 89/1000 females in the age group 45–54, compared with 160/1000 males and 147/1000 females in the age group 65–74.

The reasons for the elderly diabetic patient or his family to consult a doctor and especially to be admitted to a hospital are the chronic complications of the disease in the majority of cases. Gries and Teutloff (1985), from the Diabetesforschungsinstitut in Düsseldorf, studied the complications of chronic diabetes in 595 hospitalized diabetic patients. No chronic complications at all were found in 66.7% of the patients below age 40 and in 0% of the patients above age 60, while four or more chronic complications existed in 65.6% of the patients above age 60 and in only 5.5% of the patients below age 40.

Macroangiopathic Complications of Diabetes

Concerning the macroangiopathic complications of diabetes, we shall concentrate on the results of two prospective German Studies, one from East and one from West Germany.

Panzram (1987), from East Germany, prospectively analyzed the prognosis of diabetes in the closed and centrally registered population of the Erfurt district for a period of 11 years (1960–1970). He found that of 1694 deceased diabetic patients, of whom 97.9% were older than 40 years at diagnosis, 59.4% died from all kinds of vascular disease, or, to be more precise, 34.7% from coronary heart disease, 22% from cerebrovascular disease, and 2.7% from general atherosclerosis. From these data and the results of comparable studies it can be concluded that age- and sex-related overall mortality rates of patients with type II diabetes are approximately twice as high as those of nondiabetic subjects and that the

[1] Medizinische Klink III, Bürgerhospital, Tunzhoferstr. 14–16, D-7000 Stuttgart 1 / FRG

Gerontology
Ed. by D. Platt
© Springer-Verlag Berlin Heidelberg 1989

overall mortality rates in female type II diabetic patients are equal to or even exceed those in men, in contrast to the nondiabetic population. However, a conclusion of special interest regarding the elderly is that no significant difference in the death rates of type II diabetic patients and nondiabetic control subjects was found for patients older than 75 years at diagnosis (Panzram 1987).

The prospective Schwabinger study carried out by Prof. Mehnert's co-workers in Munich, and above all by Janka (Janka et al. 1985), is the contribution from West Germany on the subject of macroangiopathy in diabetic patients. The study was started in 1976 with 623 diabetic outpatients of all age groups. Over a 5-year period, major atherosclerotic complications (cardiovascular death, typical ECG changes for myocardial infarction, cerebrovascular insult, and ischemic gangrene) occurred in 26.5% of all patients. The proportion of diabetic patients developing these major atherosclerotic complications clearly increased with age, the elderly being at the highest risk. Higher age, hypertriglyceridemia, systolic hypertension, and a longer duration of diabetes were statistically significant risk factors for the major atherosclerotic complications in the Schwabinger study.

Concerning the risk factors for macrovascular complications in diabetes, many questions are still open or controversial, e.g., the role of hyperglycemia itself and especially of its severity and its duration, the role of hyperinsulinemia, and the role of disorders in platelet function, in coagulation, and in blood rheology.

One result from the Schwabinger study (Janka et al. 1985) is of great general interst and is very stimulating for further research. As Table 1 illustrates, the relative risk of dying from a cardiovascular disease is four to five times higher in diabetic patients starting off with vascular disease of the leg than in those without such vascular disease. Vascular disease of the leg thus appears to be a strong risk indicator for cardiovascular death.

Four hundred and eighty-five diabetic patients admitted to our clinic in 1987 showed the following age distribution (%): second decade, 1.7; third decade, 5.1; fourth decade, 1.9; fifth decade, 3.6; sixth decade, 8.0; seventh decade, 13.7; eighth decade, 33.9; ninth decade, 29.4; and tenth decade, 2.7. Of the 485 patients, 426 suffered from type II diabetes, including a minority with diabetes accompanying other diseases.

In addition to geriatric medicine and diabetology, angiology is a special discipline of the clinic. We set out to evaluate prospectively the relationship between leg vascular, cardiovascular, and cerebrovascular manifestations of atherosclerosis in diabetes, between macrovascular and microvascular as well as neuropathic complications, and between the numerous complications and the possible risk factors.

One minor aspect within the vast field of research is the evaluation of data from more than 100 patients with vascular disease of the leg according to Fontaine who were treated intra-arterially with prostaglandin E_1 in 1987 and 1988 following a standardized protocol (Hinderer, Brachmann, Nedder, Beischer 1989).

Table 1. The Schwabinger Study: percentage of patients showing vascular disease of the leg (LVD) at the beginning of the study among those still alive and those who died during a 5-year follow-up period (Janka et al. 1985)

Patients	LVD
Alive (n = 474)	12.7%
Dead (n = 68)	51.5%
Death from cardiovascular Disease (n = 46)	67.4%

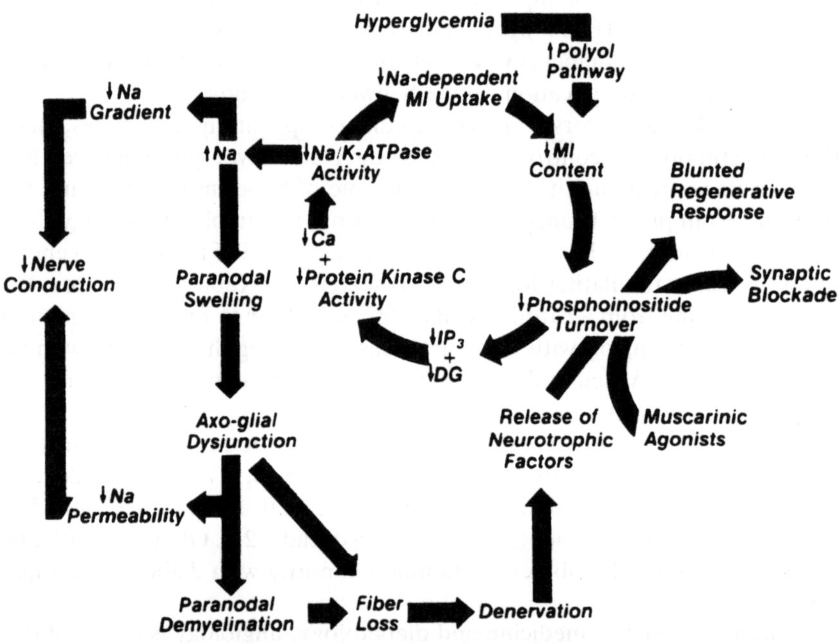

Fig. 1. Proposed pathogenetic scheme linking disturbances in nerve *myo*-inositol metabolism to slowing of nerve conduction; nerve fiber damage, demyelination, and degeneration; impaired synaptic transmission; and blunted nerve fiber repair and regeneration. The identity of neurotrophic factors is unknown, but they may include insulin-like growth factors and/or nerve growth factor. *MI, myo*-inositol. (Greene et al. 1988)

Microangiopathic and Neuropathic Complications of Diabetes

Neuropathy plays an essential and perhaps the most important role in the complaints, signs, and symptoms and the quality of life of a diabetic patient. Many neuropathic disorders have been recognized only in the last few years, and some still await full appreciation. Neuropathy occurs in both types of diabetes and often early in the course of the disease; in type II diabetes it may lead to the diagnosis of diabetes. Fascinating progress has been made most recently in elucidating the pathogenesis of diabetic neuropathy, as shown in Fig. 1. Metabolic disturbances initiated by hyperglycemia are linked with functional defects like reduced Na/K-ATPase activity and slowed nerve conduction and with morphological changes like demyelination, fiber loss, and denervation.

Diabetic peripheral neuropathies are classified as (a) distal polyneuropathies which can have a sensorimotor, a predominantly sensory, or a predominantly motor character, (b) proximal neuropathies, (c) autonomic neuropathies, and (d) focal and multifocal neuropathies concerning either cranial or limb and truncal nerves.

Autonomic neuropathy (Table 2) is an area of special interest. Most of the knowledge in this field is new, and data from the elderly in special are very rare. Disturbances of autonomic function essentially influence everyday well-being and according to Ewing and Clarke (1986) may also greatly shorten life expectancy. Progress has to be made in standardization of autonomic nerve function tests. The important cardiovascular autonomic function tests like the heart rate response to deep breathing, to the Valsalva maneuver, or to standing and the blood pressure response to standing and to sustained handgrip are among the best standardized tests and have recently been adapted to computerized evaluation (Ewing and Clarke 1986).

According to Kohner and Barry (1984), diabetic retinopathy can be subdivided into background retinopathy, maculopathy, proliferative retinopathy, and advan-

Table 2. Classification of diabetic autonomic neuropathy (Diabetic peripheral neuropathies ... 1986)

Unawareness of hypoglycemia

Pupillary and lacrimal gland dysfunction

Cardiovascular and pulmonary disturbances
- postural hypotension
- cardiac dysregulation
- vasomotor dysfunction
- respiratory dysfunction

Thermoregulatory disorders
- dyshidrosis
- vasomotor instability to changes in temperature

Alimentary tract disorders
- esophageal atony
- gastric and duodenal atony
- gallbladder atony
- diarrhea
- colonic atony

Genitourinary disturbances
- bladder atony
- impotence (erectile and/or ejaculatory)
- retrograde ejaculation

ced diabetic eye disease. Most relevant to the elderly is diabetic maculopathy, a background retinopathy located in the macular region. Diabetic patients of young, medium, and old age show a very similar prevalence and dependence on duration of diabetes for retinopathy of all kinds (Standl 1984). However, the prevalence of proliferative retinopathy, the dangerous form of the disease in the young, is much lower in the elderly (Hermann et al. 1983), who on the other hand are prone to the aforementioned dangerous maculopathy.

Körner (1988) reports that in the event of diabetic retinopathy the 5-year risk of becoming blind is 20% if diabetes began after the age of 60, but only 3% if it began before 60. Therefore retinopathy should by no means be neglected in the elderly diabetic patient.

We finally want to consider diabetic nephropathy. Much has been learned during recent years about the course and deleterious consequences of this microangiopathic complication (reviewed by Grenfell and Watkins 1986; Viberti and Wiseman 1986). In type I diabetes, which is the subject of most studies, albumin excretion in urine as determined by micromethods has been shown to be a predictor of renal insufficiency and early death. Fabre et al. (1982) and Hasslacher et al. (1987) are among the few groups who have also studied nephropathy in type II diabetes. Fabre et al. found an increased and abnormal protein excretion in 48% of 510 patients with the diagnosis of diabetes made after the age of 40. Nephropathy in type II diabetes appears to develop earlier in the course of the disease, but the progress to renal failure appears to be rarer and slower than in type I diabetes. However, microalbuminuria in type II diabetes might be a strong predictor for cardiovascular disease (reviewed by Janka 1987).

What can be done to prevent and treat diabetic nephropathy? Table 3 summarizes the current knowledge on this subject. Early intervention appears to be of great importance, especially for strict glycemic control. The data from Hasslacher et al. (1987) stress the importance of antihypertensive treatment and strict glycemic control in type II as well as type I diabetes.

We recently started a prospective study recruiting all diabetic patients newly admitted to our clinic and aiming to compare the occurrence and severity of diabetic nephropathy in young, medium aged, old, and very old diabetic patients. One of our first conclusions is that albuminuria detectable by micromethods only occurs especially often and early in the course of the disease in diabetic patients

Table 3. Effects of treatment on early renal changes in diabetic man (Viberti and Wiseman 1986)

Variable	Antihypertensive treatment	Strict glycemic control	Low protein diet
GFR	?	↓	↓
AER	↓	↓	↓
Kidney volume	?	→	?

GFR, glomerular filtration rate; AER, albumin excretion rate; → = unchanged; ↓ = reduced; ? = unknown.

of old age (Seyfferth, Nedder, Brachmann, Gloyer, Müller-Beisenhirtz, Beischer 1989).

Discussion

Frenzel

Diabetic cardiomyopathy has been discussed as a cause of heart failure in recent years. Can you comment on its frequency in your patient group?

Beischer

No, I can't yet and I think it is a very difficult problem. The cause of this heart failure is not clear. There is no doubt that diabetics have a considerably increased rate of heart failure, but it has not been established whether this is due to a microangiopathic complication or whether neuropathy plays an important role. We included in our study the heart insufficiency parameters according to the New York Heart Association, hoping that this might be of epidemiological help.

Linke

I have a heretic question. When you treat your patients, do they do better?

Beischer

I hope so: you should come and see! But it's a difficult question, really. I think one should differentiate between acute problems due to hyperglycemia and exsiccosis and chronic problems in the old patient. With acute problems it's often quite easy to change the situation. What we want to examine in our study is the extent to which clinical complaints result from objective findings, and which complaints relate to late complications. This is of special interest for the neuropathic complications which are not rare in old patients. For example, the full bladder of an old man may be mainly caused by the diabetes and neuropathy and much less by an enlarged prostate. There are several problems, especially in the neuropathic field, which I think are interesting in terms of the extent to which they influence the patient's life.

Hofecker

If we think of diabetes in old age we think of type II diabetes, but you have shown that even in the 80-year-old age group and, I think, in older age groups as well, a substantial number of patients have type I diabetes. Is there a difference between the pattern of complications in these two different groups?

Beischer

This is a very interesting question which I cannot yet answer. As you perhaps know, Gleichmann et al. published a paper in *Diabetoligia* a few years ago [Gleichmann et al. (1984) *Diabetologia* 27: 90–92] examining islet cell antibodies and HLA-DR phenotypes in adults with diabetes mellitus. The presence of islet cell antibodies and certain HLA-DR phenotypes identified a subgroup of about 20% within the adult diabetic population which can be regarded has having a retarded form of type I diabetes. I don't know in how far this applies to diabetic patients of old age. In some patients the type of diabetes is very obvious from the clinical point of view. A few months ago we admitted an 81-year-old woman with newly manifested type I diabetes. Nevertheless, such an obvious situation is rare. It is well known, however, that the older the patient at the time of manifestation of type I diabetes, the more benign the course is likely to be. Therefore I could very well imagine that even in very old patients type I diabetes cannot be neglected.

Kennedy

You did not mention in detail anything about hyperosmolar nonketotic elderly diabetics. Do they have a different pattern of complications from type II diabetics?

Beischer

That's also an intersting question, but I can't give an answer to it.

References

Diabetic peripheral neuropathies: physiopathology and clinical guidelines (1986) Diabetes Res Clin Practice 2: 183–256

Ewing DJ, Clarke BF (1986) Autonomic neuropathy: its diagnosis and prognosis. Clin Endocrinol Metab 15: 855–888

Fabre J, Balant LP, Dayer PG, Fox HM, Vernet AT (1982) The kidney in maturity onset diabetes mellitus: a clinical study of 510 patients. Kidney Int 21: 730–738

Greene DA, Lattimer SA, Sima AAF (1988) Are disturbances of sorbitol, phosphoinositide, and Na^+-K^+-ATPase regulation involved in pathogenesis of diabetic neuropathy? Diabetes 37: 688–693

Grenfell A, Watkins PJ (1986) Clinical diabetic nephropathy: natural history and complications. Clin Endocrinol Metab 15: 783–805

Gries FA, Teutloff H (1985) Zur Multimorbidität bei Typ-II-Diabetikern. In: Drost H, Gries FA, Jahnke K (eds) Der nicht insulinabhängige Diabetes mellitus (Typ II). Schattauer, Stuttgart, pp 141–148

Hasslacher C, Wolfrum M, Stech G, Wahl P, Ritz E (1987) Diabetische Nephropathie bei Typ-II-Diabetes. Dtsch Med Wochenschr 112: 1445–1449

Health and Nutrition Examination Survey, Cycle II (1976–1980) National Center for Health Statistics

Hermann WH, Teutsch SM, Sepe SJ, Sinnock P, Klein R (1983) An approach to the prevention of blindness in diabetes. Diabetes Care 6: 608

Hinderer S, Brachmann R, Nedder K-H, Beischer W (1989) Prostaglandin E_1 (Prostavasin^R) intraarteriell: bei Diabetikern erfolgreicher als bei Nichtdiabetikern. Akt Endokr Stoffw 10: 98

Janka HU (1987) Proteinurie bei Diabetes mellitus – auch beim Typ II ein prognostischer Indikator? Dtsch Med Wochenschr 112: 1443–1444

Janka HM, Standl E, Dirschedl P, Waldmann G, Grünwald P, Mehnert H (1985) Kardiovaskuläre Risikofaktoren beim Typ-II-Diabetes. Die Schwabinger Studie. In: Drost H, Gries FA, Jahnke K (eds) Der nicht insulinabhängige Diabetes mellitus (Typ II). Schattauer, Stuttgart, pp 119–127

Kohner EM, Barry PJ (1984) Prevention of blindness in diabetic retinopathy. Diabetologia 26: 173–179

Körner (1988) Diabetische Retinopathie und Photokoagulation. Enke, Stuttgart, p 22

Panzram G (1987) Mortality and survival in type 2 (non-insulin-dependent) diabetes mellitus. Diabetologia 30: 123–131

Seyfferth T, Nedder K-H, Brachmann R, Gloyer J, Müller-Beisenhirtz W, Beischer W (1989) Altersabhängige Zunahme der Nephropathiehäufigkeit beim Typ-II-Diabetiker. Akt Endokr Stoffw 10: 125

Standl E (1984) Diabetische Mikroangiopathie: Epidemiologie, Risikofaktoren und Möglichkeiten der Prävention durch gute Diabeteseinstellung. In: Lerche N (ed) Diabetische Retinopathie. Schattauer, Stuttgart, pp 1–14

Tattersal RB (1984) Diabetes in the elderly – a neglected area? Diabetologia 27: 167–173

Viberti GC, Wiseman MJ (1986) The kidney in diabetes: significance of the early abnormalities. Clin Endocrinol Metab 15: 753–782

Clinical Pharmacology and Aging

General Aspects of Pharmacokinetics in the Elderly

D. PLATT[1]

The prophylaxis, diagnosis, and therapy of diseases is a major preoccupation in advanced age. The increase in man's mean life expectancy and the multimorbidity which is demonstrably a feature of old age give added emphasis to the importance of gerontology. The fact that elderly people may have several diseases simultaneously, predominantly chronic diseases (Figs. 1, 2), necessarily entails – at least initially – treatment with a number of drugs at the same time. The rank of the different diseases, a study of our clinical hospital, is disclosed in Figs. 3 and 4.

It must be expected that, in later years, therapy will be marked by certain special features due both to age-induced physiological changes in the organs and to the pathological alterations which occur with increasing frequency in old age. It must be left to future basic research to determine to what extent old age itself causes disease and influences its course and how far senile changes are hastened by disease.

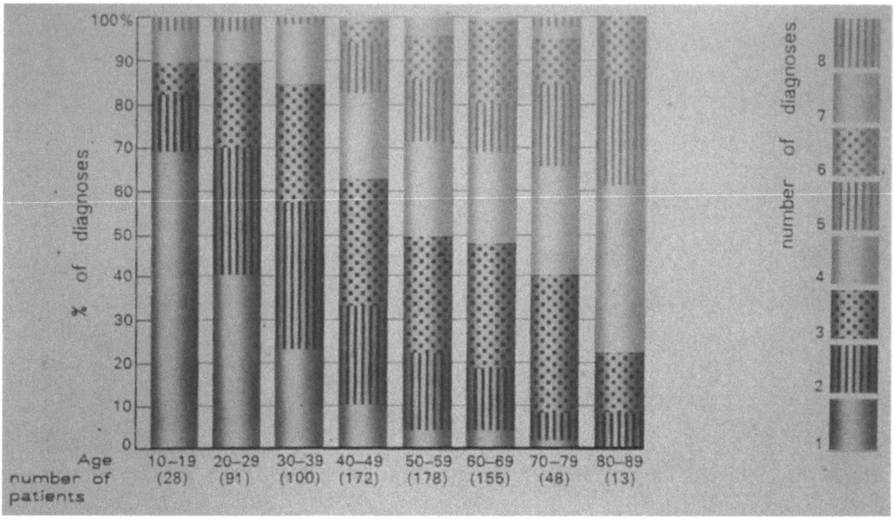

Fig. 1. Multimorbidity and age (Franke 1973)

[1] Lehrstuhl für Innere Medizin – Gerontologie der Universität Erlangen-Nürnberg
Heimerichstr. 58, D-8500 Nürnberg / FRG

Gerontology
Ed. by D. Platt
© Springer-Verlag Berlin Heidelberg 1989

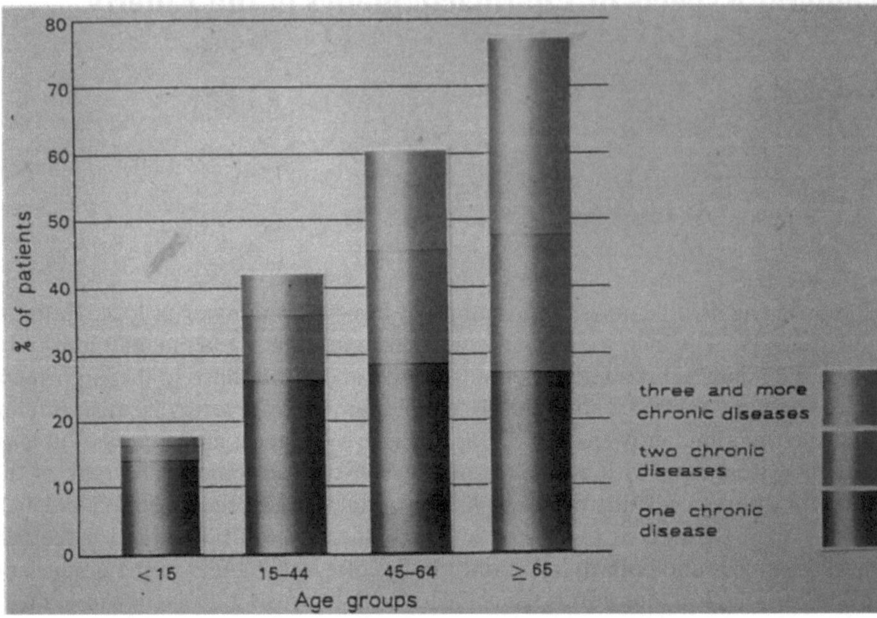

Fig. 2. Chronic diseases in geriatric patients (Vital and Health Statistics, USA 1959)

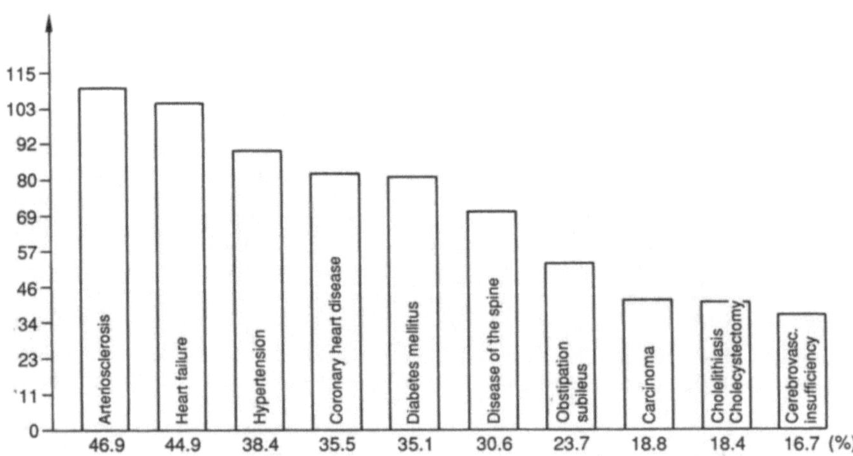

Fig. 3. Distribution of the most frequent diseases. Age group 80–90 years, $n = 245$ patients

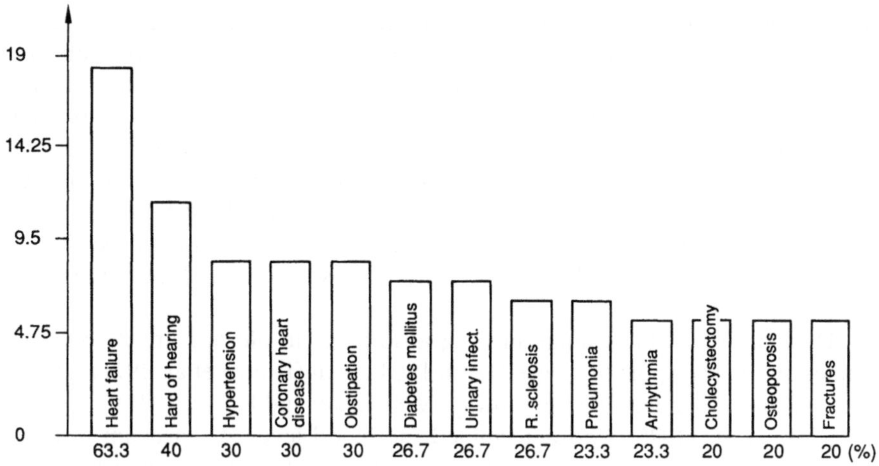

Fig. 4. Distribution of the most frequent diseases. Age group over 90 years, $n = 30$ patients

There can be no advances in the field of geriatrics without an expansion of basic research.

Pharmacokinetics

Drug therapy in the elderly requires an understanding of pharmacokinetics and pharmacodynamics. There may be crucial changes in pharmacokinetics at various stages up to and including the site of drug action (Fig. 5). The physiological age-induced changes in organs serving very different functions do not all occur at the same time and are not of equal magnitude. Since the changes which can be shown to be typically "age-induced" are almost invariably overlaid by diseases, it follows that the influence of physiological aging on pharmacokinetic and pharmacodynamic data cannot be gauged with accuracy.

Gastrointestinal Changes and Their Influence on Absorption

Elderly patients are given the majority of drugs orally and consequently senile changes in the gastrointestinal tract affecting the course of absorption may influence treatment. For example, with increasing age, both the basal and the maximum histamine-induced release of acid decreases (Baron 1963). Moreover, changes in pH values and the atrophic gastritis frequently found in advanced age affect the solubility of certain drugs. The investigations of Andreas et al. (1967) revealed that severe forms of atrophic gastritis involve a loss of the main and secondary cells and also cause a diminished secretion of hydrochloric acid and intrinsic factor. The absorption of drugs is likewise affected more especially by the motility of the stomach. Rapid emptying of the stomach, for instance, may result in increased and more rapid drug absorption in the upper portion of the small intestine. Aspirin (Schüren and Rietbrock 1982), barbiturates (Kojuma et al. 1971), and warfarin (Kekk et al. 1971) are cases in point. Studies conducted to date suggest that age-induced changes in the small intestine are not very pronounced. Compared with the stomach, the absorption of drugs from the small intestine is influenced by numerous factors such as the blood flow through the organ, motility, bacterial colonization, intensity of the digestive processes, the function and number of cells involved in drug absorption, and the rate at which the stomach empties.

Data on a possible change in drug absorption in old age are derived from studies on the transport of xylose (Guth 1968), iron (Dietze et al. 1971), glucose, and galactose (Bender 1968; Holloway 1974; Lamy and Kittler 1971).

Klotz et al. (1975) who determined the blood level of diazepam in elderly subjects, showed that oral administration in the aged led to a diminished rise in

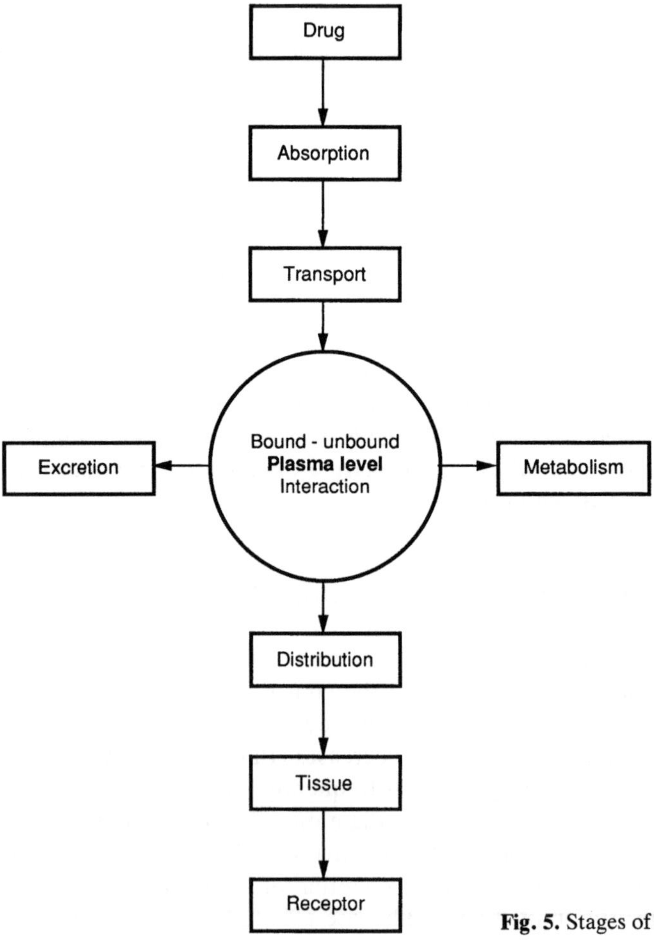

Fig. 5. Stages of drug action

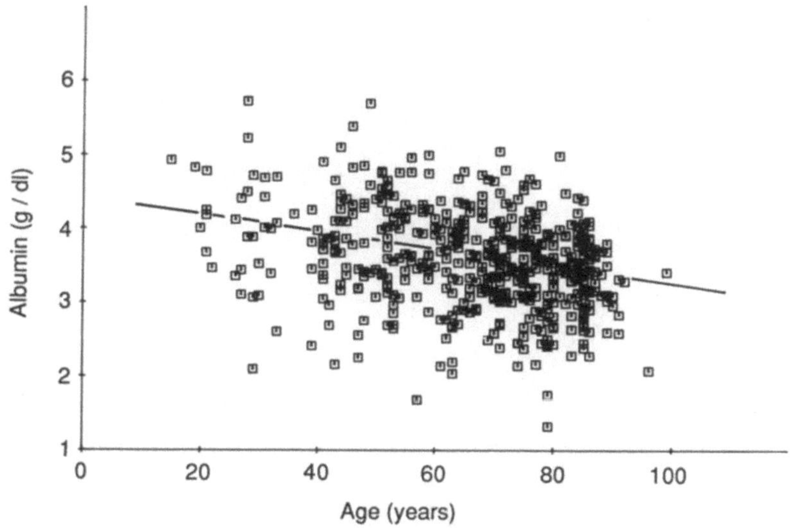

Fig. 6. Albumin concentration and aging

the drug level and a longer half-life. Physiological and pathological metaplastic processes in the heart result in a lower cardiac output in later life and hence a reduced blood flow to the organs, including the small intestine. The blood flow in the visceral nervous system is also diminished (Bender 1965). Both these age-induced changes affect drug absorption.

Drug Transport

After drugs have been absorbed and have entered the circulation, they are bound to circulating plasma proteins or cellular components. There exists a balanced relationship between the bound and the unbound fraction which is responsible for the action at the target organ receptor. Among the plasma proteins albumin plays a special role in drug binding. The concentration of blood albumin decreases with advancing age (Fig. 6). More recent work has shown that the concentration of alpha-1 acid glycoprotein also figures importantly in the transport of drugs. Chlorpromazine, tricyclic antidepressants, propranolol, and lidocaine are among the drugs which are bound to alpha-1 acid glycoprotein (Plafsky 1980; Routledge et al. 1980). Braithwaite and his team also showed that, in later life, the concentration of alpha-1 Acid glycoprotein increases and is associated, for example, with increased lidocaine and maprotiline binding (Braithwaite et al. 1978). The reduced albumin concentration explains why, in old age, protein binding is reduced in the case of certain drugs. Age-induced changes in histones in the DNA region and in collagen and elastin might be taken to suggest that structural alterations in transport proteins exert an influence on drug protein binding. However, the studies carried out so far (Bender et al. 1975; Hayes et al. 1975; Wallace et al. 1976) argue

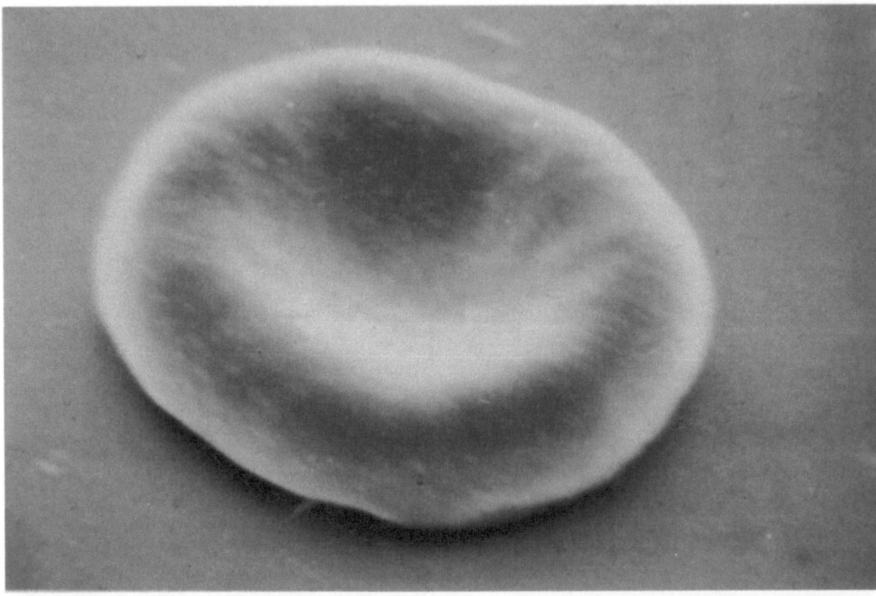
7

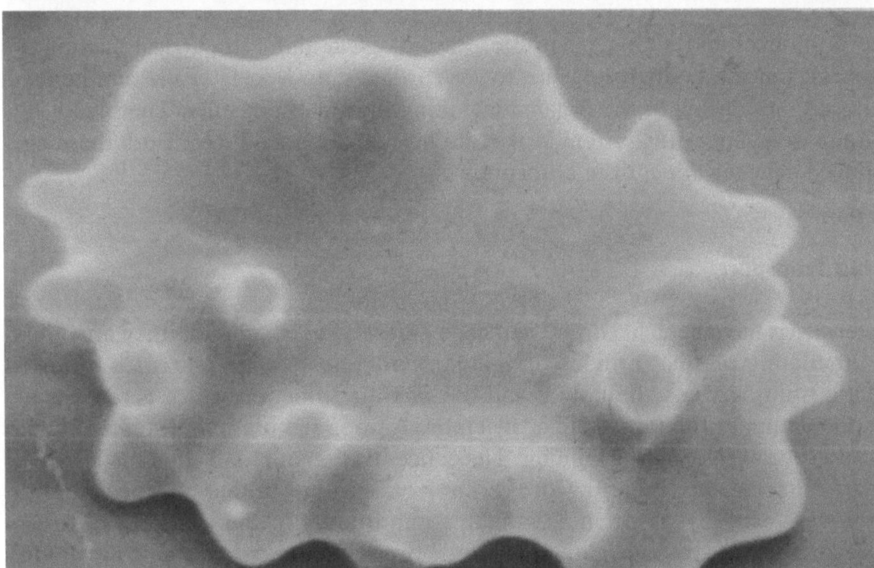
8

Fig. 7. Young human red cell
Fig. 8. Old human red cell

against this proposition. Klotz et al. (1975) found that, as age increased, the protein binding of diazepam or the metabolite desmethyldiazepam remained unchanged.

Not only plasma proteins but also erythrocytes function as instruments of drug transport. Little work has been done so far on the influence of age on the binding of drugs to erythrocytes. Age-induced changes in the membranes (Hegner et al. 1979: Platt and Norwig 1980) (Figs. 7, 8) suggest that there may be changes in the erythrocyte binding of drugs. Studies with pethidine, chlormethiazole, and piracetam show that erythrocyte binding diminishes or remains unchanged in advanced years. Other groups (Ehrenbo et al. 1974; Klotz et al. 1975) could find no age-induced differences between the bound and unbound fraction with regard to erythrocyte binding (Ehrenbo et al. 1974; Klotz et al. 1975).

Besides protein binding, age-induced changes in the transit route to the target organ also play a prominent role in drug action at the cell. There are, for instance, changes in the concentration of proteoglycans, in collagen and elastin, and in the electrolyte and water balance, which vary from one organ to another. According to Lamy and Vestal (1976), extracellular fluid decreases by 40% between the 20th and 65th year. The action of the drug on reaching the target organ may be influenced by qualitative and quantitative changes in the receptors. There have so far been few studies on the effects of aging in this field.

Influence of Hepatic and Renal Changes on Drug Metabolism

Hepatic Changes

The liver occupies a central position in drug metabolism. In advanced age deposits of the age pigment lipofuscin become more numerous (Platt 1976, 1977), the amount of scleroprotein increases, and there is a higher rate of cellular destruction. In elderly patients there are increased polyploid cell populations, chromosome aberrations, and mitochondrial changes in the liver (Table 1) (Platt 1976). Only water-soluble drugs can be excreted by the kidneys. There are not many drug possessing groups suitable for conjugation with sulfuric acid and glucuronic acid. Most drugs must first be hydroxylized. The enzymes responsible for the water solubility of drugs are located in the lipid portions of the membrane. Thus the oxidation of aliphatic and aromatic groups (phenytoin, phenothiazine, antihistamines, barbiturates, digitoxin) is catalyzed by cytochrome P_{450} and the hydrolysis of esters and alkaloids (atropine, procaine, lidocaine) is brought about by esterases, whereas binding to glucuronic acid is catalyzed by transferases (Table 2). Age-induced changes in the microsomes affecting the activities of the microsomal enzymes may thus influence the steady state of the drug level in the plasma. Most of the evidence suggesting that drug metabolism in the liver is disturbed in old age is obtained from indirect methods. Determination of the plasma half-lives or drug clearances revealed age-dependent differences. Information to date seems to show that age-induced changes affect solely phase I metabolism. Phase II

Table 1. Morphological and functional alterations in the liver with aging

Morphological changes		Functional Changes	
Liver weight	V	Hepatic blood flow	V ?
Number of cells	V	Endocytic capacity	
Number of mitochondria	V	of Kupffer cells	V
Surface area of		Cellular regeneration	V
Golgi apparatus	V ?	Enzyme adaptability	V
Size of cells	V	Enzyme inducibility	V
Size and number of nuclei		Transformation	
(Polyploidy of nuclei)	V	(phase II) step	V =
Size of mitochondria	V	Mono-oxygenase	
Number of lysosomes	V	cytochrome P_{450}	V
Lipofuscin	V	Hydrolytic enzymes	V
Rough and smooth			
Endoplasmatic reticulum	V ?		

Table 2. Biotransformation of some drugs in old age

Metabolism/substance	In old age
Hydroxylation	
Phenazone	Prolonged half-life
Quinidine	Prolonged half-life
Warfarin	No change
Phenylbutazone	No change
N-dealkylation, N-demethylation	
Pethidine	No change
Lidocaine	Prolonged half-life, increased distribution volume
Imipramine	Higher steady-state plasma level
Diazepam	Prolonged half-life, increased distribution volume
Glucuronide conjugation	
Lorazepam	No Change or reduced distribution volume, reduced clearance
Oxazepam	No change
Paracetamol	Prolonged half-life

metabolism is apparently not affected by aging. Apart from the changes in the enzyme systems responsible for drug metabolism, the hepatic blood flow is also of primary importance. Thus the elimination rate of drugs excreted via the biliary tract is limited by the hepatic blood flow rather than by the pattern of activity of drug-metabolizing enzymes (Gilette 1971).

Renal Changes

Specific age-induced changes in the kidney are difficult to assess because they are overlaid by pathological changes. Thus, to take an example, Kapides and Zierdt (1967) see no relationship between renal function and age but believe that the reduced function known to occur in old age is due primarily to the increased incidence of disease. Reduction in the weight of the kidneys in advanced years, the smaller number of glomeruli and nephrons, the diminished renal blood flow, and the increase in pyelonephritic lesions must invitably result in functional alterations. The upshot is a reduction in the clearance of creatinine, insulin, and PAH. At the same time the concentration power of the kidneys diminishes. The reduction in the glomerular filtration rate may be due, on the one hand, to a reduced renal blood flow or, on the other, to a diminution in the number or function of glomeruli, or to both together. This restricted function is of primary importance for pharmacotherapy in old age. Thus drugs predominantly eliminated via the renal pathway appear in the blood in higher concentration and hence may provoke earlier side-effects. To reduce such side-effects to a minimum, endogenous creatinine clearance tests (Fig. 9) should be performed so that the dose may be modified where necessary. Drugs with high liposolubility are turned into a water-soluble form by hydroxylation processes in the liver so as to permit excretion via the kidneys. Thus age-induced changes in the liver involving modified hydroxylation may in themselves be enough to limit renal elimination. The dearance of drug metabolites is dependent essentially on the glomeruli, since these substances can as a rule no longer be reabsorbed in the tubular system. A number of studies in which higher drug plasma levels were measured in elderly subjects and attributed to reduced renal excretion do not hold up against critical evaluation. For instance, the "urine recovery" was not determined or the possibility was not ruled out that the increased plasma concentrations were due to derangements in the distribution. In this context, for example, drug displacements into erythrocytes are a factor. In our own studies (Mühlberg and Platt 1982; Mühlberg et al. 1986; Platt and Mühlberg 1982) drugs from groups with different actions were investigated with regard to their kinetics and the effects of aging. The results given in Figs. 10–12 show that higher blood levels can be demonstrated in elderly patients. A point of interest in this connection is that, compared with healthy elderly subjects, the data obtained from those with multiple diseases display a greater range of variation. This might be evidence that it is not old age per se but the increasing number of diseases afflicting the elderly which primarily affects their pharmacokinetics.

Multimorbidity and Multiple Drug Therapy

Multiple diseases frequently invite multiple drug therapies in order to treat the individual diseases simultaneously. The ingestion of a number of drugs incurs a risk of early and more frequent side-effects as well as of interactions between the

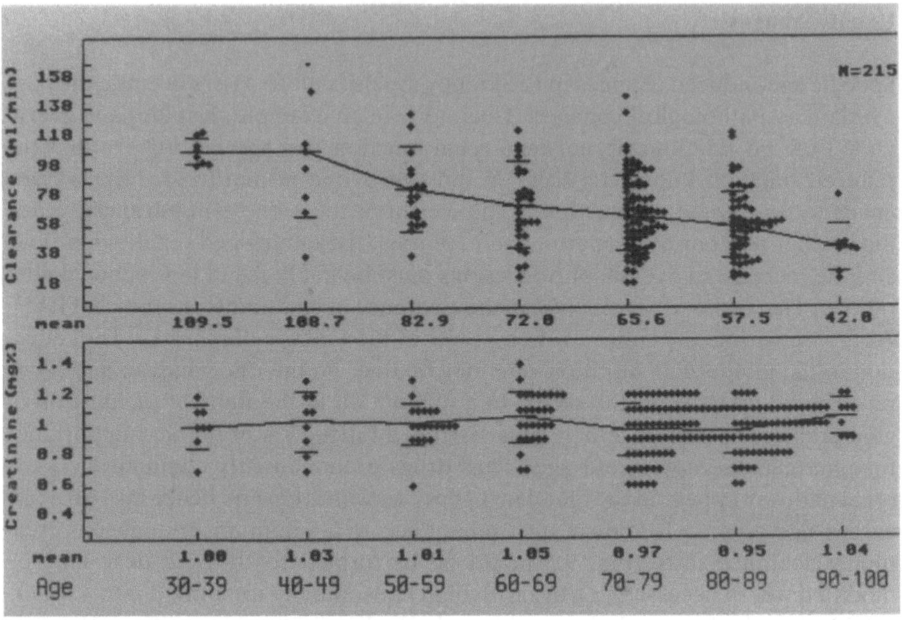

Fig. 9. Changes in creatinine clearance and aging

drugs taken. In a study of 3000 persons aged 65 years and above, Van Zonnefeld (1972) found that 37.9% of the women and 26.6% of the men were on drugs prescribed by their doctors. The rate of side-effects rises pari passu with the increase in the drugs taken. Thus Burger et al. (1977) found, in prospective studies, unwanted effects of drug therapy in 20.6% of all patients admitted to a general medical hospital and treated. The number of fatalities due to drug side-effects also increases with age. A study by Jansen et al. (1976) on "unwanted drug side-effects in old age from the viewpoint of pathological anatomy" with reference to 10000 autopsies at the Heidelberg and Darmstadt Institute of Pathology revealed morphological manifestations of drug damage in 2.57%. In 34.6% of these 257 cases drug damage was the principal cause of death, in 17.5% of them it represented a major finding, and in 26,8% a minor finding. In 20.6% the drug damage could not be separated from the underlying disease. The incidence in percent of the various forms of drug damage was as follows: corticoid damage (31.5%), hemorrhage after anticoagulants (19,8%), damage to the hematopoietic system (12.8%), phenacetin kidneys (12,8%), postantibiotic enterocolitis (10.9%), and other forms (12.1%).

Elderly patients with multiple diseases are often more sensitive to the effects of drugs than younger ones. The simultaneous ingestion of various drugs can invite drug interactions. Moreover, age-induced physiological and pathological changes can influences pharmacokinetics and pharmacodynamics. Table 3 gives a number of points which may favor drug interactions (Blaschke et al. 1981). Since compared with earlier periods of life, we still know very little about pharmacokinetics and

10
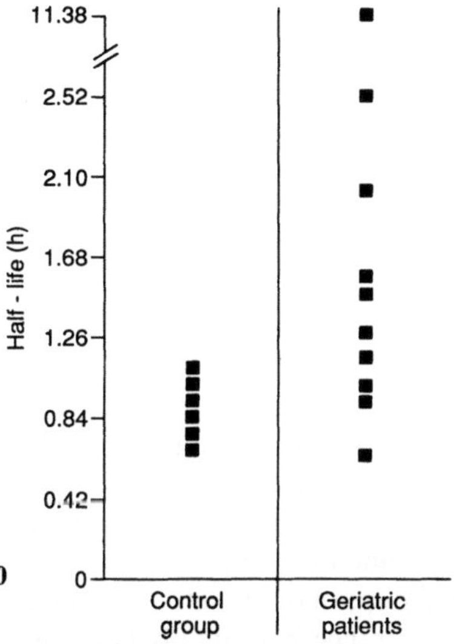

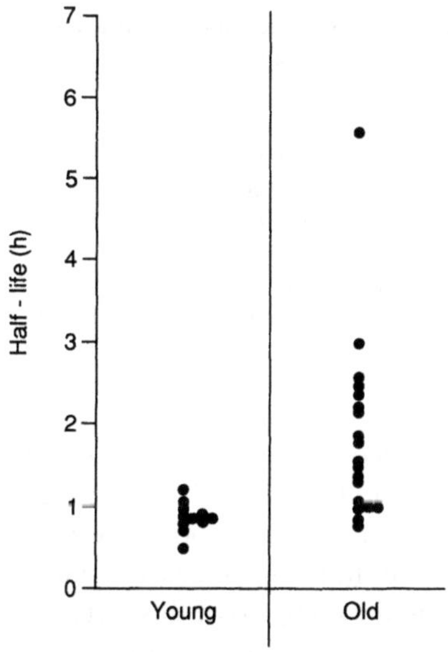

11

Fig. 10. Comparison of half-life in geriatric patients ($n = 10$) and age-matched controls ($n = 6$) after administration of 2 g cefotaxime i.v.

Fig. 11. Comparison of half-life in young subjects ($n = 12$) and geriatric patients ($n = 20$) after administration of 40 mg furosemide i.v.

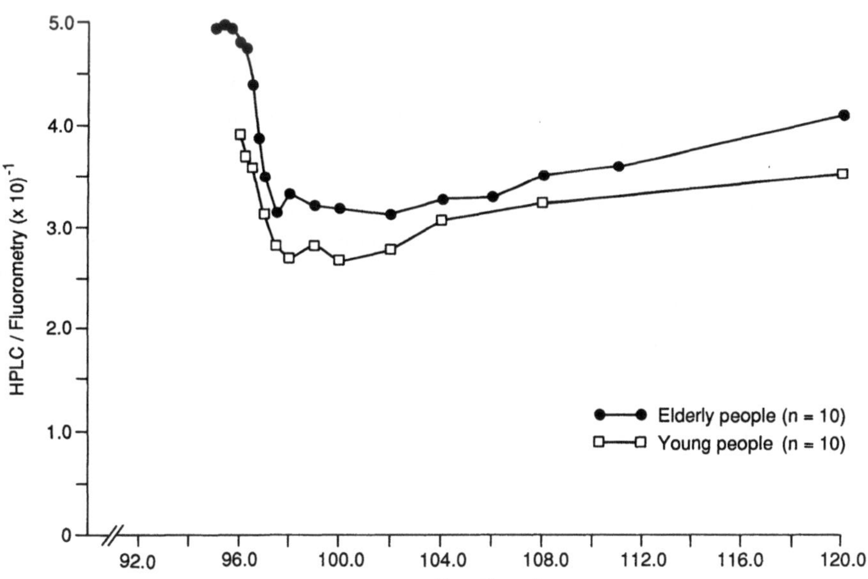

Fig. 12. Serum concentration curves (means ± SE) for canrenone as determined by HPLC in elderly and young people

Table 3. Factors predisposing to drug interactions in geriatric patients (Blaschke et al. 1981)

Reduced renal function
Altered hepatic metabolism
Deranged distribution in the tissue
Changes in binding
Increasing receptor sensitivity
Reduction of compensatory mechanisms

pharmacodynamics in old age, it follows that, in patients with multiple pathology, closer monitoring and a more accurate diagnosis before drug therapy is instituted are of far greater importance than wholesale prescription and the isolated treatment of individual diseases against the background of multiple diseases. Clearly, within the compass of this article, only a few groups of drugs among the multitude used in advanced age can be referred to. Reference has already been made to digoxin in our discussion of the limiting effects of the kidneys on the elimination of drugs in old age. Clinicians and practitioners are regularly confronted with the question – prompted among other factors by the divergent promotions of the drug companies – whether they should give preference to digitoxin or digoxin in advanced age. Certainly, the maxim "once digitalis, always digitalis," which used to have the force of dogma, is no longer valid in this form. Quite apart from the fact that more discriminate digitalization would help substantially to reduce health costs (Schüren and Rietbrock 1982), the risk of side-effects would also be distinctly lower. Numerous studies have been published on the question of digoxin or digitoxin therapy in old age (Kaufmann et al. 1981; Kolenda et al. 1978; Kuhlmann and Pabst 1982; Ochs et al. 1982). Signs of intoxication may also appear individually in patients on "normal" digitalis concentrations. In elderly patients additional factors – the simultaneous administration of other drugs (β-blockers, diuretics, quinidine) – play a considerable role. At the same time it must be remembered that in later years the potassium concentration in the plasma and the heart diminishes. Arrhythmias are a common symptom in old age arising in association with glycoside intoxication or independently of it. According to Wiese et al. (1981), in 30% – 40% of the tachyarrhythmias occurring in old age there are also bradycardiac abnormalities. Therapy to control arrhythmias can therefore easily provoke side-effects which lead to a worsening of the clinical picture. Treatment with antiarrhythmic agents may produce interactions between digoxin and quinidine or digoxin and amiodarone – to give only two examples. Quinidine clearance diminishes in later life (Smith 1978). Quinidine itself, however, leads to an elevation of the digoxin blood level by as much as 50% . Thus both the elevated quinidine and digoxin levels may cause specific side-effects in geriatric patients. The administration of amiodarone as part of digoxin therapy (Nademanee et al. 1984) produced a significant increase in the serum digoxin level. The influence of phenylbutazone, phenobarbital, or rifampicin on liver metabolism may speed up the hydroxylation of digitoxin through the induction of mixed functional hydroxylases. In a poorly compliant patient this mechanism may lead to digitalis intoxication upon his discharge from hospital.

For the treatment of senile ulcers H_2-receptor antagonists are used. As cimetidine has been on the market for some years longer than ranitidine, the literature on cimetidine is understandably very much larger and its possible side-effects have been better identified. The age-induced changes in phase I metabolism mentioned above and the known data on essential differences between cimetidine and ranitidine – specifically, that cimetidine interferes in the liver with a number of drugs whose metabolism is catalyzed by cytochrome P_{450} oxygenases – should be borne in mind when treating geriatric patients with multiple pathology. During cimetidine medication there may be drug interactions when diazepam, desmethyldiazepam, warfarin, propranolol, metoprolol, lidocaine, antipyrine, aminopyrine, etc. are administered at the same time. In the case of ranitidine the influence on the metabolism in the liver appears to be less marked (Kirch et al. 1983). The β-blockers, which are being increasingly used to control hypertension in the elderly, may possibly be given along with an H_2-receptor antagonist. In this connection a study by Kirch et al. (1982) is of interest. These authors were able to show that combined administration with cimetidine of metoprolol, propranolol, or atenolol over 7 days resulted in different pharmacokinetics for each β-blocker. For example, the medication with cimetidine produced no change in the kinetics of atenolol. In contrast to this, it was followed by an increase in the maximum metoprolol plasma level of 70% and one of 85% in the case of propranolol, compared with the levels attained when these two β-blockers were given alone.

It is becoming an increasingly common practice to give geriatric patients anticoagulants because of the higher incidence of venous thrombosis and consequent pulmonary embolism in advanced age. Quite apart from the direct side-effects (bleeding) in old age, hemorrhage may be provoked by interactions as, for example, via the induction of hydroxylases in the liver by barbiturates. When elderly patients with multiple pathology who have been satisfactorily stabilized in hospital on combined therapy (barbiturate and anticoagulants) are discharged, they may well sleep better in their wanted surroundings and, if so, may dispense with the hypnotic and thereby reduce induction. This results in a reduced degradation of dicoumarol. If there is no simultaneous reduction in the dose of anticoagulant and the same quantity as before is taken, hemorrhage may rapidly ensue. Simultaneous administration of heparin and digitoxin or digoxin may affect the kinetics of the cardiac glycosides. An increase in free fatty acids following the administration of heparin may cause digitoxin to be displaced from the binding sites on albumin, thereby increasing the unbound portion.

Patient Compliance

There is a tendency among patients of all age groups not to take their medication, by either accident or design. Among elderly patients regularity in taking medication constitutes a special problem. There are a number of understandable reasons for this. The geriatric patient, who in any case tolerates drugs less well than younger people, is frequently required, because of his multiple pathology, to take several drugs at a time and more than once a day. If only because of the memory defects that accompany old age, the patient may have difficulty in taking several drugs as laid down in his regimen. The more complex the dosage instructions, the more irregular and uncontrolled the ingestion of medication becomes (Werner 1975). Elderly patients often have difficulty even in reading the label on the pack because of failing eyesight. Understandably the probability of error increases with the number of drugs to be taken.

Summary

Elderly patients with multiple diseases are often more sensitive to the effects of drugs than younger ones. The simultaneous ingestion of various drugs can produce drug interactions. Moreover age-induced physiological and pathological changes can influence pharmacokinetics and pharmacodynamics. Since compared with earlier periods of life, we still know very little about pharmacokinetics and pharmacodynamics, it follows that, in patients with multimorbidity, closer monitoring and a more accurate diagnosis before drug therapy is instituted are of far greater importance than wholesale prescription and the isolated treatment of individual diseases against the background of multiple diseases.

Research Perspectives

More basic research is necessary in pharmacokinetics and pharmacodynamics. In the circulating blood there is competition between blood cells and plasma proteins. The binding to red cells is generally rapid for lipophilic substances. Age-dependent changes of red cell membranes may influence the binding of drugs. Future research will provide more information on the distribution properties of drugs.

Discussion

Klotz

I would like to refer to your example of the red blood cells. Do you have any data for cyclosporine, because this drug is taken up by the red blood cells and therefore it would be a good model drug.

Platt

We never measured the concentration of drugs inside red cells. We only found a direct statistical correlation of several drugs with the number of red cells. That doesn't say anything but a common study between Völker, Abshagen and our group revealed that spironolactone can be found inside red cells. We have measured this compound, and I think triamterene has also been proved inside red cells.

Brocklehurst

One different aspect of the problem of drugs in old people is the question of compliance. We insist that the patients coming to our clinics always bring all the drugs with them and we begin the consultation by going through all the drugs and finding out what they are taking, which is very often not what we expect them to be taking or what their general practitioners expect them to be taking. They do take so many and communication is sometimes difficult. I think the single drug that is most abused in the United Kingdom is prochlorperazine. This is almost universally prescribed for dizziness and any old person, if you ask them positively, will agree that they suffer from dizziness.

References

Andreas GR, Haneman B, Arnold BJ, Booth J, Taylor K (1967) Atrophic gastritis in the aged. Australas Ann Med 16: 230

Baron JH (1963) Studies of basal peak acid output with an augmented histamine test. Gut 4: 136

Bender AD (1965) The effect of increasing age on the distribution of peripheral blood flow in man. J Am Geriatr Soc 13: 192

Bender AD (1968) Effect of age on intestinal absorption: implications for drug absorption in the elderly. J Am Geriatr Soc 16: 1131

Bender AG, Post A, Meier JP, Higson JE, Reichard G (1975) Plasma protein binding of drugs as a function of age in adult human subjects. J. Pharm Sci 64: 1711

Blaschke TF, Cohen SN, Tatro DS, Rubin PG (1981) In: Javic LF et al. (eds) Clinical pharmacology and the aged patient. Raven, New York, pp 4–26

Braithwaite RA, Heard R, Snape A (1978) Plasma protein binding of maprotiline in geriatric patients-influence of alpha, acid glycoprotein. Br J Clin Pharmacol 6: 448

Burger R, Schmehe G, Strothmann G, Engelhardt K (1977) Arzneimittelnebenwirkungen bei Patienten einer Medizinischen Klinik. Med Klin 72: 21

Dietze VF, Kalbe J, Kranz D, Broschke G, Richter H (1971) Geriatrische Aspekte der Eisenresorption. Z Alternsforsch 24: 229

Ehrenbo M, Agurell S, Borens LO, Gordonie, Lonroth U (1974) Pentazocine binding to blood cells and plasma proteins. Clin Pharmacol Ther 16: 424

Gilette JR (1971) Factors affecting drug metabolism. Ann NY Acad Sci 179: 43

Guth PH (1968) Physiologic alterations in small bowel function. Am J Digest Dis 13: 565

Hayes MJ, Langmann MJS, Short AG (1975) Changes in drug metabolism with increasing age: 1. Warfarin binding and plasma proteins. Br J Clin Pharmacol 2: 69

Hegner D, Platt D, Heckers H, Schloeder U, Breuninger V (1979) Age-dependent physiochemical and biochemical studies of red cell membranes. Mech Ageing Dev 10: 117

Holloway DA (1974) Drug problems in the geriatric patient. Drug Intell Clin Pharm 8: 632

Jansen HW, Höpker W, Dörnberger V, Fauser U (1976) Unerwünschte medikamentöse Nebenwirkungen im Alter aus pathologisch-anatomischer Sicht. Z Gerontol 8: 339

Kapides J, Zierdt D (1967) Compatibility of normal renal function with aging. JAMA 201: 778

Kaufmann B, Olcay A, Schaumann W, Teufel W, Weih W (1981) Pharmacokinetics of metildigoxin and digoxin in geriatric patients with normal and elevated serum creatinine levels. Clin Pharmacokinet 6: 463

Kekk M, Pyorala K, Mustala O, Salmi H, Jussila J, Siurala M (1971) Multicompartment analysis of the absorption kinetics of warfarin from the stomach and small intestine. Int J Clin Pharmacol Res 2: 209

Kirch W, Spahn H, Köhler H, Ohnhaus EE, Mutschler E (1982) Interaction of metoprolol, propranolol and atenolol with concurrent administration of cimetidine, Klin Wochenschr 60: 1401

Kirch W, Janisch HD, Heidemann H, Rämisch K, Ohnhaus EE (1983) Einfluß von Cimetidin und Ranitidin auf Pharmakokinetik und antihypertensiven Effect von Nifedipin. Dtsch Med Wochenschr 108: 1757

Klotz U, Avant GR, Hoyumpa A, Schneker S, Wilkinson GR (1975) The effects of age and liver disease on the disposition and elimination of diazepam in adult man. J Clin Invest 55: 347
Kojuma S, Smith RB, Doluisio JT (1971) Drug absorption, V: influence of food on oral absorption of phenobarbital in rats. J Pharm Sci 60: 1639
Kolenda KD, Jost ST, Kogenge F (1978) Digoxin oder Digitoxin? Therapiewoche 28: 8726
Kuhlmann J, Pabst J (1982) Eiweißbindung und Hydroxylierungsrate von Digitoxin bei Niereninsuffizienz. Dtsch Med Wochenschr 107: 1551
Lamy PP, Kittler ME (1971) Drugs and the geriatric patient. J Am Geriat Soc 19: 23
Lamy PP, Vestal RE (1976) Drug prescribing for the elderly. Hosp Pract 11: 111
Mühlberg W, Platt D (1982) Elimination von Desacetyl-Cefotaxime bei geriatrischen Patienten mit Multimorbidität. Klin Wochenschr 60: 1497
Mühlberg W, Platt D, Neubig E (1986) Pharmacokinetics and pharmacodynamics of furosemide in geriatric patients. Arch Gerontol Geriatr 5: 249
Nademanee K, Kannan R, Handrickson J, Ookhtens M, Kay J, Singh BN (1984) IACC 4: 11
Ochs HR, Greenblatt DJ, Bodem G, Denler HJ (1982) Disease related alterations in cardiac glycoside disposition. Clin Pharmacokinet 7: 434
Plafsky KM (1980) Disease-induced changes in plasma binding of basic drugs. Clin Pharmacokinet 5: 246
Platt D (1976) Biologie des Alterns. Quelle & Meyer, Heidelberg
Platt D (1977) Liver and ageing. Schattauer, Stuttgart
Platt D, Mühlberg W (1982) Pharmacokinetics of active drug metabolites and liver metabolism in elderly patients. In: Kitani K (ed) Liver and aging. Elsevier, Amsterdam
Platt D, Norwig P (1980) Biochemical studies of membrane glycoproteins during red cell aging. Mech Ageing Dev 14: 119
Routledge PA, Barchowsky A, Bjornson TD, Kitchell BG, Shand DG (1980) Lidocaine plasma protein binding. Clin Pharmacol Ther 27: 347
Schüren KG, Rietbrock N (1982) Digitalisbehandlung in Deutschland. Dtsch Med Wochenschr 107: 1935
Smith TW (1978) Reduced quinidine clearance in the elderly persons. Am J Cardiol 42–481
Van Zonnefeld RJ (1972) Arzneimittelverbrauch im Alter. Scriptum Geriatricum
Wallace S, Whiting G, Runge J (1976) Factors affecting drug binding in plasma of elderly patients. Br J Clin Pharmacol 3: 327
Werner V (1975) Pharmakotherapie in der Gerontopsychiatrie. Geriatrie 3: 70
Wiese KH, Walter J, Schramm A, Gärner FR, Bracharz M (1981) Art und Häufigkeit von Herzrhythmusstörungen und Abhängigkeit vom Patientenalter, therapeutische Aspekte. Z Kardiol 70: 516

Drug-Drug Interactions in Geriatric Patients

J.-J. L. KONDO and T. F. BLASCHKE[1]

The geriatric group comprises the fastest growing segment of the current U.S. population. It has been projected that one in six Americans will be over age 65 by the year 2030 (Kane and Kane 1982). As a result, issues related to medication use are assuming even greater importance in this expanding subpopulation. Our focus here will be drug-drug interactions and their clinical significance in aging patients. Although the subject is important from the pharmacist's perspective, our discussion will not include pharmaceutical incompatibilities.

Drug-Drug Interactions

When drugs are administered concurrently or in close sequence, they may or may not interact. When drug interactions do occur, the resultant effect may be beneficial or undesirable. Usually, a beneficial drug interaction is an intended outcome of a treatment strategy. It is the unwanted, adverse effect of a drug-drug interaction, which may manifest itself as a decrease in or loss of therapeutic effect, an increase in drug toxicity, or an unexpected pharmacological action, that complicates clinical management when multiple drugs are used. During the past two decades, the subject of adverse drug interactions has received a considerable amount of attention from clinicians and other health care professionals. This is due to several factors: more new drugs are being introduced; patients commonly take multiple medications concomitantly; and an increasing number of case reports and clinical investigations in the literature have documented serious therapeutic consequences of drug-drug interactions.

Magnitude of the Problem

When more than one drug is administered to a patient, the number of possible combinations of any two drugs may be expressed by the following equation:

$$\text{number of combinations} = (\text{number of drugs})!/\,2!(\text{number of drugs} - 2)!$$

[1] Division of Clinical Pharmacology, Stanford University School of Medicine, Stanford, California 94305, USA

Gerontology
Ed. by D. Platt
© Springer-Verlag Berlin Heidelberg 1989

As the equation illustrates, as the number of drugs given concurrently increases, the number of possible drug-drug combinations increases sharply. For example, there are only three possible combinations for a patient taking three drugs, but 45 combinations for a patient taking ten drugs. Fortunately, only a small subset of all possible drug-drug combinations have the potential to interact and not every potential drug interaction will be experienced by every individual given the same drug combination. When experienced, the magnitude of a drug-drug interaction will vary among different patients, such that only a small percentage of the potential drug interactions will have significant clinical consequences (Puckett and Visconti 1971; Kurfees and Dotson 1987; Ford et al. 1977; Mitchell et al. 1979; Brown et al. 1977). However, the true incidence of clinically relevant adverse drug-drug interactions is uncertain. The low reported incidence of clinically important drug-drug interactions may be an underestimate, due at least in part to methodological limitations. Retrospective review of patient medical records, employed by most investigators in this field, is very insensitive when trying to confirm the occurrence of an adverse drug interaction because of insufficient clinical/laboratory data; moreover, an interaction which results in a decrease in or loss of therapeutic effect is often attributed to disease progression or lack of response to a drug rather than to a drug interaction. The average number of drugs received by both hospitalized and ambulatory elderly patients ranges from 2.8 to 8.3 in various studies (Foxall 1982; Cooper et al. 1975; Mitchell et al. 1979; Blaschke et al. 1981). In the vast majority of patients, the use of multiple, concurrent drugs is necessary for optimal therapy. Since most drug interactions are predictable and, thus, avoidable, it is imperative that efficient and effective means of monitoring and advising physicians about potential drug interactions be implemented so that adverse drug-drug interaction can be minimized.

Mechanisms of Drug-Drug Interactions

Drugs may interact by several mechanisms. A brief review of these mechanisms provides a basis for understanding how factors common in the aging patient could predispose this group to more clinically important drug-drug interactions:

Pharmacokinetic Interactions

1. Interactions Affecting Drug Absorption

a) One drug may affect the absorption of another drug by altering its disintegration, dissolution, and/or ionization. For example, the absorption of ketoconazole is reduced when cimetidine is administered concomitantly (Van Der Meer et al. 1980; Lelawongs et al. 1988).
b) A drug may change gastrointestinal motility and thereby change the rate and/or extent of absorption of another drug. A possible example is reduced oral absorption of digoxin due to an increase in gastrointestinal motility caused by metoclopramide (Johnson et al. 1984).

c) A drug may be an adsorbent (e.g., kaolin), an ion exchange resin (e.g., cholestyramine), or a bi- or polyvalent cation (e.g., aluminum) which binds or forms a complex with another drug and renders it insoluble. Reduced absorption of tetracycline due to formation of a poorly soluble chelate with calcium is a classic example.

2. *Interactions Affecting Drug Distribution*

a) A drug may compete for plasma protein or tissue binding sites with another drug, which may result in an altered volume of distribution. Displacement of digoxin from tissues by quinidine is one of the mechanisms involved in the digoxin-quinidine interaction (Fichtl and Doering 1983).
b) When a drug displaces another drug from its binding sites on plasma proteins, this results in an alteration in the free fraction and a possible transient increase in the intensity of its pharmacological effect. This is the acute mechanism of interaction when chloral hydrate is added to the regimen of a patient receiving coumarin. However, displacement interactions are complex, and acute and chronic effects may differ (Rowland 1980; Koch-Weser and Sellers 1976).

3. *Interactions Affecting Drug Elimination*

a) Some drugs induce hepatic microsomal enzyme activities and increase the metabolism of other drugs, resulting in loss of therapeutic effect. Rifampin and oral anticoagulants represent such a drug combination.
b) Some drugs inhibit the metabolism of other drugs and therefore increase plasma levels and risk of toxicity. Excessive theophylline levels, associated with toxic symptoms, have been reported when cimetidine is added to the regimen of patients receiving theophylline.
c) Renal clearance of a drug may be affected by another drug when there is competition for active secretion (e.g., methotrexate and probenecid), or when the tubular reabsorption is modified due to a change in urine pH (e.g., decrease in urinary excretion of chlorpropamide by urinary acidifiers).

Pharmacodynamic Interactions

Examples of various mechanisms responsible for pharmacodynamic interactions include competition at the receptor site (epinephrine and β-adrenergic blockers, epinephrine and phenothiazines), alteration of receptor affinity (oral anticoagulants and dextrothyroxine), modification of responses at a site of action (potassium-wasting diuretics and digoxin), and mediation of additive or synergistic effects through different biological systems which augment or diminish the total pharmacological response (aspirin and oral anticoagulants). Pharmacodynamic interactions are more difficult to identify than pharmacokinetic interactions, but are probably responsible for many clinically important interactions.

Factors in the Elderly Predisposing to Drug-Drug Interactions

Aging patients are more likely to experience adverse drug-drug interactions than other age groups. They suffer from more illnesses, therefore receiving more drugs, and in addition exhibit physiological changes associated with aging which alter responses to drugs. Factors which contribute to the increased risk of the elderly for adverse drug-drug interactions are summarized below.

Pharmacokinetic Changes with Aging

Based on the premise that the magnitude of most pharmacological responses depends on the drug concentration at the site of action, drug disposition in the elderly has been the subject of a number of studies (Greenblatt et al. 1982; Morgan and Furst 1986). Table 1 illustrates current understanding of the physiological changes associated with aging that may affect pharmacokinetics.

Pharmacodynamic Changes with Aging

Both increases and decreases in "receptor sensitivity" have been reported. Some of the benzodiazepine derivatives were shown to produce more CNS depression in the elderly than in the young (Riedenberg et al. 1978; Giles et al 1978; Castleden et al. 1977). Although not conclusive, there are studies suggesting a greater anticoagulant effect of warfarin in older patients (Husted and Andreasen 1977; Shepherd et al. 1977; Hotraphinyo et al. 1978). In contrast, reduced responses to

Table 1. Physiological changes associated with aging that may affect pharmacokinetics

Absorption[a]	Increased gastric pH Decreased rate of gastric emptying Decreased intestinal motility
Distribution[b]	Decreased total body water Decreased lean body mass Increased body fat Decreased plasma albumin
Elimination	Decreased renal blood flow Decreased glomerular filtration rate Decreased tubular function Decreased hepatic blood flow Decreased liver mass Decreased enzyme activity

[a] Since most orally administered drugs are absorbed by passive diffusion, the effect of aging on drug absorption has been considered minimal.
[b] Altered distribution influences volume of distribution and elimination half-life.

β-adrenergic agonists and antagonists were found (Vestal et al. 1979; Pan et al. 1986). In the presence of altered sensitivity, pharmacokinetic interactions are more likely to lead to toxicity or loss of efficacy.

Compromised Homeostasis

The ability to maintain homeostasis declines with age (Collins 1983). Compensatory mechanisms are much less effective, for instance, when a combination of hypotensive agents is given to the elderly (Vestal 1978; Jackson et al. 1976). Another example is higher morbidity and mortality associated with drug interactions (e.g., warfarin and NSAIDs) causing bleeding. Although systematic studies are lacking, the implication is that the impaired homeostatic responses found in the elderly increase the risk of significant clinical consequences resulting from adverse drug interactions.

Prescribing Habits / Drug-Taking Behavior

A study of elderly residents of an urban apartment building revealed that the average numbers of prescribed and over-the-counter drugs being taken were 4.5 and 3.4 respectively, for a total of 7.9 drugs per resident. This study also reported that 29.1% of the respondents had experienced adverse drug reactions, including drug-drug interactions (Darnell et al. 1986). Another study of elderly subjects from two residential homes found that the average number of prescribed drugs was 5.75 per patient (Brown et al. 1977). Blaschke et al. (1981) found that nearly 10% of 1965 nursing home patients whose drug profiles were screened with a computer system took 12 or more drugs. As the number of prescriptions per patient increased, the percentage of patients with potentially interacting combinations also increased to the point that 56% of patients receiving 12 drugs had a potentially interacting combination. Older patients in acute care hospitals generally receive an even higher number of drugs. The phenomenon of polypharmacy is well known in the geriatric age group and is particularly worrisome because a high percentage (38%–75%) of drugs used by elderly patients are equivocal or unnecessary (Bruce 1982; Tulloch 1981). In addition, appropriate adjustment of doses due to changes associated with aging is infrequent (Campion et al. 1987; Sjoqvist 1981). Although various mandatory and voluntary quality assurance programs have been implemented by acute care hospitals and long-term, skilled nursing facilities in the United States, a large proportion of the older population taking multiple drugs remains ambulatory and has minimal monitoring of drug use. The use of over-the-counter drugs, the receipt of health care from more than one physician, and the frequent purchase of prescription drugs from different pharmacies make detection of clinically important drug interactions very difficult with current approaches.

Significance of the Drug-Drug Interaction Problem in the Elderly

A number of investigators have studied the incidence of potential drug-drug interactions in various patient populations (Blaschke et al. 1981; Cohen et al. 1981; Durrence et al. 1985; Cooper et al. 1975; Mitchell et al. 1979; Ford et al. 1977; Greenlaw and Zellers 1978; Foxall 1982; Kurfees and Dotson 1987; Brown et al. 1977; Armstrong et al. 1980). In these studies, either manual checking or computerized screening (on-line or in batch mode) was used to analyze patients' drug profiles. Different sources of information defining potential drug-drug interactions were employed in the studies cited, which implies different criteria for estimating the incidence of potential drug interactions. Additionally, the length of study or period of data collection as well as number of patients included varies considerably from study to study. Thus, direct comparison of the reported frequencies of potential drug-drug interactions is difficult and only broad conclusions can be drawn. Table 2 displays the characteristics and results of a number of recent studies of drug-drug interactions. It is worth noting that only a few studies attempted to verify whether an identified potential drug-drug interaction resulted in an adverse drug reaction. As discussed earlier, underreporting of actual adverse drug-drug interactions is likely due to the difficulty in documenting a decrease or loss of therapeutic affect, or attribution of an adverse effect to the underlying disease.

Despite the differences among the study results, the data suggest that, overall, a higher percentage of geriatric patients receives drug combinations that can potentially interact. Based on the predisposing factors discussed earlier, one could speculate that the actual occurrence of adverse drug interactions in the elderly is more frequent and the clinical consequences are more severe, although this was not demonstrated in any of these studies. There is evidence from epidemiological studies that the incidence of adverse drug reactions is higher in the elderly (Hurwitz 1969). Of interest is that the most frequent interacting combinations observed in the studies of elderly patients differ considerably. Nevertheless, hypoglycemic agents, anticoagulants, diuretics, CNS-active drugs, and cardiovascular agents appear to be the major pharmacological classes involved.

Approaches to Avoid Adverse Effects of Drug-Drug Interactions

An interacting drug combination is not synonymous with a contraindicated combination; such combinations are often required for optimal patient care. Nevertheless, physicians and other health care professionals are responsible for detecting and preventing the adverse effects of potential drug-drug interactions. The following approaches may be helpful in dealing with this problem:

1. Minimize the Number of Drugs a Patient Is Taking by Establishing and Then Regularly Reviewing the Indications for All Medications. In planning a drug regi-

Table 2. Characteristics and results of epidemiological studies of drug-drug interactions

Investigator	Patient population/size	Length of study or period of data collection	Method/Source	% of PTS with PDI[a]	% of PTS who EDI[b]
Patient age not specified					
Cohen et al. (1981)	5 acute care hospitals/63663	12 m–3 y	Computer, online/MEDIPHOR	16	–
Durrence et al. (1985)	Surgical/1825	12 m	Manual/Drug Interactions (Hansten)/The Med Letter	17	–
Greenlaw and Zellers (1978)	Acute care hospital/–	–	Computer, batch/PADIS	g[c]	–
Ford et al. (1977)	Acute care hospital/1004	43 d	Computer, batch/The Med Letter	8	0.7
Mitchell et al. (1979)	Outpatients, medical/662	2 m	Manual/Drug Interactions (Hansten), Evualations of Drug Interactions (APhA)	24	0.3
Puckett and Visconti (1971)	Community hospital/2422	2 m	Computer, batch/self-generated	4.7	0.3
Patient age 60 and older					
Blaschke et al. (1981)	Nursing home/1965	3 y	Computer, batch/ MEDIPHOR	20	–
Cooper et al. (1975)	Nursing home/562	–	Manual/Drug Interactions (Hansten), Evaluations of Drug Interactions (APhA)	23	–
Armstrong et al. (1980)	Nursing home/11173	–	Computer, batch/Evaluations of Drug Interactions (APhA)	2.7	–
Brown et al. (1977)	Nursing home/188	–	Computer, batch/Bouchard et al.	53.2	0
Kurfees and Dotson (1987)	Outpatients, fam. medical/400	–	Computer, batch/Drug Master	42	0
Foxall (1982)	Nursing home/106	7 d	Computer, batch/MEDIPHOR	41	–

[a] potential drug-drug interactions; [b] experienced drug-drug interactions; [c] expressed in patient / day.

men, the physician should obviously try to avoid chronic use of drugs for symptomatic relief. This is especially important with the geriatrics since chronic drug use is prevalent. The benefit of multiple drug therapy need not be compromised because of a potential drug interaction. If therapeutically equivalent drug alternatives are not available and drug combinations are therefore essential, the manipulation of dose, route, and administration schedule may be all that is needed to reduce the risk of adverse drug interactions. Appropriate clinical and laboratory monitoring should be used to help detect early signs of certain drug interactions and prevent serious consequences. Although aging is associated with declines in many physiological functions, the extent of decline varies widely among different individuals. Individualizing dosing regimens and maintaining a high level of vigilance throughout the treatment course is essential in optimizing drug therapy.

2. Increase Practitioners' As Well as Patients' Awareness of the Significance of Clinically Important Drug-Drug Interactions. The subject of drug interactions should be included in curricula and continuing education programs for all health practitioners (physicians, nurses, pharmacists). Patients taking medications, whether ambulatory, in a nursing home, or in an acute care hospital, should receive appropriate counseling from prescribing physicians and dispensing pharmacists with regard to possible drug interactions and early reporting of any untoward drug reactions.

3. Make Effective Tools for Detecting Drug Interactions Readily Available. All potentially important drug interactions cannot be remembered even by the most conscientious physician or pharmacist. Therefore tools are needed to assist in monitoring. Examples of such tools include drug-drug interaction references and, particularly, computer-based sources of drug-drug interaction data. An important attribute of these tools is the quality of the database. Few practitioners can devote sufficient time to or have the expertise in scrutinizing drug interaction literature. Monitoring effectiveness will be jeopardized when the knowledge base is not built on critical analysis of the interaction literature and when the knowledge base is not properly updated. Drug interaction databases must therefore include only drug interactions which are well documented and must be revised and updated periodically to reflect current knowledge. An "online" system is also highly desirable. Such a system, called MEDIPHOR, has been implemented at Stanford Hospital for the last 15 years. The MEDIPHOR system not only monitors hospitalized patients for drug interactions on a real time basis, it also serves as an educational resource for medical students and house staff. Although definitive data demonstrating the cost-effectiveness of such an online drug interaction monitoring system are lacking, the reduction in cost and increased power of computer hardware make this potentially an effective and economically feasible way of handling the drug interaction problem. A number of computer-based drug interaction programs designed for different clinical settings (physician's office, retail pharmacy, multispecialty clinic, and hospital pharmacy service) are now available on the market. Ambulatory patients should be greatly encouraged to utilize the same pharmacy so that the pharmacist may have a complete patient drug profile for checking drug interactions. An alternative to this is to share patient drug profiles among all pharmacies. In July 1988, Medicare (the health insurance segment of the U.S. Social Security System for citizens age 65 and older) decided to equip 52000 pharmacies (approximately 95% of the total in the nation) with computer terminals connected to a central computer. In addition to handling the administrative needs of Medicare, the computer system will be able to provide drug-drug interaction checking for 32 million Medicare beneficiaries who will be obtaining prescription drugs from any of these participating pharmacies. This represents an important new development and resource for the study of drug-drug interactions in the elderly.

Acknowledgements. This work was supported by grants from the National Institute of General Medical Sciences (GM22209) and the National Center for Health Services Research and Technology Assessment (HS05263).

Discussion

Mühlberg

Although we performed some 20 studies investigating age-dependent changes of pharmacokinetics in geriatric patients, interactions were observed only in one study (on the influence of concomitant piretanide and hydrochlorothiazide on the kinetics of triamterene). For this study (carried out together with Prof. Mutschler and his co-workers) two different methods (or study designs) were used: a crossover comparison and a comparison between two independent groups (each with ten geriatric patients, and each with different concomitant diuretic therapy, i.e., piretanide or hydrochlorothiazide). Mean plasma levels of triamterene were significantly increased in the patients with concomitant hydrochlorothiazide (as compared with piretanide). This influence of different concomitant diuretics was shown by the crossover comparison as well as by the comparison between two independent groups; however, it could be proved much better in the crossover comparison, since all of the patients had increased triamterene levels when receiving concomitant hydrochlorothiazide. The main problem of interaction studies in geriatric patients is caused by the fact that so many different additional factors affect the pharmacokinetics and pharmacodynamics of a drug (i.e., multiple diseases). Even if your results show statistically significant differences, it is difficult to decide whether these differences are really caused by an interaction between two drugs. A crossover comparison seems to be the best method because the number of other disturbing factors or influences is rather small.

Blaschke

I agree with you entirely. I think it's very difficult to perform interaction studies in older patients; certainly the design that you're describing, crossover studies in older patients, is the most sensitive in detecting interactions and identifying those situations in which further monitoring would be necessary. Your example is a good one. Combinations of thiazide diuretics and potassium-sparing diuretics are useful in many patients, and what is needed is to identify the adjustments that are necessary to individualize the doses in older patients. One other thing that we would like to do with our system is to carry out studies in the clinical environment. One of the potential advantages of the real-time interface that we are establishing between our computer system and the hospital information system is that we will be able to identify particular patients at the time when they are about to begin receiving a particular combination that might be of interest for study. As a result we can perform prospective studies. We can get a blood sample just before the new drug is started or we can follow certain clinical or laboratory parameters if we suspect a pharmacodynamic interaction rather than a pharmacokinetic interaction. I agree with Professor Platt that we need to carry out interaction studies in the clinical environment. It's important to do studies not just in healthy older subjects, but also in older patients who have concurrent diseases and who are receiving drugs other than those being studied. It's very easy to imagine, particularly with potassium supplements and potassium-sparing diuretics, that such patients might also be receiving ACE inhibitors. It's quite possible for a patient to be taking five drugs that are all influencing the serum potassium and it's going to be extraordinarily difficult to sort out some of these questions. Although it may not be possible to sort out all drug-drug interaction questions even in an experimental environment, interesting data can be generated in the clinical setting. But such studies are very difficult and I certainly agree with your comment.

Kennedy

One of the areas which seems to be attracting interest is the role of drug nutrient interactions, particularly in the long-stay patient. Do you have any information about how frequent such interactions are in the elderly, and secondly does your system pick it up?

Blaschke

We have no data. Our system could potentially identify some nutrients, for example, those in total parenteral nutrition. It might be interesting to see if we could correlate drug kinetics with diet. We have dietary information on the hospital information computer but at the moment we do not have any studies going on in that area. It's a very important area, as we heard yesterday, and I think it certainly deserves some attention.

Linke

Certain drugs have an adverse effect by themselves, without any interactions with other drugs. How do you exclude those actions? You have mentioned penicillin and rashes. I am asking, because from the title of your talk one can assume that you are dealing only with interactions of drugs.

Blaschke

Our computer monitoring system can deal with individual drugs as well as drug combinations. The original system which was first developed at Stanford dealt only with the monitoring of drug-drug interactions, but now we are moving forward with monitoring single drugs and monitoring many other aspects of drug therapy.

Mühlberg

If your computer system and its processing speed and memory capacity are large enough, it will be not too difficult to list all of the drugs that were administered to the patients (and also the time of administration). As a next step, you can look for all drug combinations that are known from the literature to cause interactions. Using an appropriate data base, the computer will do this for you automatically. If the computer system has access to another data base (storing the time course of the clinical and biochemical parameters of the patients) it will be easy to find out (and list) all the patients with known dangerous drug combinations who *really show* unwanted side-effects – you may find out the real frequency of unwanted side-effects caused by an interaction that is described as dangerous in the literature. And, most preferable, your computer system may look for a lot of other drug combinations which are not known to be dangerous, perhaps just because nobody has investigated a possible interaction. However, you will need a great number of patients.

Blaschke

Absolutely correct. The approach you are describing is the type of population analysis that's been promoted in the field of pharmacoepidemiology. I think a computer-based system that is capturing specific laboratory test data in combination with patient prescriptions has the potential to allow that kind of analysis to also be carried out. That is certainly something that we hope to do.
The nice thing about a fully integrated hospital information system is that nobody gets a drug that is not entered in the system. We eliminate the issue of compliance in the inpatient environment. Obviously one of the things that we'd love to do in the future is to extend this kind of approach into the outpatient environment. Another thing which I failed to mention, which may generate a lot of interesting information, is that the Medicare system in the United States has announced within the last few weeks that they plan to install computer terminals in 35000 pharmacies in the United States and that every Medicare patient who gets a prescription will have a drug profile maintained centrally on large mainframe computers. This is being done mainly for billing purposes, which is the driving force for much of the computerization in health care, but again it offers a potentially useful tool for monitoring drug interactions, for looking at patterns of drug use among elderly patients, and ultimately for expanding the approach to other forms of monitoring that could be done with computer systems. That's a new government plan which I think is fascinating and one that may really revolutionize what we know about drug use in older patients.

Schlierf

Dr. Blaschke, I don't share your optimism that in hospital you know what's going on in the hospital. Professor Weger, I think, 10 years ago studied the intake of drugs which were put in front of patients in the hospital, and only about 30% compliance was noted. Thus you will not get interactions of drugs which are not taken; your information system will be deceived.

Blaschke

You're right. There is a significant discrepancy between what is prescribed and what is actually taken. But most systems, hospital information systems for example, will also eventually include a medication administration record so I'm more optimistic.

Schlierf

There's also the other side of the coin. It's our custom to tell the patient when he enters the hospital that he will recieve the medication he needs and should not take previously prescribed medication. But a sizeable proportion of patients think that we don't know what they need: A patient has been on a drug for many years; he has a good family physician who gave him this drug and what are we hospital doctors doing to take it away from him. So he takes it surreptitiously and we don't know.

Blaschke

I'm sure you are right. I think patient attitudes certainly differ from one place to another. Therefore, I believe that it is less likely to happen in our hospital but maybe I'm wrong, maybe I'm naive.

Vömel

Have you any information about alcohol interactions? About 15% of the elderly have alcohol problems and a lot of drug preparations contain alcohol.

Blaschke

We are looking at some interactions but I don't have any data. I agree with you; I think it's a very important area. There may be some significant interactions.

References

Armstrong WA Jr, Driever CW, Hays RL (1980) Analysis of drug-drug interactions in a geriatric population. Am J Hosp Pharm 37: 385–387

Blaschke TF, Cohen SN, Tatro DS, Rubin PC (1981) Drug-drug interactions and aging. In: Jarvik LF, Greenblatt DJ, Harman D (eds) Clinical pharmacology and the aged patient. Raven Press, New York, pp 11–26

Brown MM, Boosinger JK, Henderson M, Rife SS, Rustia JK, Taylor O, Young WW (1977) Drug-drug interactions among residents in homes for the elderly: a pilot study. Nurs Res 26: 47–52

Bruce SA (1982) Regular prescribing in a residential home for elderly women. Br Med J 284: 1235–1238

Campion EW, Avorn J, Reder VA, Olins NJ (1987) Overmedication of the low-weight elderly. Arch Intern Med 147: 945–947

Castleden CM, George CF, Marcer D, Hallett C (1977) Increased sensitivity to nitrazepam in old age. Br Med J I: 10–12

Cohen SN, Flood AB, Himmelberger DU, Mangini RJ, Moore TN (1981) Development, implementation, and evaluation of the monitoring and evaluation of drug interaction by a pharmacy oriented reporting system (MEDIPHOR). A final report to the National Center for Health Services Research

Collins KJ (1983) Autonomic failure and the elderly. In: Babbusterm R (ed) Autonomoic failure. Oxford University, Oxford, pp 489–507

Cooper JW Jr, Wellins I, Fish KH Jr, Loomis ME (1975) Frequency of potential drug-drug interactions. J Am Pharm Assoc 15: 24–31

Darnell JC, Murray MD, Martz BL, Weinberger M (1986) Medication use by ambulatory elderly, an in-home survey. J Am Geriatr Soc 34: 1–4

Durrence CW, DiPiro JT, May JR, Nesbit RR Jr, Sisley JF, Cooper JW (1985) Potential drug interactions in surgical patients. Am J Hosp Pharm 42: 1553–1556

Fichtl B, Doering W (1983) The quindine-digoxin interaction in perspective. Clin Pharmacokinet 8: 137–154

Ford DR Jr, Nelson PR, Wood GC (1977) A computerized detection system for potentially significant adverse drug-drug interactions. J Am Pharm Assoc 17: 354–357

Foxall MJH (1982) Elderly patient at risk of potential drug interactions in long-term care facilities. West J Nurs Res 4: 133–151

Giles HG, MacLeod SM, Wright JR, Sellers EM (1978) Influence of age and previous use on diazepam dosage required for endoscopy. CMA Journal 118: 513–514

Greenblatt DJ, Sellers EM, Shader RI (1982) Drug disposition in old age. N Engl J Med 3: 1081–1088

Greenlaw CW, Zellers DD (1978) Computerized drug-drug interaction screening system. Am J Hosp Pharm 35: 567–570

Hotraphinyo K, Triggs EJ, Maybloom B, Maclaine-Cross A (1978) Warfarin sodium: steady-state plasma levels and patient age. Clin Exp Pharmacol Physiol 5: 143–149

Hurwitz N (1969) Predisposing factors in reactions to drugs. Br Med J I: 536–539

Husted S, Andreasen F (1977) The influence of age on the response to anticoagulants. Br J Clin Pharmacol 4: 559–565

Jackson G, Pierscianowski TA, Mahon W, Condon J (1976) Inappropriate antihypertensive therapy in the elderly. Lancet 1317–1318

Johnson BF, Bustrack JA, Urbach DR, Hull JH, Marwaha R (1984) Effects of metoclopramide on digoxin absorption from tablets and capsules. Clin Pharmacol Ther 36: 724–730

Kane RL, Kane RA (eds) (1982) Values and long-term care. Lexington Books, Lexington, MA, p 10

Koch-Weser J, Sellers EM (1976) Binding of drugs to serum albumin. N Engl J Med 294: 526–531

Kurfess JF, Dotson RL (1987) Drug interactions in the elderly. J Fam Pract 25: 477–488

Lelawongs P, Barone JA, Colaizzi JL, Hsuan ATM, Mechlinski W, Legendre R, Guarnieri J (1988) Effect of food and gastric acidity on absorption of orally administered ketoconazole. Clin Pharm 7: 228–235

Mitchell GW, Stanaszek WF, Nichols NB (1979) Documenting drug-drug interactions in ambulatory patients. Am J Hosp Pharm 36: 653–657

Morgan J, Furst DE (1986) Implications of drug therapy in the elderly. Clin Rheum Dis 12: 227–244

Pan HYM, Hoffman BB, Pershe RA, Blaschke TF (1986) Decline in beta adrenergic receptor-mediated vascular relaxation with aging in man. J Pharmacol Exp Ther 239: 802–807

Puckett WH Jr, Visconti JA (1971) an epidemiological study of the clinical significance of drug-drug interactions in a private community hospital. Am J Hosp Pharm 28: 247–253

Reidenberg MM, Levy M, Warner H, Coutinho CB, Schwartz MA, Yu G, Cheripko J (1978) Relationship between diazepam dose, plasma level, age, and central nervous system depression. Clin Pharmacol Ther 23: 371–374

Rowland M (1980) Plasma protein binding and therapeutic drug monitoring. Ther Drug Monit 2: 29–37

Shepherd AMM, Hewick DS, Moreland TA, Stevenson IH (1977) Age as a determinant of sensitivity to warfarin. Br J Clin Pharmacol 4: 315–320

Sjoqvist F (1981) General issues related to age and the pharmacology of psychoactive drugs. In: Raskin A, Robinson D, Levine J (eds) Age and the pharmacology of psychoacitve drugs. Elsevier, New York, pp 195–204

Tulloch AJ (1981) Repeat prescribing for elderly patients. Br J Med 282: 1669–1672

Van Der Meer JWM, Keuning JJ, Sheijgrond HW (1980) The influence of gastric acidity on the bioavailability of ketoconazole. J Antimicrob Chemother 6: 552–554

Vestal RE (1978) Drug use in the elderly: a review of problems and special considerations. Drugs 16: 358–382
Vestal RE, Wood AJJ, Shand DG (1979) Reduced beta-adrenoceptor sensitivity in the elderly. Clin Pharmacol Ther 26: 181–186

Altered Response to Benzodiazepines in the Elderly

U. KLOTZ[1]

Introduction

In the Federal Republic of Germany the elderly (defined as subjects over 65 years of age) constitute about 15% of the general population and they consume more than 30% of all drugs (WHO 1985). Benzodiazepines (BZDs) are among the most widely used drugs in the elderly and this population at risk demonstrates an approximately two- to threefold higher incidence of side-effects to various BZDs (for review see Klotz 1986). The increased frequency of adverse reactions to BZDs in the elderly has stimulated basic and clinical research in investigating the mechanism(s) of altered drug response with age. Several studies have evaluated the clinically important problem by a combined pharmacokinetic and pharmacodynamic approach. In general, age-dependent alterations could occur at different levels (see Fig. 1).

Pharmacokinetic Considerations

Following the administration of a certain dose of a BZD the pharmacokinetics (or drug disposition) of this particular drug could be different in the elderly. Whereas absorption of BZDs exhibits no age-related changes, there are many examples showing that the distribution and elimination of BZDs are age dependent. In the elderly the apparent volume of distribution (Vd) of bromazepam, chlordiazepoxide, clobazam, desmethyldiazepam (and its prodrugs), diazepam, midazolam, and nitrazepam is larger than in younger control subjects. In addition, the total body clearance (CL) of alprazolam, brotizolam, chlordiazepoxide, and desmethyldiazepam is reduced in older patients. Consequently, the elimination half-life ($t\frac{1}{2}$), which is related to CL and Vd ($t\frac{1}{2} = \frac{0.69 \cdot Vd}{CL}$), can be prolonged in the elderly, as has been demonstrated for alprazolam, bromazepam, brotizolam, chlordiazepoxide, clobazam, desalkylflurazepam, desmethyldiazepam, diazepam, loprazolam, midazolam, and quazepam. However, there are also BZDs such as oxazepam, temazepam, and lorazepam (which are eliminated by glucuronidation)

[1] Dr. Margarete Fischer-Bosch-Institut für Klinische Pharmakologie, D-7000 Stuttgart 50 / FRG

Gerontology
Ed. by D. Platt
© Springer-Verlag Berlin Heidelberg 1989

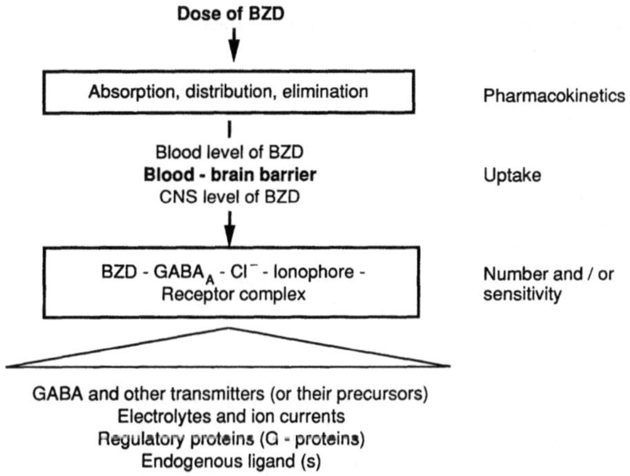

Fig. 1. Different factors which can modify the GABA- and receptor-mediated actions of BZDs

exhibiting no pharmacokinetic changes in the elderly (Klotz 1986). Since the elderly population is also more sensitive to those BZDs, age-dependent pharmacokinetic changes cannot solely explain the altered response to this group of CNS-active drugs.

Pharmacokinetic studies in man rely on measuring concentration of BZDs (and their active metabolites) in blood or plasma. Since BZDs exert their action in the CNS, monitoring of CNS levels would be more meaningful but is not feasible in man. Therefore it could be possible that brain uptake or penetration of BZDs through the blood-brain barrier (BBB) is facilitated in the elderly. Some indirect hints for such a hypothesis could be derived from the increase of Vd with aging. However, the barrier and carrier function of BBB apparently demonstrates only subtle changes with aging (Mooradian 1988).

Pharmacodynamic Considerations

For several BZDs (e.g., diazepam, loprazolam, midazolam, nitrazepam) the elderly demonstrate an increased sensitivity. In these pharmacological studies with geriatric patients the pharmacodynamic action (response) of BZDs was assessed by various methods (see Table 1). If the standard drug diazepam was administered as a single dose to different older patients it became evident that these subjects needed lower doses for a certain clinical effect, such as a defined degree of CNS depression (Reidenberg et al. 1978; Cook et al. 1984). The greater responsiveness of the elderly to an oral dose of 10 mg diazepam (Swift et al. 1985a) was associated with lower effective plasma levels for total and free diazepam (Cook et al. 1984). However, it should be realized that independent of drug treatment, cognitive performance and psychomotor skills decline with age (Hinrichs and Ghoneim 1987).

The relatively new and short-acting midazolam also has to be given in considerably lower doses (e.g., 2.5–3 mg) in older patients (from 60 years onwards)

Table 1. Methods for assessing pharmacodynamic response to BZDs in the elderly

Critical flicker fusion frequency
Visual analogue scales
Choice reaction time
Postural sway
Digit symbol substitution test
"Letter e" cancellation test
Defined CNS depression/muscle relaxation

than in younger patients (range 15–60 years) to achieve the same standardized degree of sedation (Bell et al. 1987). Since pharmacokinetic parameters and plasma concentrations following a single dose were similar between two age groups (Castleden et al. 1987); Kanto et al. 1986), it could be concluded that mainly pharmacodynamic alterations occur in older patients.

Likewise, despite similar plasma concentrations of nitrazepam and loprazolam, psychomotor testing indicated an increased sensitivity of the aging brain to the action of both BZDs (Castleden et al. 1977; Swift et al. 1985b). However, the often poor comprehension in elderly patients should also be taken into consideration (Cook et al. 1983).

Similarly, in the absence of pharmacokinetic changes a single oral dose of temazepam (20 mg) induced more pronounced CNS effects in the elderly (age range 68–79 years) than in a group of subjects aged 20–27 years (Swift et al. 1981).

The exact mechanism(s) involved in the higher sensitivity of the aging brain to BZDs have not yet been determined, because in man there is no direct information on the status of the specific central BZD receptors.

(Patho-) Physiological Considerations

With age, one would expect a decrease in cellular brain mass, sensory conduction time, and cerebral blood flow. There is also a decline in the homeostatic response. All these "normal" alterations can be exaggerated by drug therapy and might contribute to the higher sensitivity of the aging brain to BZDs (Lamy 1987). Since the action of BZDs is mediated by the inhibitory neurotransmitter GABA, synaptic regulation and neurotransmitter function involving different electrolytes and local ion currents both might demonstrate age-related alterations (Severson 1987) which could contribute to the increased response to BZDs (see Fig. 1).

Positron emission tomography (PET) scans following injection of flumazenil visualized in man an age-dependent cortex/blood concentration ratio of this specific BZD antagonist (Yamasaki et al. 1986). This may indicate either changes in the disposition, uptake mechanism(s), or receptor density for BZDs or just alterations in CNS blood flow.

Experimental Studies

Most such in vivo and in vitro experiments have been performed with rats. Similarly to man, this species demonstrates an age-associated increase in Vd for diazepam (Klotz 1979; Tsang and Wilkinson 1982). Following a single intravenous injection of diazepam, the brain of the senescent male Fischer 344 rat (29–31 months old) is exposed to more diazepam and active metabolites than that of young and mature control rats (Rahman et al. 1986). Thus, aging can affect the disposition of diazepam in rats, too.

In most of the in vitro binding studies with crude BZD receptor preparations from different rat brain areas no significant changes in the binding characteristics (receptor density or affinity) of BZDs to their corresponding recognition sites at the BZD-$GABA_A$-chloride channel receptor complex could be found (see Table 2). Recently, ex vivo binding of labeled flunitrazepam following a single intravenous injection of diazepam was decreased in senescent rats (Komiskey 1987). As a different brain content of diazepam (and its active metabolites) at the time of sacrifice cannot be ruled out completely (see also Rahman et al. 1986), the exact mechanism(s) of this observation needs to be delineated.

Whereas no solid evidence for age-related changes of the BZD receptors is apparent, GABA levels in the brain might change with age. Another working hypothesis might be generated if endogenous ligands to the BZD receptor complex could be identified. Putative candidates are a peptide with anxiogenic and diazepam binding inhibiting properties (Alho et al. 1985) and/or perhaps natural BZDs which could be identified recently in the brain of different species (Klotz 1989).

Conclusions

The elderly represent a population at risk when exposed to the "normal standard" dose of drugs, including BZDs. Since older patients can suffer from an exaggerated

Table 2. Influence of age on BZD receptors

In vitro effects described in old rats	Reference
Decrease in receptor density only in hippocampus	Memo et al. 1981
No changes in binding characteristics	Pedigo et al. 1981
No changes in binding characteristics	Tsang et al. 1982
No difference in total receptor density	Reeves and Schweizer 1983
Decrease in ex vivo FNP binding (5' following diazepam i.v.)	Komiskey 1987
Higher brain levels of diazepam and active metabolites	Rahman et al. 1986

and prolonged response to BZDs the dosage of this group of drugs should be reduced by at least a factor of 2. Numerous clinical studies have revealed that age-related pharmacokinetic changes can only partly contribute or explain this actual problem. Several other pharmacodynamically orientated factors might be involved, such as changes in:

1. Permeability of the blood-brain barrier
2. Rate of synthesis of receptors (receptor density)
3. (Super)sensitivity of receptors
4. Neurotransmitter levels and functions
5. Homeostatic mechanisms
6. Predrug conditions
7. Endogenous ligands

Additional investigations and research activities in the area of geriatric pharmacology are necessary to improve our understanding of this pertinent clinical problem.

Acknowledgments. The secretarial help of Mrs. B. Grözinger is gratefully acknowledged. The work was supported by the Robert Bosch Foundation Stuttgart, FRG.

Discussion

Hofecker

I think you should look more closely into the blood-brain barrier. Dr. Bubna-Littitz at my institute has looked into the blood-brain barrier of rats during maturation and aging. He studied the brain uptake index according to the Oldendorf method using amino acids and a highly lipophilic drug, *N*-methyl-nitrosourea, which is a carcinogen. He found that during maturation the passage of lipophilic drugs decreases but in senescence, from 12 to 36 months, the passage increases. Perhaps this finding could contribute to a solution of your problem.

Klotz

One problem is the blood-brain barrier, as you indicated; it has two functions, and for amino acids and some biological substrates there are special carrier systems while for lipophilic drugs there is just transport by passive diffusion. But you are right and I know of ongoing experiments by Dr. Wilkinson's group in Nashville at the Vanderbilt University to investigate this uptake mechanism in young and old rats. So far no data have been published. I think consideration of the uptake mechanism or the blood-brain barrier is a crucial point which so far has been neglected.

Böhm

I have a question concerning the receptor complex and its regulation. Is it possible to induce up- or downregulation by application or withdrawal of the drugs?

Klotz

Yes, there is a very recent paper in the *Journal of Pharmacology and Experimental Therapeutics* (246: 170–182, 1988) from Greenblatt's group. They used chronic treatment with lorazepam in rats and explained the phenomena of tolerance and withdrawal symptoms after chronic treatment by up- and downregulation of the receptors. It's the first study indicating that tolerance to benzodiazepines is due to a downregulation of the receptors and that withdrawal symptoms after stopping benzodiazepines are associated with the upregulation of the receptors. This might happen in man too. But there are indications that tolerance also develops in the elderly; some authors claim it develops somewhat slower, but there are no hard data.

Kennedy

One of the clinical problems we sometimes meet in the very old on benzodiazepines is the paradoxical effect of very low doses in people who had previously been cognitively intact. Do you have any information on whether there are any changes in receptor affinity or anything else in the pharmacodynamics in these people that can help us to detect such individuals?

Klotz

No. It was always claimed that such paradoxical reactions occur more often in very young patients and in the elderly. I remember a review in *British Journal of Clinical Pharmacology* 3 or 4 years ago. The author collected all the data on so-called paradoxical reactions and tried unsuccessfully to identify one factor common to all of them. If they don't know the reason for a drug reaction, pharmacologists call it idiosyncratic. If such a paradoxical reaction is seen, the new benzodiazepine antagonist flumazenil can be used to block it.

Mutschler

In my opinion it has not yet been clearly shown that the sensitivity of the receptor molecule itself can be changed. If a higher or lower sensitivity was observed it was believed to be caused by a receptor down- or upregulation, i.e., by a change in the receptor density.

Klotz

I was puzzled 2 days ago when I heard the talk on glycosylation. In rats glycosylation does not happen. And it came to my mind that all the receptor studies in connection with age have been performed in rats. One year ago the structure and amino acid sequence of this receptor complex was published in *Nature* (328: 221, 1987). The authors also included some marks in the chain where there are the so-called glycosylation sites, and perhaps the fact that the rat is insensitive in terms of receptor changes has somthing to do with glycosylation. Maybe one should look at another species and not rats.

Mutschler

May I ask one more question? If I understood you correctly, there was a discrepancy during your talk. In the middle of it you told us that there are no important pharmacokinetic changes which are responsible for the alteration in sensitivity. However, at the end of your talk, you made the statement that blood levels or other pharmacokinetic changes are more important than pharmacodynamic alterations. Is this true or did I not understand you correctly?

Klotz

If you go through the literature there are some phamacokinetic changes like a prolongation of half-life. There are also studies in which the plasma levels have been monitored and concomitantly the pharmacodynamics have been assessed, and no changes in the pharmacokinetics have been observed. There seems to be no influence or effect of the pharmacokinetics on the action of the drug because the blood levels during the monitored phase were similar in young and old subjects.

Mutschler

But do blood levels give the correct information?

Klotz

That blood levels were about the same could be due to changes in the distribution volume and the clearance at the same time. This is correct.

Mutschler

In my opinion pharmacokinetic changes are much more important than pharmacodynamic changes.

Klotz

I don't believe it, because there are studies which show no pharmacokinetic changes with the so-called glucuronidated benzodiazepines. But still you have a higher sensitivity in the elderly.

Formerly, I was also more in favour of pharmacokinetic changes, but nowadays I think that pharmacodynamic changes are more important. Pharmacokinetic changes could be of some signifcance, but I think pharmacokinetics have been overemphasized in the past.

Beischer

I would like to ask a question on behalf of the clinician. Is it correct that you recommend being careful not only with the hepatically oxidized preparations but in general with the dosage of all benzodiazepines?

Klotz

That's right, yes.

Böhm

What is known about endogenous modulators of the benzodiazepine receptor complex. Which substances are involved? Do adenosine receptors or adenosine uptake mechanisms play a role?

Klotz

So far no endogenous substrate to this natural occurring receptor complex has been identified. Right now the most likely candidate as an endogenous ligand is the so-called diazepine-binding inhibitor, isolated from the brain of different species, including man, by the group of Costa and Guidotti at the NIH in Washington. This is a large peptide or it can be broken down to a peptide of 18 amino acids; this endogenous compound can induce anxiety, it's a kind of inverse agonist. As the name suggests it can displace benzodiazepines from their binding sites. This would be one endogenous ligand, but so far there is no proof that we have an endogenous ligand.

Blaschke

I think we have to distinguish between the two uses of benzodiazepines in the elderly, both of which are very common. One is to combat anxiety, the other is to induce sedation and amnesia prior to procedures. I think that the differences in indication may be important in terms of whether the pharmacokinetics or the pharmacodynamics are more important. You are probably aware of the work that Dr. Donald Stanski has done investigating the acute distribution of sedative/hypnotic drugs in the central nervous system and how the distribution processes differ when the drug is used as a rapid infusion or bolus dose in older patients. Older patients differ in terms of the fraction of their cardiac output that goes to the central nervous system, and apparent increases in sensitivity in this age group are in part related to the larger fraction of the cardiac output that goes to the central nervous system. Thus there is no true increase in "sensitivity" but rather a pharmacokinetic difference in terms of distribution of cardiac output.

Klotz

You are right. One has to distinguish between the acute dosing under different test conditions and, for instance, in a gastroenterology setting where benzodiazepines are given for sedation or muscle relaxation. On the other hand under chronic treatment, the slight changes in the pharmacokinetics become more effective. But I still think that even during chronic treatment in a clinical setting one should carefully titrate the drug, because of the danger of accumulation.

References

Alho H, Costa E, Ferrero P, Fujimoto M, Consenza-Morphy D, Guidotti A (1985) Diazepam-binding inhibitor: a neuropeptide located in selected neuronal populations of rat brain. Science 229: 179–182

Bell GD, Spickett GP, Reeve PA, Morden A, Logan RFA (1987) Intravenous midazolam for upper gastrointestinal endoscopy: a study of 800 consecutive cases relating dose to age and sex of patient. Br J Clin Pharmacol 23: 241–243

Castleden CM, George CF, Marcer D, Hallett C (1977) Increased sensitivity to nitrazepam in old age. Br Med J I: 10–12

Castleden CM, Allen JG, Altman J, John-Smith P St (1987) A comparison of oral midazolam, nitrazepam and placebo in young and elderly subjects. Eur J Clin Pharmacol 32: 253–257

Cook PJ, Huggett A, Graham-Pole R, Savage IT, James IM (1983) Hypnotic accumulation and hangover in elderly inpatients: a controlled double–blind study of temazepam and nitrazepam. Br Med J 286: 100–102

Cook PJ, Flanagan R, James IM (1984) Diazepam tolerance: effect of age, regular sedation, and alcohol. Br Med J 289: 351–353

Hinrichs JV, Ghoneim MM (1987) Diazepam, behavior, and aging: increased sensitivity or lower baseline performance? Psychopharmacology 92: 100–105

Kanto J, Aaltonen L, Himberg J-J, Hovi-Viander M (1986) Midazolam as an intravenous induction agent in the elderly: a clinical and pharmacokinetic study. Anesth Analg 65: 15–20

Klotz U (1979) Effect of age on levels of diazepam in plasma and brain of rats. Naunyn-Schmiedebergs Arch Pharmacol 307: 167–169

Klotz U (1986) Age-dependent actions of benzodiazepines. In: Platt D (ed) Drugs and aging, Springer Berlin Heidelberg New York pp 131–139

Klotz U (1989) Stellen Benzodiazepine »natürliche« Arzneimittel dar? Klin Wochenschr 67: 93–94

Komiskey HL (1987) Aging: effect on ex-vivo benzodiazepine binding after a diazepam injection. Neurochem Res 12: 754–749

Lamy PP (1987) Age-associated pharmacodynamic changes. Methods Find Exp Clin Pharmacol 9: 153–159

Memo M, Spano PF, Trabucchi M (1981) Brain benzodiazepine receptor changes during aging. J Pharm Pharmacol 33: 64

Mooradian AD (1988) Effect of aging on the blood-brain barrier. Neurobiol Aging 9: 31–39

Pedigo NW, Schoemaker H, Morelli M, McDougal JN, Malick JB, Burks TF, Yamamura HI (1981) Benzodiazepine receptor binding in young, mature and senescent rat brain and kidney. Neurobiol Aging 2: 83–88

Rahman A, Komiskey HL, Hayton WL, Weisenburger WP (1986) Aging: changes in distribution of diazepam and metabolites in the rat. Drug Metab Dispos 14: 299–302

Reeves PM, Schweizer MP (1983) Aging, diazepam exposure and benzodiazepine receptors in rat cortex. Brain Res 270: 376–379

Reidenberg MM, Levy M, Warner H, Coutinho CB, Schwartz MA, Yu G, Cheripko J (1978) Relationship between diazepam dose, plasma level, age, and central nervous system depression. Clin Pharmacol Ther 23: 371–374

Severson JA (1987) Synaptic regulation of neurotransmitter function in aging. Rev Biol Aging 3: 191–206

Swift CG, Haythorne JM, Clarke P, Stevenson IH (1981) The effect of aging on measured responses to single doses of oral temazepam. Br J Pharmacol 73: 413P–414P

Swift CG, Ewen JM, Clarke P, Stevenson IH (1985a) Responsiveness to oral diazepam in the elderly: relationship to total and free plasma concentrations. Br J Clin Pharmacol 20: 111–118

Swift CG, Swift MR, Ankier SI, Pidgen A, Robinson J (1985b) Single dose pharmacokinetics and pharmacodynamics of oral loprazolam in the elderly. Br J Clin Pharmacol 20: 119–128

Tsang C-FC, Wilkinson GR (1982) Diazepam disposition in mature and aged rabbits and rats. Drug Metab Dispos 10: 413–416

Tsang CC, Speeg Jr KV, Wilkonson GR (1982) Aging and benzodiazepine binding in the rat cerebral cortex. Life Sci 30: 343–346

WHO Regional Office for Europe (1985) Drugs for the elderly. Copenhagen

Yamasaki T, Inoue O, Shinotoh H et al. (1986) Benzodiazepine receptor study in the elderly using PET and clinical application of a new tracer, C-11-α–methyl-N-methylbenzylamine. In: Kitani K (ed) Liver and aging – 1986, liver and brain, Elsevier Scientific Amsterdam, pp 265–276

Treatment with Diuretics in the Elderly

E. MUTSCHLER, W. MÖHRKE, H. SPAHN, and K.-D. VÖLGER[1]

Diuretics are used alone or in combination with other drugs to eliminate edema and increasingly in patients with arterial hypertension and/or heart failure. This explains the increasing prescription of drugs from this group of agents in elderly patients. Thus about two-thirds of all diuretic prescriptions are for patients over 65 years old (Table 1). After the cardiac glycosides, diuretics are the second most frequently prescribed agents in West Germany.

Groups of Diuretics

In accordance with their site of action in the nephron, diuretics are subdivided into:

1. Loop diuretics
2. Thiazides and analogous compounds
3. Potassium-sparing diuretics

In principle, all groups are suitable for use in the elderly. However, as described below, selection of an agent from one of the groups must be based on the indication and both kidney and liver function.

Table 1. Prescription of diuretics in the elderly in 1981 (after Hyams 1984)

Country	Percentage of all prescriptions for the age group 65 years and older
West Germany	57
Great Britain	60
Netherlands	51
Belgium	54

[1] Pharmakologisches Institut der Universität Frankfurt, Theodor-Stern-Kai, D-6000 Frankfurt / FRG

Gerontology
Ed. by D. Platt
© Springer-Verlag Berlin Heidelberg 1989

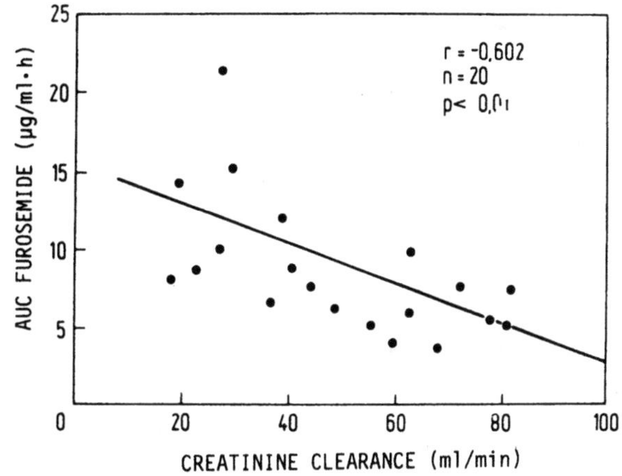

Fig. 1. Negative (inverse) correlation between the creatinine clearance (ml/min) and the total area under the concentration-time curve of furosemide (AUC_O – infinity, µg/ml × hours) (Neubig et al. 1984)

Loop Diuretics

A brief, but very intensive action is characteristic for these agents. With high doses of these compounds, elimination of edema can be attained even when thiazides are no longer active. Only loop diuretics are indicated in patients with renal insufficiency.

In acute left ventricular heart failure, these compounds are hemodynamically active in patients with intact kidney function even before onset of a diuretic effect. The action arises in that prostaglandins or prostacyclin are released in increased amounts from the kidney: these then lead to venous pooling and thus to a lowering of the preload. Not a direct but an indirect effect is thus involved.

After oral administration, substances with a furosemide-like action are absorbed quickly, but with different rates and extents of absorption. The bioavailability of furosemide, the most commonly used substance, is about 50%–60%. A higher fraction of the loop diuretics bumetanide and piretanide is absorbed. The transport in the kidney mainly takes place by active proximal tubular secretion. In renal insufficiency, in which processes of secretion are impaired, high doses are therefore necessary. Furthermore, the onset of action is delayed. In elderly patients, the kinetics of furosemide are altered compared to those in younger patients (Kerremans et al. 1983; Andreasen et al. 1984; Neubig et al. 1984; Traeger et al. 1984): the plasma half-life is prolonged to about 2–3 h and the renal clearance is lowered depending on the creatinine clearance (Figs. 1, 2). On the other hand, the proportion of unbound furosemide may be raised in patients with reduced total protein, so that the renal excretion will be accelerated. However, as a general rule this effect is less significant for the processes of elimination than are the loss of functional nephrons and the reduced renal and hepatic blood flow.

The reduced hepatic blood flow also appears to be the reason for the less pronounced glucuronidation of furosemide in elderly patients. The pharmaco-

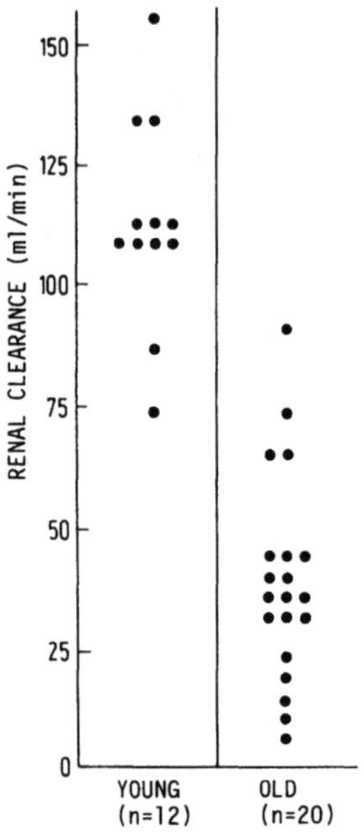

Fig. 2. Comparison of the renal clearance (ml/min) of furosemide in geriatric patients with the renal clearance in the group of younger healthy subjects. The average renal clearance is considerably lowered in the geriatric patients (Neubig et al. 1984)

dynamic and pharmacokinetic alterations described result in the following clinical consequences for pharmacotherapy with furosemide in the elderly: Although higher doses than in younger patients tend to be required to attain an adequate diuretic effect owing to the frequently restricted kidney function, cautious administration of furosemide is indicated in the elderly, particularly in multimorbid patients, since side-effects may be especially pronounced after administration of high doses (Hyams 1986). Caution with regard to the dosage is also required for the presence of highly raised blood levels of uric acid because of the competition for the acid carriers and the consequently raised levels of furosemide in the plasma (Neubig et al. 1984). An individually adapted dosage is also necessary in patients with reduced cardiac performance.

Thiazides and Analogous Compounds

Thiazides (dihydrobenzothiadiazines) are bicyclic sulfonamide derivatives acting on the early distal tubule. Some of these substances are listed in Table 2. Besides thiazides in the narrower sense, there are further agents with the same activity profile, thiazide-analogous sulfonamide diuretics, which are listed in Table 3. Thiazides increase the excretion of sodium and chloride ions. Potassium and magnesium ions are also excreted to an increased extent. On the other hand, the excretion of calcium and phosphate ions decreases after administration of thiazides. The thiazides differ qualitatively from the loop diuretics in this respect, since the latter increase calcium excretion. The glomerular filtration rate is reduced by

Table 2. Dihydrobenzothiadizine derivatives

Generic name	Trade name (registered trademark in West Germany)	Mean daily dose (mg)
Hydrochlorothiazide	Di-Chlotride, Esidrix	25
Trichloromethiazide	Esmarin	2
Butizide	Saltucin	5
Polythiazide	Drenusil	2
Bendroflumethiazide	Sinesalin	5

Table 3. Thiazide-analogous sulfonamide diuretics

Generic name	Trade name (registered trademark in West Germany)	Mean daily dose (mg)
Mefruside	Baycaron	25
Clopamide	Brinaldix	20
Chlortalidone	Hygroton	25
Xipamide	Aquaphor	20

thiazides. However, this reduction is not very pronounced and mostly only occurs at the beginning of drug therapy.

The substances specified in Tables 2 and 3 are absorbed rapidly and well from the gastrointestinal tract after oral administration. However, their biotransformation differs considerably. Whereas, for example, hydrochlorothiazide is practically not biotransformed at all, bendroflumethiazide is metabolized to about 70% (Hyams 1986). There are also marked differences in the plasma half-lifes. For example, these are 6.5 h for hydrochlorothiazide and 26 h for polythiazide (Niemeyer et al. 1983; Hobbs and Twomey 1987). For chlortalidone, a half-life of 50 h was determined (Fleuren and van Rossum 1977). The excretion is mainly renal by glomerular filtration and tubular secretion.

Because of their relatively slow onset of action (so that there is less stress for the patients), the lower danger of exsiccosis, the long duration of action, and consequently the possibility of giving a single dose per day, thiazides are used especially frequently in geriatric patients.

The dose-effect curve for the diuretic and antihypertensive effect is flat, so that it is of little benefit to increase the dose when the effect is not adequate, especially since there is a marked increase in the side-effects. Since in addition the renal clearance of thiazides is lowered physiologically in elderly patients, a low dose treatment is also to be recommended with these agents (McMahon 1984). Accordingly, the normal daily dose of hydrochlorothiazide should be 12.5 mg in patients over 65 years old, and 25 mg should not be exceeded. Furthermore, it is to be pointed out that thiazides no longer have an adequate effect with a creatinine clearance of less than 30 ml/min, and should be replaced by loop diuretics in such cases.

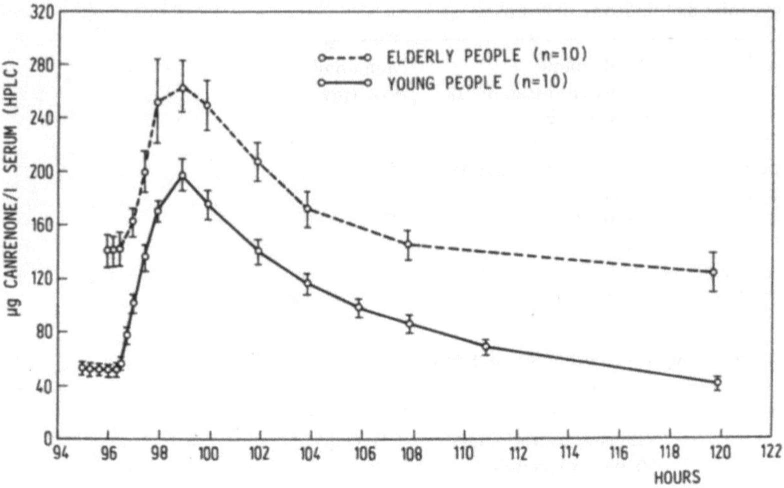

Fig. 3. Serum concentration curves (means ± SE) for canrenone determined by HPLC (Platt et al. 1984)

Potassium-Sparing Diuretics

Loop diuretics and thiazides have their enhanced potassium elimination in common. To avoid this deleterious effect, potassium-retaining diuretics are administered concomitantly. Two groups of such diuretics are distinguished the aldosterone antagonists and the cycloamidines.

Spironolactone and Potassium Canrenoate

The aldosterone antagonists available at present are spironolactone (e.g., Aldactone, Aldopur, Osyrol) and potassium canrenoate (Aldactone, Osyrol for injection). Their onset of action only occurs after a latency of a few hours, but on the other hand the duration of action is relatively long.

After oral administration, spironolactone is absorbed rapidly and almost completely. As a steroid, it is subject to a pronounced metabolism. One of the numerous (in some cases still active) metabolites is canrenone, which is transformed by opening the lactone ring into the potassium salt, potassium canrenoate, which has a good water solubility and is thus injectable. The excretion by spironolactone or of its metabolites takes place about 45% via the kidneys and about 35% via the bile in healthy subjects (Abshagen et al. 1979).

Pharmacokinetic investigations of spironolactone in elderly patients (Platt et al. 1984) showed that compared to younger persons the serum concentrations are about twice as high in geriatric patients (Fig. 3). The same study group (Abshagen et al. 1981) also demonstrated that the metabolic pattern does not change even in old age. Ho et al. (1984) arrived at similar results. The authors conclude from these investigations that spironolactone should be used with caution in old age.

Table 4. Level and time of the maximum plasma concentrations, terminal half-lives, area under the plasma time-concentration curves, and AUC ratios of TA and OH-TA esters after administration of 100 mg TA in young test subjects ($n = 6$, mean age 29.5 years) and in elderly patients ($n = 10$, mean age 73.7 years)

	Triamterene				OH-TA-ester				$AUC_{OH\text{-}TA\text{-}ester}$
	C_{max} (ng/ml)	t_{max} (h)	t/2 (h)	AUC (μg/ml · min)	C_{max} (ng/ml)	t_{max} (h)	t/2 (h)	AUC (μg/ml · min)	AUC_{TA}
Young volunteers ($n = 6$)	46.5	2.25	4.32	18.1	722.5	2.33	5.13	252.4	17.35
Elderly patients ($n = 10$)	235.0	2.45	6.50	118.2	1140.3	3.50	7.69	652.9	13.91
Significance $P =$	0.0012	0.25	0.16	0.0017	0.11	0.02	0.33	0.01	0.06

Triamterene and Amiloride

The cycloamidine derivatives triamterene (Jatropur) and amiloride (Arumil) directly inhibit the reabsorption of sodium and secretion of potassium in the late distal tubule. They hence act much more rapidly than spironolactone.

After oral administration, the two substances are rapidly absorbed from the intestine. The diuretic action begins after about 1 h and reaches its maximum after about 3–4 h. Triamterene is very rapidly biotransformed via hydroxytriamterene into the phase II metabolite hydroxytriamterene sulfuric acid ester (Knauf et al. 1987), which, interestingly, is still biologically active, and mainly excreted as such by the kidneys and the liver. On the other hand, amiloride is only metabolized to a small extent. The half-life of triamterene is 4–6 h and that of amiloride 18–20 h.

Investigations on the pharmacokinetics of triamterene in elderly patients (Möhrke et al. 1983) provided the following results (cf. Table 4): The maximum plasma levels (C_{max}) after a single dose of triamterene were five times higher in the elderly patients than in healthy subjects, whereas the time up to attaining of the maximum plasma level (t_{max}) was not changed. The area under the plasma level time curve (AUC) increased to a highly significant extent, and the metabolism to the phase II metabolite, as well as its excretion, was also delayed. Corresponding investigations are not yet available for amiloride, but a markedly slower excretion in geriatric patients is also to be expected for this agent because of the markedly delayed excretion in renal insufficiency (Knauf et al. 1985). As with spironolactone, the clinical consequence of this is that the dose of triamterene and amiloride must be reduced in geriatric patients.

Indications

Indications to be specified (also for geriatric patients) are:

1. Acute and chronic edema
2. Hypertension
3. Acute as well as chronic heart failure

Use of diuretics is logical in edema, since an agent is designated as a diuretic especially when it induces the increased excretion of sodium chloride and water, which is necessary to eliminate edema. However, in the treatment of edema diuretics are able only to supplement a therapy directed specifically against the underlying disease, not to replace it. Thus in edema of renal origin, the edema can be eliminated more or less well with diuretics, but this does not affect the cause of the edema, the loss of protein due to the defective renal filter. In ascites of hepatogenic origin, diuretics can eliminate neither the inadequate albumin synthesis nor the portal hypertension. Not every edema may or should be treated with diuretics. Thus diuretics should be administered at the most temporarily in edema in the context of venous insufficiency, which is especially frequent in elderly patients. It is to be emphasized that they are not able to replace physical measures, e.g., compression treatment.

In the treatment of hypertension, diuretics are still the agents of first choice (Empfehlungen der Hochdruckliga 1987). Although the precise mechanism of action has not yet been established, it can be assumed that their blood pressure-lowering effect arises initially by reduction of the circulating blood volume and in long-term therapy by reduction of the responsiveness of the vessels to endogenous pressor stimuli. Consequently the vascular tone and thus the peripheral arterial resistance are lowered. In addition, the venous return to the heart decreases (lowering of preload and afterload). Apart from their use as monotherapeutics, diuretics are also especially suitable for administration in combination with other hypertensives to lower blood pressure.

The decrease in the preload and afterload of the heart under diuretic treatment is also the reason for their use in heart failure. In contrast to the cardiac glycosides, they do not have a positive inotropic effect, but improve cardiac performance by increased economy of cardiac work (Bolte 1982). For this reason, cardiac glycosides and diuretics can be combined well in this indication. According to Roos (1981), diuretics should be given preference in:

1. Mild forms of heart failure with normal sinoatrial rhythm
2. Moderate forms of heart failure with normal sinoatrial rhythm in which edema is most prominent
3. "High output failure", e.g., in cor pulmonale

In English-speaking countries, they are quite commonly used before administration of digitalis glycosides (Schüren 1982). The stepped treatment scheme according to Bertel (1983) for various forms of heart failure with or without arrhythmias is shown in Fig. 4.

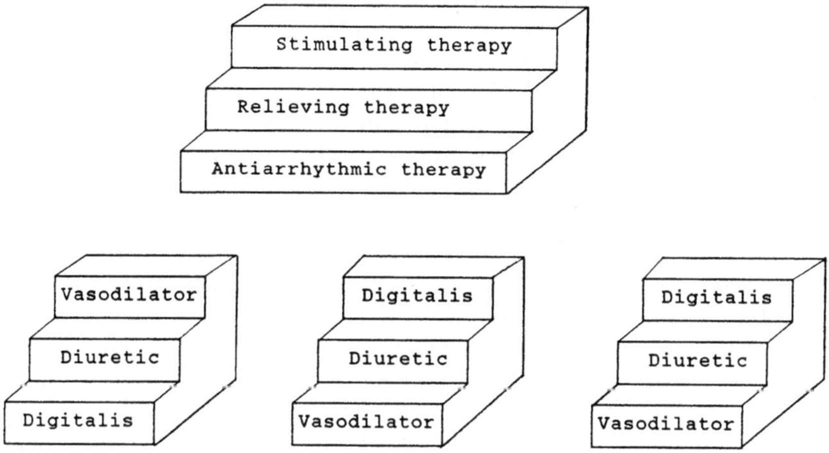

Fig. 4. Stepped treatment scheme according to Bertel (1983) for various forms of heart failure with or without arrhythmias

Side-effects

Like other active drugs, diuretics are subject to the danger of adverse effects (side-effects). An important adverse effect of loop diuretics and thiazides is the already mentioned loss of potassium; besides this, magnesium excretion is increased. These disturbing effects are attributable on the one hand to an enhanced exchange of cations in the late distal tubule (owing to the reduced reabsorption of sodium in the more proximal sections of the tubule, the late distal sodium concentration is raised) and on the other hand to the activation of the renin-angiotensin-aldosterone system.

In rapid elimination of edema (especially with loop diuretics in higher dosage), there is an increase in the hematocrit due to losses of intravascular fluid which cannot be replaced quickly enough from the extravascular space, and thus an increase in the viscosity of the blood. As a consequence of this, the perfusion in the terminal vascular bed is worsened and the tendency for thrombosis to occur is increased. The loss of circulating plasma volume under diuretic therapy may lead to orthostatic dysregulation.

Loop diuretics and thiazides also result in a deterioration of glucose tolerance. As a consequence of this, a latent diabetes may become manifest, or in the case of an existing diabetes a patient compensated with oral antidiabetics may develop a requirement for insulin. In insulin-dependent diabetics, the insulin requirement may increase. Further side-effects of the two groups of diuretics involve lipid metabolism: the plasma concentration of the triglycerides as well as that of the low density and very low density lipoproteins may increase in the plasma. Finally, there may be an attack of gout in predisposed patients owing to an increase in the blood level of uric acid.

With potassium-sparing diuretics, the most important side-effect is the potassium retention with a danger of hyperkalemia. Gastrointestinal disorders, exanthema, in men gynecomastia and disorders of sexual function, in women amenorrhea, hirsutism, and a feeling of tension in the breasts as well as alterations in the voice characteristics in men and women may occur after administration of spironolactone or of potassium canrenoate. Gastrointestinal symptoms and vertigo are observed after administration of triamterene and amiloride.

The most important of the side-effects described are highly dose-dependent. If a lower dosage than that commonly applied is given in accordance with present-day knowledge these side-effects are mostly not very significant and result only in slight impairment of the value of these substances in the indications specified. However, especially in geriatric patients, attention is to be paid to these side-effects, since these disorders of homeostasis can be compensated less quickly and less well in elderly patients, and, as has been shown, accumulation can occur even after "normal" dosage with a series of substances owing to the lower elimination capacity. In this connection, the physiologically reduced kidney function in old age (decrease of the GFR in 70 year olds to about half of the value in 20 year olds with healthy kidneys) and the reduced capacity of the liver for oxidative biotransformation should be especially pointed out once more. It may not be overlooked that in many elderly patients there is already a deficiency of potassium (mostly due to inadequate potassium intake with the food), and this is additionally intensified by administration of saluretics. Consequently, the danger of hypokalemia is especially high in elderly patients (McCarthy 1982). According to Edmonds and Jasani (1972), a decrease of the serum potassium level by 1 mmol/l entails a 20% reduction in the total body potassium. Monitoring of the serum potassium level as well as appropriate measurement of potassium loss under administration of saluretics are hence necessary. This applies particularly in patients who receive digitalis glycosides at the same time.

Contraindications

With the exception of the loop diuretics, groups of diuretics are contraindicated in patients with renal insufficiency, as already described above. Further contraindications for loop diuretics and thiazides are hepatic coma and therapy-resistant hypokalemia because of their potassium ion-eliminating action. Attention is to be paid to hyperkalemia when using potassium-sparing diuretics.

Interactions

When loop diuretics were combined with aminoglycoside antibiotics as well as cefalotin, as raised nephrotoxicity was found. The risk of ototoxicity is increased with simultaneous administration of a rapidly administered high dose loop diuretic together with an aminoglycoside antibiotic. Analgesics or antirheumatics which act via inhibition of prostaglandin biosynthesis lower the effect of most diuretics. Simultaneous administration of triamterene and indomethacin (Amuno) resulted in a deterioration in kidney function (Weinberg et al. 1985), whereas a corresponding effect was not observed with spironolactone (Favre et al. 1983). However, indomethacin reduced the natriuretic action of spironolactone by about 50%.

Owing to the increased potassium excretion, loop diuretics and thiazides intensify the action (and side-effects) of cardiac glycosides and muscle relaxants of the curare type. Glucocorticoids or laxatives raise the danger of hypokalemia when there is simultaneous administration of a loop or thiazide diuretic.

Benefit of Diuretic Therapy in Geriatric Patients

In a comparison of the therapeutic value of diuretics with their potential risk when administered to elderly patients, results of numerous studies show that the benefit clearly predominates, so long as the dose is appropriate and the indication has been clearly established.

In patients with heart failure, not only the quality of life but probably also the prognosis is improved.

A treatment in which above all thiazides were used in patients with hypertension reduced the number of strokes (The Australien Therapeutic Trial in Mild Hypertension 1980; Hypertension Detection and Follow-up Program Results 1982; Veterans Administration Cooperative Study Group on Antihypertensive Agents 1970, 1972). In the EWPHE study (Amery et al. 1985), which was carried out with a combination of hydrochlorothiazide and triamterene against placebo, a decrease in apoplectic insults (strokes) by 32% (not statistically significant) as well as a statistically significant decrease in the number of deaths owing to cardiovascular events was also found in the verum group.

To summarize, diuretics are widely administered on a large scale in geriatric patients. As long as they are administered properly, they will retain their value in this group of patients in the future.

Discussion

Blaschke

I have a question about interactions and side-effects particularly involving the loop diuretics furosemide and ethacrynic acid. With regard to your comment on hearing loss in older patients, I wonder whether it is more common with the loop diuretics, what the mechanism might be, and whether there is potentiation of the hearing loss by loop diuretics in patients also receiving aminoglycoside antibiotics?

Mutschler

First of all one has to distinguish between the hearing loss due to furosemide and that due to ethacrynic acid. If there is hearing loss caused by ethacrynic acid in most cases it is irreversible, and therefore we believe that ethacrynic acid no longer should be administered to older patients. Kidney function is ameliorated only for a short time by ethacrynic acid and then there is an additional loss of kidney function. Therefore, this diuretic should only be administered with caution. Loop diuretics of the furosemide type are preferable because their mode of action is now well established, whereas the action of ethacrynic acid in the cells of the kidney is still unclear. Furthermore, a reversible hearing loss occurs with furosemide only at very high intravenous doses. The reason for this side-effect is that furosemide has the same mode of action in the inner ear as in the kidney. The potassium content is altered in the inner ear fluid, changing the endocochlear potential.
Your second question concerned the interaction of aminoglycosides and loop diuretics of the furosemide type. We both know that a severe interaction may arise and that this interaction is most pronounced if there is a reduction in blood volume. If the patient's water intake and water loss are balanced, these severe interactions and side-effects are attenuated. The same holds true for the interaction of furosemide and cis-platinum.

Schlierf

Another severe interaction may occur between furosemide and nonsteroidal antiphlogistic drugs. I recall one patient in our hospital who was treated by the urologists: he had heart failure and was taking furosemide and they gave him high doses of nonsteroidal antiphlogistics to prevent edema in the area where surgery had been performed. This patient went into intractable heart failure and actually died.

Mutschler

I also remember a patient treated for endocarditis with aminoglycoside antibiotics. Concurrently he received indomethacin 200 mg/day and furosemide. The result was a total loss of hearing and acute renal failure. One of the reasons for this interaction was that nonsteroidal antirheumatics inhibit prostaglandin biosynthesis and therefore reduce renal blood flow.

Zeeh

There is still an ongoing discussion on whether routine potassium supplements are justified in patients under diuretic therapy with normal potassium levels at the onset of therapy. Could you comment on this?

Mutschler

We do not recommend potassium supplementation. If saluretics are given a loss of potassium with or without potassium supplement can occur. In such cases we prefer potassium-retaining diuretics. I believe it is much more logical to avoid potassium loss than to substitute potassium. In addition when patients are treated with low doses of saluretics, hypokalemia is seldom seen. In the MRFIT study the patients received a daily dose of 100 mg hydrochlorothiazide. This dose is 4–8 times too high. We recommend a maximum dosage of 25 mg/day for older as well as for younger patients. Increasing the dose does not produce further improvement of the effect because of the flat dose-response curve of thiazides.

Kennedy

One of the reasons why thiazides are perhaps meeting with less favor in the United States is the hypercholesterolemic effect and the increase in low density lipoproteins when they're used for hypertension. Would you still advocate their use as antihypertensive agents in middle-aged people and the young elderly, as opposed to the old elderly, where these risk factors are not so dominant?

Mutschler

First of all if the daily dose is reduced, the influence on lipid metabolism is minimal. Even with the doses used in the past, after 2 or 3 years of treatment the initial enhancement of lipids in the blood returned to pretreatment levels. Especially in combination with other antihypertensives, e.g., ACE inhibitors or beta-blockers, diuretics are still very useful drugs for treating hypertensive patients.

References

Abshagen U, Besenfelder E, Endele R, Koch K, Neubert B (1979) Kinetics of canrenone after single and multiple doses of spironolactone. Eur J Clin Pharmacol 16: 255–262

Abshagen U, Platt D, Horn HJ (1981) Zur Pharmakokinetik von Spironolacton im Alter. Klin Wochenschr 59: 909–910

Amery A, Brixko P, Clement D, et al. (1985) Mortality and morbidity results from the European working party on high blood pressure in the elderly trial. Lancet I: 1349–1354

Andreasen F, Hansen U, Husted SE, Mogensen CE, Pedersen EB (1984) The influence of age on renal and extrarenal effects of frusemide. BR J Clin Pharmacol 18: 65–74

Bertel O (1983) Neuere Aspekte der medikamentösen Behandlung von herzinsuffizienten Patienten. Schweiz Med Wochenschr 113: 739–745

Bolte HD (1982) Typische Risiken bei der Behandlung der chronischen Herzinsuffizienz. Internist 23: 133–137

Edmonds CJ, Jasani B (1972) Total body potassium in hypertensive patients during prolonged diuretic-therapy. Lancet I: 8–12

Empfehlung der Hochdruckliga (1987) Behandlung von Patienten mit milder Hypertonie. Münch Med Wochenschr 129: 92–95

Favre L, Glasson Ph, Riondel A, Vallotton MB (1983) Interaction of diuretics and non-steroidal anti-inflammatory drugs in man. Clin Sci 64: 407–415

Fleuren HLJM, van Rossum JM (1977) Nonlinear relationship between plasma and red blood cell pharmacokinetics of chlorthalidone in man. J Pharmcokinet Biopharm 5: 359–375

Ho PC, Bourne DWA, Triggs EJ, Smithurst BA (1984) Comparison of plasma levels of canrenone and metabolites after base hydrolysis in young and elderly subjects following single and multiple doses of spironolactone. Eur J Clin Pharmacol 27: 415–419

Hobbs DC, Twomey TM (1987) Kinetics of polythiazide. Clin Pharmacol Ther 23: 241–246

Hyams DE (1984) Drug usage by the elderly. In: Roe DA (ed) Drugs and nutrition in the geriatric patient. Churchill Livingstone, New York, pp 1–26

Hyams DE (1986) The elderly patient. A special case for diuretic therapy. Drugs 31 [Suppl 4]: 138–153

Hypertension Detection and Follow-up Program Results (1982) The effect of treatment on mortality in "mild" hypertension. N Engl J Med 307: 976–980

Kerremans Ad LM, van Baars YTH, van Ginneken CAM, Gribnan FWJ (1983) Furosemide kinetics and dynamics in aged patients. Clin Pharmacol Ther 34: 181–189

Knauf H, Mutschler E, Völger KD (1978) Pharmakologische Wirksamkeit von Phase-I- und Phase-II-Metaboliten des Triamteren. Arzneimittelforschung 28: 1417–1420

Knauf H, Reuter K, Mutschler E (1985) Limitation on the use of amiloride in early renal failure. Eur J Clin Pharmacol 28: 61–66

McCarthy ST (1982) Body fluid, electrolytes and diuretics. Curr Med Res Opin 7 [Suppl 1]: 87–95

McMahon FG (1984) Diuretics: the thiazide, thiazide-like, and loop diuretics. In: McMahon FG (ed) The management of essential hypertension: the new low dose era, 2nd edn. Futura, Mt. Kisco, New York, pp 75–155

Möhrke W, Mutschler E, Völger KD, Mühlberg W, Platt D (1983) Triamterene kinetics in the higher age. In: Platt E (ed) Cardiology and ageing. Schattauer, Stuttgart, pp 367–375

Neubig E, Mühlberg W, Platt D (1984) Furosemid-Pharmakokinetik bei geriatrischem multimorbiden Patienten. Z Gerontol 17: 251–260

Niemeyer C, Hasenfuß G, Wais U, Knauf H, Schäfer-Korting M, Mutschler E (1983) Pharmacokinetics of hydrochlorothiazide in relation to renal function. Eur J Clin Pharmacol 24: 661–665

Platt D, Abshagen U, Mühlberg W, Horn HJ, Schmitt-Ruth R, Vollmar J (1984) The influence of age and multimorbidity on the pharmacokinetics and metabolism of spironolactone. Arch Gerontol Geriatr 3: 147–159

Roos JP (1981) Behandlung der Herzinsuffizienz: Stimulation oder Herzentlastung? Therapiewoche 31: 4099–4104

Schüren KP (1982) Die Behandlung der Herzinsuffizienz mit Diuretika. In: Schaper W, Gottwik MG (ed) Fortschritte in der Kardiologie – Therapie der Myokardinsuffizienz – Reperfusion und Revaskularisation des Myokards. Steinkopff, Darmstadt, pp 124–138

The Australian Therapeutic Trial in Mild Hypertension (1980) Lancet I: 1261–1267

Traeger A, Oelzner P, Stein G (1984) Pharmakokinetik und diuretische Wirkung von Furosemid bei alten Menschen. Dt Gesundh Wesen 39: 956–960

Veterans Administration Cooperative Study Group on Antihypertensive Agents (1970) Effects of treatment on morbidity – II. Results in patients with diastolic blood pressure averaging 90 through 114 mmHg. Jama 213: 1143–1152

Veterans Administration Cooperative Study Group Antihypertensive Agents (1972) Influence of age, diastolic pressure and prior cardiovasular disease; further analysis of side effects. Circulation 45: 991–1004

Weinberg MS, Cenigg RJ, Salant DJ, Bernard DB (1985) Anuric renal failure precipitated by indomethacin and triamterene. Nephron 40: 216–218

Prevention and Rehabilitation

Role of the Day Hospital in Rehabilitation and Resettlement at Home

J.C. BROCKLEHURST

Geriatric day hospitals are gradually becoming a recognised part of geriatric practice throughout the world, having being pioneered in the United Kingdom. The first purpose-built day hospital was at Cowley Road Hospital, Oxford, where the emphasis was on the management of confused old people.

In the United Kingdom there are now 600 consultant physicians in geriatric medicine and a further 150 in psychogeriatrics. The geriatric hospital services are based on health districts with an average population ob about 250 000 people. Each district supports a geriatric service and a psychogeriatric service and each of these is now linked with a separate day hospital. The psychogeriatric day hospital is particularly concerned with respite care of old people with dementia, thus sharing their management with relatives. Geriatric day hospitals, on the other hand, have their major concern with old people who are physically disabled (although inevitably many of them also have symptoms of confusion).

The day hospital is situated either in a general hospital or in a specialised geriatric hospital. Patients are brought in by ambulance transport in the morning, have a midday meal and go home in the afternoon. The average day hospital has rather fewer than 40 places. Most patients attend only 1 day a week, but others attend more frequently and the average weekly attendance is rather fewer than 100 patients. Day hospitals are run in parallel with social day centres. The latter, however, are part of the social services of the local municipality, whereas the day hospital is part of the district health service within the National Health Service. The day hospital is staffed with doctors, nurses, therapists and social workers. The social day centre has no professional staff (other than possibly a social worker). Its role is social and recreational whereas that of the day hospital is therapeutic.

The day hospital is managed rather like a hospital ward. All patients are examined by the physician on first attendance and then reviewed at a case conference every 2 or 3 weeks. Case conferences are attended by the rehabilitation team, chaired by the geriatrician. Patients' progress is reviewed, altering treatment programmes where necessary, and leading to ultimate discharge with the possibility of transferring to a social day centre for further recreational purposes.

[1] University of Manchester, Department of Geriatric Medicine, University Hospital of South Manchester, Nell Lane, Manchester M20 8LR, UK

Gerontology
Ed. by D. Platt
© Springer-Verlag Berlin Heidelberg 1989

About 50% of the patients attending the average day hospital have been in-patients and the other 50% come to the day hospital without the need for admission. In the latter case part of the intention is to avoid the necessity of admission as an in-patient.

The most common diagnosis for a day hospital referral is stroke (37%), followed by arthritis (22%), Parkinsonism (4.5%), amputation, paraplegia and dementia (each 4%), depression (3.5%) and respiratory disorder (3%) (Brocklehurst and Tucker 1980).

Patients attend a geriatric day hospital for one or more of five main reasons as follows:

1. Rehabilitation (this may start at 3–5 days weekly and gradually be diminished until rehabilitation is complete)
2. Physical maintenance following rehabilitation to monitor progress and prevent deterioration (this often on a once weekly attendance)
3. Special care of physically disabled old people (respite care)
4. Medical and nursing procedures
5. Functional assessment

Table 1 shows the reason for attendance at the time of first referral to the day hospital and this is compared with the reason for attendance of a cross-section of 233 patients actually attending. The differences between the two columns are the changes in reason for attendance between first attendance and a later date during attendance. It is seen that more than half are referred for rehabilitation and 12% for maintenance, whereas a cross-section of those attending indicates fewer for rehabilitation and more for maintenance. Similarly, there are more for social attendances and none for assessment since assessment is only likely to involve one or two attendances. At all times, however, rehabilitation predominates as the major function of the day hospital.

Patients may be referred from a variety of hospital wards (acute and rehabilitation geriatric wards, orthopaedic wards, surgical wards). In-patients are most likely to be referred for continuing rehabilitation on the understanding that this allows earlier discharge from hospital than might otherwise be possible. Those referred for maintenance and social reasons come in for supervision in an endeavour to prevent breakdown following discharge. The extent to which the day

Table 1. Geriatric day hospital patients: main reason for attendance (Brocklehurst and Tucker 1980)

	At referral (n = 456)	Cross-section of attendees (n = 233)
Rehabilitation	54%	43%
Maintenance	12%	21%
Medical-nursing	9%	19%
Social-relief	5%	17%
Assessment	20%	–

Table 2. Arrangements following in-patient discharge (n = 267) (Andrews and Brocklehurst 1987)

No follow-up	39%
Outpatient clinic	21%
Day hospital	33%
Relief admission	5%

hospital serves for this purpose in the UK is shown in Table 2, which shows the follow-up arrangements made for 267 patients discharged from 54 geriatric units during a 2-week period. This shows that one-third of patients discharged from geriatric units in the UK attend the day hospital for a period of follow-up and, as was seen from Table 1, this is partly for continuing rehabilitation and partly for maintenance and social reasons.

Thus in Great Britain the geriatric day hospital plays a prominent role both in rehabilitation and in the attempt to facilitate discharge and prevent readmission to hospital. Unfortunately, no scientific studies have been undertaken comparing the effectiveness of this management with a controlled group who do not attend the day hospital. This is the kind of research which is difficult to undertake in relation to a service which is well established. In an area where a day hospital is being newly opened it could be possible to do a comparative trial with a similar service without a day hospital.

Discussion

Schlierf

Just a brief comment. Four years ago we set up a day hospital in Heidelberg and there was no difficulty at all within the German medical system. The only difficulty which we experienced concerned transport to and from the hospital and this is probably the main difficulty with all day hospitals. I think, as you said, that the communication between the hospital and practising physician is very important; it's even more important in our setting, because we don't have a geriatrician who can go out and continue the care. But on the other hand this lack of a geriatrician gives rise to the need for contact with the admitting physician, the family physician; it gives us the chance to disseminate the idea of geriatric medicine and to provide physicians with some knowledge about drug treatment in the elderly, possibilities of maintaining rehabilitation, and so forth. So I think the day hospital can be used in Germany just as well and we are grateful for what we can learn from Great Britain.

Blaschke

What is your average census? How many patients would attend your facility on a day-to-day basis? What would be the approximate staff ratio of nurses, physicians, social workers, and so forth for the unit you described?

Brocklehurst

Well let me just give you a few figures. We run a geriatric service which is based at the moment on 230 beds in a general hospital of 1400 beds altogether. We serve a catchment area of 220000 people, of whom 15% are over the age of 65. Our average attendance at the day hospital is about 30 people a day from their own homes. And as I mentioned, the average length of attendance is about 17 different days. Those are the numbers of patients coming. As far as staff is concerned, our department operates on three clinical teams. So we have three consultants each with the junior staff, and so the 230 beds are divided by three and the day hospital is divided into three. Thus each of us has a day hospital clinic, which may have about 40 different patients. Some of them are only attending 1 day a week, some of them twice a week. In each team headed by a consultant, there would be one social worker for the inpatients and the day hospital patients. There would be one physiotherapist for the inpatients and one physiotherapist for the day hospital patients, one occupational therapist for each group and half a speech therapist, I suppose, for the whole lot. And then there are auxiliaries, untrained aides to all of these people.

Blaschke

I presume that the continuity you mentioned before is a consequence of the fact that the same two or three consultants who are working in the inpatient geriatric wards are also attending the outpatient day-care facilities and trying to coordinate their patients' visits on the days that they are in the day-care facility.

Brocklehurst

Each consultant has his own patients and he sees them in the acute wards on his ward rounds. He sees them in the rehabilitation wards on a case conference; he sees them in the day hospital on a case conference and he has a outpatient clinic as well. In addition he occasionally may be asked to do a domiciliary consultation. The patients he sees at home may be the same patients; but if he sees somebody at home and takes them on for treatment then they would remain with him throughout the whole course of treatment.

References

Andrews K, Brocklehurst JC (1987) British geriatric medicine in the 1980s. King Edward's Hospital Fund for London

Brocklehurst JC, Tucker JS (1980) Progress in geriatric day care. King Edward's Hospital Fund for London

Geriatric Rehabilitation – The Present State and Further Developments

J. RUSTEMEYER[1]

Geriatric rehabilitation is the basic term for a whole series of procedures attempting to improve the health and social setting of older people who are ill and/or disabled. As a clinician, I shall dwell on those aspects with which I deal daily in my work as chief physician of a geriatric rehabilitation hospital. A geriatric rehabilitation hospital in West Germany is a special hospital for older patients with the task of providing both geriatric general care and specific measures for chlinical rehabilitation. These hospitals are subdivided into:

1. Geriatric rehabilitation hospitals for acute care with an average hospital stay of about 40 days
2. Geriatric rehabilitation hospitals for longer term patients with an average stay exceeding 60 days

I shall limit my remarks to the geriatric rehabilitation hospitals for acute care.

The reduction in the total population of Europe as well as in that of West Germany, which resulted in a larger percentage of older people, led to empty beds in general hospitals and to a severe shortage of hospital beds in the geriatric hospitals. This led to a trend toward the use of older, dilapidated general hospitals for geriatric care, in accordance with the saying "the old belongs to the old." [In 1977 50% of the German geriatric hospital buildings had been constructed prior to 1918 (Clemens 1979)].

Because of this undesirable trend there are now some geriatric hospitals which do not really qualify for definition as such. Obviously, good geriatric rehabilitation, more than other medical disciplines, requires top quality as regards size of buildings and available equipment. Buildings used for geriatric rehabilitation must be designed to deal with:

1. The high average age of patients (73 years)
2. Multiple illnesses (four or five illnesses at once)
3. Mental impairment

Therefore, the geriatric rehabilitation buildings must provide:

1. Easy orientation

[1] Klinik für medizinische Rehabilitation und Geriatrie, Schwemannstr. 19, D-3000 Hannover 71 / FRG

Gerontology
Ed. by D. Platt
© Springer-Verlag Berlin Heidelberg 1989

2. Good lighting
3. Firm floors (avoiding slipping)
4. Wheelchair access
5. Automatic door openers
6. A large number of elevators (which can be serviced easily)
7. Extremely safe stairs
8. Control of doors to the outside

The use of wheelchairs requires larger rooms compared to conventional hospitals (Table 1).

In addition, rooms are needed for speech therapists, psychologists, and social workers, as well as for therapeutic baths and mobile occupational therapy. The rooms needed for toilets and baths also exceed what is required in a general hospital, since 75% of patients in geriatric hospitals require assistance with their bodily care (in the hospital in Hannover the figure is 40% – 50%). Older hospital buildings therefore rarely permit ideal geriatric care.

Recently I studied the present requirements for an ideal rehabilitation hospital (Rustemeyer 1988). In the course of my studies I found that only 40% of German geriatric rehabilitation hospitals satisfy the requirements for ideal area (size) and equipment. (Behrends in 1973, Clemens in 1979, and Rembeck in 1988 reached similar conclusions.)

Table 2 shows the average staffing levels for a group of recognized German rehabilitation hospitals, while Table 3 shows figures based on a review of 13

Table 1. Space required – a comparison between geriatric rehabilitation hospitals and general hospitals

	Geriatric rehabilitation hospitals	General hospitals
Bed area	14.2 m^2/inpatient	10.0 m^2/inpatient
Physiotherapy	2.5 m^2/inpatient	0.38 m^2/inpatient
Occupational therapy	2.3 m^2/inpatient	0.37 m^2/inpatient

Table 2. Average number of inpatients per member of staff in clinical geriatric rehabilitation units in West Germany

Physician	1:12.6
Physiotherapist	1:13.0
Occupational therapist	1:15.0
Speech therapist	1:41.7
Masseur	1:72.2
Social worker	1:91.3
Psychologist	1:105
Mobile occupational therapist	1:105
Nurse	1:2.0

Table 3. Number of beds and staff-inpatient ratios in 13 West German geriatric hospitals

Hospitals	1	2	3	4	5	6	7	8	9	10	11	12	13
Number of beds	84	125	64	105	120	80	96	105	130	103	81	42	82
Staff member – inpatient ratios													
Physician	1:16.6	1:15.4	*1:10.6*	*1:12.3*	1:20.0	*1:10.0*	1:16.0	*1:11.6*	1:21.6	*1:13.7*	*1:10.1*	*1:10.5*	*1:12.5*
Nurse	*1:2.0*	*1:2.3*	*1:1.5*	1:2.8	*1:2.0*	1:2.5	1:2.5	*1:2.3*	1:2.8	*1:2.0*	1:2.6	1:3.4	*1:2.1*
Physiotherapist	1:27.0	1:16.6	1:32.0	1:26.2	1:120	1:26.6	1:16.0	*1:11.6*	1:43.3	*1:14.7*	*1:12.4*	1:21.0	1:36.2
Occupational therapist	1:27.0	1:50.0	1:64.0	1:35.0	*1:17.1*	0	1:48.0	*1:16.7*	1:52.0	*1:17.1*	*1:10.8*	1:42.0	1:62.1
Speech therapist	1:54.0	1:150	0	0	*1:40.0*	1:160	0	1:52.5	*1:43.3*	*1:34.3*	*1:40.5*	0	1:94.0
Masseur	*1:54.0*	*1:60.0*	*1:64.0*	*1:42.0*	*1:12.0*	0	*1:32.0*	1:105	*1:32.5*	*1:41.2*	*1:82.0*	0	0
Social worker	1:270	*1:100*	0	1:131.2	1:120	0	*1:96.0*	*1:105*	1:960	1:128	*1:40.5*	0	0
Psychologist	0	0	1:320	0	0	0	0	*1:105*	0	*1:128*	*1:81.0*	0	0
Mobile occupational Therapist	0	0	0	0	0	0	0	*1:105*	0	0	*1:81.0*	0	0

German geriatric hospitals by Meier-Baumgartner, published in 1988. As Table 3 suggests, only a few of the geriatric hospitals satisfy quality requirements (see the italicized numbers!). The table furthermore shows that only eight hospitals have a physician-to-patient ratio of about 1:12.6. The situation is worse as regards the nursing staff, (only seven hospitals meet the requirements), and worse still in respect of physiotherapists, occupational therapists, and speech therapists. German rehabilitation hospitals seem to do better with massage therapists. Social work and psychology fare poorly. Only two institutions provide a department of *mobile* occupational therapy, i.e. a department which sends a worker to the house or apartment of patients to inspect their homes and recommend adaptation. To summarize the Figures , only 44 of my 117 quality demands are being met, which is 37.6%.

Staffing requirements are, of course, modified by the conditions and experiences at each geriatric rehabilitation hospital. For instance, a hospital such as that in Hannover with a high percentage of stroke patients needs more speech therapists than does a hospital with fewer stroke patients. The optimal size for a geriatric rehabilitation hospital appears to be about 100 beds (80 – 120). This seems to be the size of all the institutions in the Meier-Baumgartner 1988 survey, previously mentioned.

So much for the present condition of geriatric acute-care rehabilitation hospitals in West Germany. Rembeck found in 1988 that in Switzerland, Great Britain, and Scandinavia, the present need for geriatric rehabilitative care is about equal to the care offered. This is true in West Germany in certain high density populated areas, but not for the whole of the country. Therefore, West Germany continues to have a shortage of geriatric hospital beds (while Great Britain plans for 82 000 beds by 1990).

In 1979 I found a need for 50 beds for a population of 100 000. Translated to the whole of West Germany, this would mean a total geriatric bed requirement of 31 000. In 1988 Rembeck postulated a need for 39 900 beds. There are currently 14 800 geriatric beds available in West Germany (Fr. Dr. Dieck, Deutsches Zentrum f. Altersfragen, personal communication, 1988). When only the approved institutions which nearly meet the aforementioned criteria are considered, only 10% of the need is being met.

Because of this, the bulk of our old patients who require institutional geriatric rehabilitation find themselves in acute regular hospitals, where their treatment is lacking in terms of the specifics of geriatric care as well as not being cost-efficient. According to data from the German Hospital Institute, 28.7% of the acute hospital beds were occupied by geriatric patients in 1983 (Rembeck 1988). If it is agreed that perhaps half of this group would have done better in special geriatric rehabilitation hospitals, we reach the postulated total of 30 000 – 40 000. A corresponding percentage of present regular acute hospital beds should be converted to regular geriatric rehabilitation beds for medical, economic, and humanitarian reasons. The longer average hospital stay of a geriatric patient in a nongeriatric acute care hospital increases the cost without benefit. Since the geriatric patient has multiple illnesses, he or she does not fit the present pattern of acute care hospitals, which are arranged by specialities and subspecialities.

To summarize; the present state of geriatric rehabilitation in West Germany is characterized by:

1. A shortfall in the number of both geriatric rehabilitative institutions and number of beds
2. Insufficient support countrywide to establish further geriatric rehabilitative institutions (in some of our districts such institutions even receive no mention in the district-wide need plan, an exception being Nordrhein-Westfalen, which has an excellent plan)
3. Lack of professionally qualified personnel, due to an insufficient number of training places in gerontology for initial training as well as for continued education.

This lack of opportunity for training is apparent both at the medical school level as well as at the paramedical schools for physiotherapy, occupational therapy, speech therapy, and nursing. At present, in 1988, we have only *one* German medical school which has a formal department for gerontology (the department of Prof. Platt). This is in contrast to France, Belgium, the Netherlands, Denmark, Sweden, and Great Britain. Italy, in 1971, already had six such departments. All these countries recognize a specialist for geriatrics who requires a specialized training period of 4 – 7 years (an EEC recommendation), which underscores the amount of specialized knowledge needed.

The lack of training in geriatric rehabilitation in medical and paramedical schools forces the geriatric rehabilitation hospitals in West Germany to resort to on-the-job training. Obviously, such methods are troublesome and poorly coordinated. At present there are only two German formal training centers for geriatric rehabilitation, the Albertine House in Hamburg and the geriatric rehabilitation hospital at the Henrietten Foundation in Hannover, under my direction. Both institutions provide a 1-year course, with both didactic and practical application aspects. They end with formal examinations, after which a certificate is awarded.

The urgent need for both more geriatric rehabilitation beds and more geriatric rehabilitation personnel in Germany is illustrated by the fact that the German geriatric rehabilitation hospitals have a bed occupancy rate of 96.5% while the overall German hospital average is 85% . Most geriatric rehabilitation hospitals are plagued by long waiting lists; our patients presently wait 5 weeks.

In spite of the deficiencies, the standard of German geriatric rehabilitation seems higher than the international average: The percentage of inpatients who return to their homes after rehabilitation at German geriatric hospitals ranges from 62% to 90% with a mean of 77% (Rembeck 1988). The rate for the Hannover hospital is 82%. The international average is 75%. [Those hospitals with lower rates of return to normal life-style (between 62% and 67%) are those with the worst space conditions and the worst overall personnel situation (Meier-Baumgartner 1988).]

The transfer rate from German geriatric rehabilitation hospitals to nursing homes is presently 5.4% , with a range from 4.5% to 7.2% (Rembeck 1988). The average lenght of stay for inpatients in geriatric rehabilitation hospitals is 39.5

days in Germany (Meier-Baumgartner 1988), 40 days in Austria (Lachnit 1983), and 46 days in Great Britain, according to Professor Brocklehurst.

The improvement both in diagnostic methods and in treatment methods has raised the international standard of present-day geriatric rehabilitation considerably. In this respect one need mention only the modern imaging techniques and improved techniques for cardiovascular and orthopedic surgery. The improved climate in our specialty, of course, leads to an increased number of patients who qualify for geriatric rehabilitation. Institutions and especially funds and resources cannot keep pace with this development, at least not in West Germany. I consider it an urgent requirement that we look for new ways and means of allowing a larger segment of our population access to geriatric rehabilitation, in the sense of both individual help and a reduction in the social and economic burdens that often accompany old age. This, however, requires a greater number of specialist geriatric rehabilitation units and, to relieve them of less ill patients, a greater number of geriatric day hospitals, which is being pioneered by Professor Brocklehurst. In West Germany considerably more effort needs to be devoted to outpatient geriatric rehabilitation at day care facilities and to home visits for geriatric domiciliary rehabilitation. Again, such expansion is hindered by the lack of physicians and paramedical personnel. The German system of service reimbursement has, for instance, not established a satisfactory fee schedule for outpatient occupational therapy, and occupational therapists are therefore found only in hospitals.

There are four significant advantages of geriatric rehabilitation at the patient's home:

1. The therapist diagnoses the problems and treats the patient on the spot.
2. The older patient does not lose his habitual environment and there are consequently less problems with disorientation.
3. The treatment is cheaper than in hospitals.
4. Domiciliary rehabilitation relieves geriatric hospitals.

Especially with clear orders from the general practitioner plus coordination of therapeutic, nursing, and rehabilitation measures, home care can provide a significant measure of rehabilitation services for older patients.

Below I shall discuss practical step-by-step geriatric rehabilitation procedures as practiced in Hannover at present. Figure 1 deals with only two areas of our work, namely physiotherapy and occupational therapy, in order to point out the close relationship between these two areas.

Upon admission 90% of patients are bedridden. In such cases we at once start with early mobilization. Both physiotherapists and occupational therapists work together on this. Even at an early stage some of the occupational therapy exercises involve training for self-help and daily living. As the patient progresses, physiotherapy will entail sitting and standing exercises. Daily living exercises, in occupational therapy, deal with eating, washing, and dressing. The first walking exercises are often very difficult, requiring two or three therapists at the same time.

As the patient improves his walking, occupational therapy involves activity in the hospital's adjustable practice kitchen and in the practice bathroom, with emphasis being placed on what needs adapting to fit the patient's disability. At

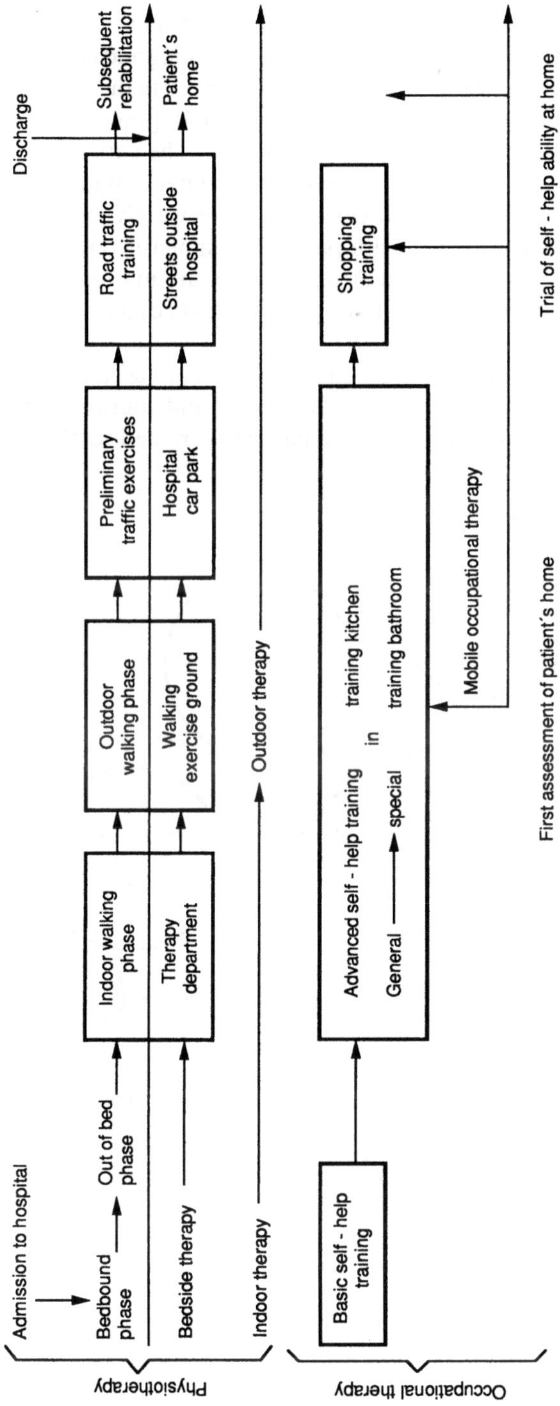

Fig. 1. The treatment phases in geriatric rehabilitation

this point, a mobile occupational therapist visits the patient's home, usually together with the physiotherapist. Emphasis is now shifted to goal-directed rehabilitation, which means that all further exercises focus on the return of the patient to his actual home. Once the patient more or less masters safe walking and climbing stairs in the geriatric hospital setting, walking exercises will be given in the outdoor walking exercise area using paths made from paving stones, sand, gravel, and so on, some of which have gradients, or stairs without rail support. The patient must regain the courage and confidence to leave his home environment. With some patients, we add exercises within the hospital car park. Here we give patients practice at being passengers in a car or bus, with particular emphasis on getting in and out of the vehicle. Once entering and leaving a vehicle are mastered, the patient and his therapist go to a normal street. Each patient practices individually how to cross the street and to use transport safely.

The next step is called "city training." The occupational therapist accompanies the patient shopping, allowing a gradual return of confidence and courage, e.g., when dealing with sales staff. At the same time the patient is trained to choose

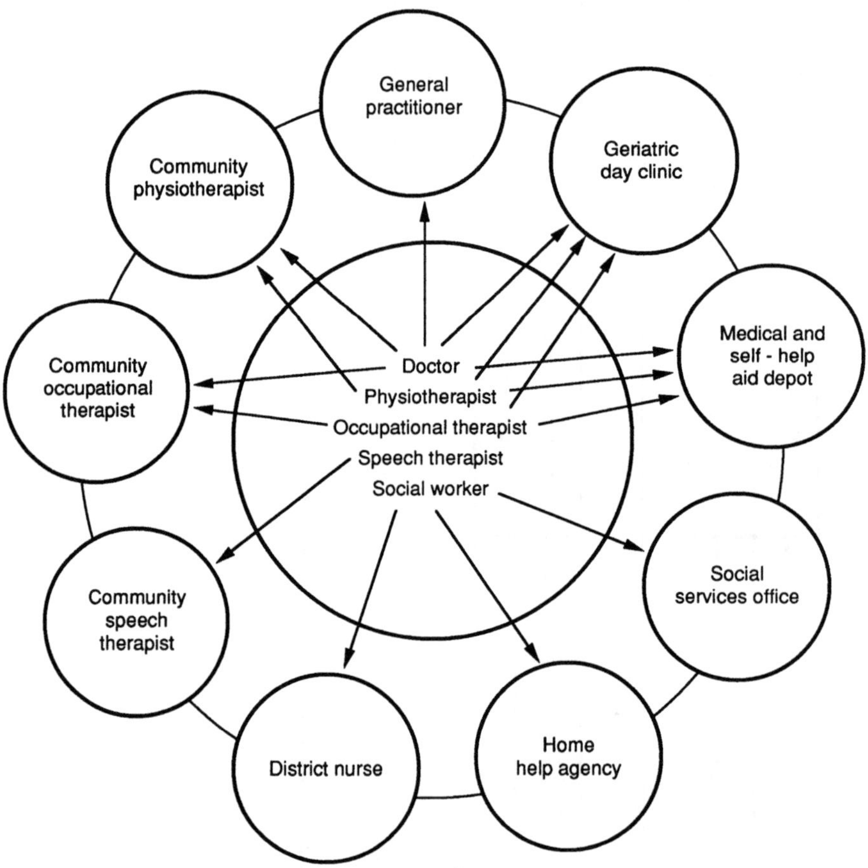

Fig. 2. The geriatric rehabilitation clinic and its cooperation with other agencies

the most appropriate food and the most suitable clothes. Finally, the patient, together with his mobile occupational therapist, spends some time "test-living at home." Attention is paid to all important steps and procedures. This is the time when changes and adaptations in the home can be proposed by the therapist, such as guard rails, special holding rails, and various devices. A decision is then made on what else is needed and the duration of the required treatment. Continued treatment at a day hospital may be considered. If necessary, "test-living at home" is repeated a second time. Assuming that the patient does well during the test-living at home phase, he or she is discharged from the hospital but is not abandoned. Within 1–4 days after hospital discharge, the mobile occupational therapist visits the patient at home again, to clear up any problems which have occurred. If necessary, the mobile occupational therapist continues to treat the patient at home, until self-reliance and reintegration have reached their optimal state. Moreover, the hospital rehabilitation team will have prepared plans for the continuation of the rehabilitative care of discharged patients at their homes, by involving all members of an outdoor team of the residential district of each patient (Fig. 2).

The method described has allowed us to achieve a reintegration rate of 82% for our inpatients, reducing repeat admissions – the so-called revolving-door patients – to 3%. To repeat, as far as we are concerned geriatric rehabilitation does not stop with hospital discharge but is continued as needed at the day hospital or at home.

Future developments should involve increasing our outpatient geriatric rehabilitation, both at home and at day hospitals, allowing us to shorten the period of hospital rehabilitation or – in many cases – to avoid it altogether.

Discussion

Brocklehurst

In your rehabilitation hospital do you transfer patients from other hospitals or are they nearly all admitted directly from home?

Rustemeyer

About 60% come from other hospitals and about 40% from home – we are the acute form of rehabilitation hospital.

Brocklehurst

When you say that there are 29% acute beds occupied by geriatric patients, do you mean that these are patients awaiting rehabilitation or are these patients who are needing nursing home care?

Rustemeyer

Both.

Brocklehurst

One of the current developments in the UK within geriatric rehabilitation is the creation of a number of specialist rehabilitation words for stroke rehabilitation and for fracture of the neck of the femur. The latter is called the "ortho" geriatric rehabilitation unit. And we have found especially for stroke, which is such a complex illness, that to have a specialist team managing the rehabilitation of stroke patients is an advantage. I wonder whether in your acute hospitals, where probably quite a lot of stroke patients are awaiting rehabilitation, it might not be possible to set up a small stroke rehabilitation unit actually within the hospital.

Rustemeyer

We intend to do that in the near future.

Beischer

What are the conditions of admission to your hospital?

Rustemeyer

The normal conditions which apply to every hospital. We need a referral from a general practitioner, and our costs are met by each of the health insurance companies in the Federal Republic. The system is just the same as in every other hospital.

Beischer

You don't cover the entire field of geriatric acute care; rather you select your patients according to their capacity for rehabilitation? This seems to be the big difference from England. In England geriatrics is practiced as a unit comprising acute care, rehabilitation, and day hospital; in contrast here the structures are quite distinct, many factors admittedly playing a role in this situation. I think that in the Federal Republic rehabilitative measures tend to be taken in specialist geriatric hospitals.

Rustemeyer

Yes, that is correct. Normally we do not accept cases that require intensive care, although we do have the necessary facilities. However, we do attach importance to patients coming to us directly after they have overcome this acute phase, which still requires intensive care.

Beischer

Mental disturbed patients are not admitted at all; this really limits the situation from my point of view.

Rustemeyer

Yes, that's right. Our hospital is open and unprotected; for this reason alone there are juridical grounds for not admitting disoriented patients, namely the danger that they will abscond. This does, however, constitute a sensitive restriction.

Vömel

I have a question concerning the number of physicians and physiotherapists. I think you presented the ideal figures and not the normal ones. For acute hospital therapy the accepted physician/patient ratio is 1:17 and the physiotherapist/patient ratio, 1:65. The ratios for more chronic rehabilitation are 1:40 and 1:24 respectively.

Rustemeyer

We must distinguish between general geriatric hospital which cater predominantly for internal medical care, and rehabilitative geriatric hospitals which concentrate overwhelmingly on clinical rehabilitative therapy. The acute form of rehabilitation hospital requires a certain physician/patient ratio, as I have indicated.

Vömel

In a rehabilitation hospital that is run in accordance with § 184a RVO, the physician/patient ratio is 1:40 – at least, this is the case in North Rhine-Westphalia.

Rustemeyer

There are no guidelines on ratios in geriatric clinical rehabilitation. In West Germany "geriatrics" is broken down only into "general geriatrics" and "acute level geriatrics." Rehabilitative measures are taken in both areas. The clinical facilities for geriatric rehabilitation that I have described in my presentation relate to the acute level and are staffed with the physician and physiotherapist to patient ratios that I have cited. In my opinion a worse ratio would make it impossible to carry out clinical rehabilitation within an average time span of ca. 42 days.

References

Behrends H (1973) Rehabilitation im Alter. Acta Gerontol 3: 493–497

Clemens W (1979) Analyse klinischer geriatrischer Einrichtungen in der BRD. Deutsches Zentrum f. Altersfragen, Berlin

Lachnit K (1983) Möglichkeiten der Rehabilitation im geriatrischen Krankenhaus und in geriatrischen Pflegehäusern. Österr Krankenhauszeitung 24: 279–282

Meier-Baumgartner HP (1988) Übersicht über geriatrische Kliniken und Tageskliniken in Deutschland. Z Gerontol 1: 28–32

Rembeck W (1988) Die geriatrische Klinik. KDA Forum, Köln

Rustemeyer J (1988) Organisation und Durchführung der klinischen Rehabilitation im Spezialkrankenhaus. Z Gerontol 5

Subject Index

The international standard

D. Platt, University of Erlangen-Nuremberg (Ed.)

Geriatrics 1

Cardiology and Vascular System Central Nervous System

1982. XXII, 488 pp. 88 figs. Hardcover
ISBN 3-540-10981-1

"This volume is an excellent contribution to geriatric medicine. It is well written, the illustrations are of high quality, the references extensive, and the subject index is comprehensive. **I recommend it highly to both practitioners and specialists in the field.**" *Journal of Gerontology*

D. Platt, University of Erlangen-Nuremberg (Ed.)

Geriatrics 2

Digestive System – Endocrine System – Kidney and Urogenital System – Haematological System – Respiratory System – Rehabilitation – Nutrition – Drug Treatment

1983. XXIII, 490 pp. 67 figs. Hardcover
ISBN 3-540-10982-X

"Undoubtedly an authoritative, well written, comprehensive text of this sort should prove a great asset in a library of a geriatric department. When faced with a difficult case, or the need arises to review a particular topic, this is an excellent text to turn to for the required information, as well as for introduction to the relevant literature." *Gerontology*

D. Platt, University of Erlangen-Nuremberg (Ed.)

Geriatrics 3

Gynecology – Orthopaedics – Anesthesiology – Surgery – Otorhinolaryngology – Ophthalmology – Dermatology

1984. XXIV, 482 pp. 150 figs. Hardcover
ISBN 3-540-12220-6

"This book is recommended to all those interested in obtaining complete information about the various aspects of geriatrics in surgical disciplines." *ORL*

Springer-Verlag Berlin
Heidelberg New York London
Paris Tokyo Hong Kong

Springer

D. Platt, University of Erlangen-Nuremberg (Ed.)

Drugs and Aging

1986. XI, 216 pp. 105 figs. 49 tabs. Hardcover
ISBN 3-540-15913-4

Gerontological research is necessary to obtain optimal information and thus ensure proper drug therapy for the elderly.
The contributions compiled in this book cover drug actions and interactions at the molecular, cellular, organic, and organismic level. They are based on the lectures and discussions of the 2nd international Erlangen-Nuremberg Symposium on Experimental Gerontology in which many distinguished scientists in the fields of biology, biochemistry, pharmacology, pathology, and medicine participated.
This book will expand the knowledge of drug therapy in the elderly and will provide a firm foundation for future work on clinical and experimental pharmacology in the aged.

D. Platt, University of Erlangen-Nuremberg (Ed.)

Blood Cells, Rheology, and Aging

1988. XII, 217 pp. 67 figs. 47 tabs. Hardcover
ISBN 3-540-17401-X

This volume on experimental gerontology deals with the effects of aging on blood cells and rheology. Since gerontology is an interdisciplinary science, numerous experts engaged in various disciplines present their up-to-date results related to aging.
The detailed accounts compiled in this book will augment the knowledge of red cells, immunology, receptors, blood coagulation, and rheology. The volume provides a valuable basis for future scientific work in gerontological research.

Springer-Verlag
Berlin Heidelberg
New York London Paris
Tokyo Hong Kong

Springer

MIX
Papier aus verantwortungsvollen Quellen
Paper from responsible sources
FSC® C105338

FSC
www.fsc.org

If you have any concerns about our products,
you can contact us on
ProductSafety@springernature.com

In case Publisher is established outside the EU,
the EU authorized representative is:
Springer Nature Customer Service Center GmbH
Europaplatz 3, 69115 Heidelberg, Germany

Printed by Libri Plureos GmbH
in Hamburg, Germany

Criminal Justice
Recent Scholarship

Edited by
Marilyn McShane and Frank P. Williams III

A Series from LFB Scholarly

54692215
02/07

CAMERON UNIVERSITY LIBRARY
2800 W. GORE BLVD.
LAWTON, OK 73505-6377

KF
1307
.A97
2004

Police Accountability, Risk Management, and Legal Advising

Carol A. Archbold

LFB Scholarly Publishing LLC
New York 2004

Copyright © 2004 by LFB Scholarly Publishing LLC

All rights reserved.

Library of Congress Cataloging-in-Publication Data

Archbold, Carol.
Police accountability, risk management, and legal advising / Carol A. Archbold.
p. cm. -- (Criminal justice)
Includes bibliographical references and index.
ISBN 1-59332-038-8 (acid-free paper)
1. Tort liability of police--United States. 2. Police legal advisors--United States. 3. Police misconduct--United States. 4. Risk management--United States. I. Title. II. Series: Criminal justice (LFB Scholarly Publishing LLC)
KF1307.A97 2004
344.7305'2--dc22

2004005486

ISBN 1-59332-038-8

Printed on acid-free 250-year-life paper.

Manufactured in the United States of America.

Table of Contents

Acknowledgements

I would like to thank all of the law enforcement agencies that participated in this study. The completion of this research project would not have been possible without their cooperation. I am especially grateful to all of the people that took time out of their busy schedules to allow me to visit their agencies. Those individuals include: Roger Haven and Michael Palmer of the Police Liability Management Division of the Portland Police Bureau; Michael Stairiker of the Bureau of Risk Management for the city of Portland; Lt. Scott Johnson and Lori Douglas from the Los Angeles Sheriffs Department; Kevin Brazile of the Legal Advisory Unit for the County of Los Angeles; Lt. Ted Moody and Trish Diamond from the Risk Management Division of the Las Vegas Metropolitan Police Department; Walt Cannon of Rawlings, Olson, Cannon, Gormley, & Desruisseaux; Deputy District Attorney Mitch Cohen of Las Vegas; Judy Pitts of the Risk Management Office for Charlotte-Mecklenburg, and Mark Newbold, police attorney for the Charlotte-Mecklenburg Police Department.

I am grateful to the Dean of the Arts and Sciences, Dr. Michael McKinney, for providing me with summer support to continue working on this book. I am also grateful for the travel funds and research support awarded to me from the Committee on Research in the Office of Research and Sponsored Programs. My fellow colleagues in the Social and Cultural Sciences Department have also provided unending support and encouragement as I was writing this book (thanks Melissa, Jane, Mary Ann and Jim). A special thanks to Dr. Melissa Schrift for reviewing an early draft of this book.

I would also like to thank my mentor and friend, Dr. Samuel Walker of the University of Nebraska-Omaha. During the time that I worked with Sam, I learned how important it is to believe wholeheartedly in every research project that I decide to take on. Sam's numerous projects and writings on police accountability issues have inspired me to explore similar issues. The completion of this research project, and ultimately, this book would not have been possible without Dr. Walker's support and advice.

And finally, I would like to thank my husband Jason for his patience and understanding during the time that I was working on this research project and book. Your support means the world to me.

A Foreword *by Dr. Samuel Walker*

This book represents a pioneering exploration of important but largely neglected aspects of policing and police accountability. The problem of police misconduct has been with us since the first American police departments were established about 170 years ago. Use of excessive force, unjustifiable fatal shootings of citizens, and other acts of misconduct continue to plague our society. They are also an important part of the racial and ethnic tensions that pervade our communities. While we have long known that these problems exist, we have only recently begun to address them in a serious fashion.

The question before us is not whether we should do something about police misconduct, but which remedy or combination of remedies is most effective. In recent years we have made significant progress in developing administrative controls over police use of force and other aspects of policing that pose a threat to the life, liberty, and well being of citizens. We have also developed a new tool, early intervention systems, to identify patterns of misconduct and do something about them. Finally, new forms of citizen oversight are bringing an important element of external citizen perspective to misconduct issues.

This book explores two important but long neglected accountability mechanisms. As Carol Archbold's research indicates, the concept of police legal advisors first appeared more than thirty years ago. But as she explains, the idea never fully developed. At the same time, the idea of risk management is well established in other areas of American life, particularly private industry and health care. But it has never taken hold in American policing.

Carol Archbold's book is an important contribution to the literature on police accountability. It not only explains the concepts of police legal advisors and risk management, but also provides valuable data on what mechanisms currently exist in American police departments - and even more important, what does not exist. I fully expect that this pioneering work will spark a new body of research and policy development in policing. And I also expect that the resulting policy developments will make a significant contribution to the professionalization of the American police.

Professor Samuel Walker
Department of Criminal Justice
University of Nebraska at Omaha
Omaha, NE 68182-0149

CHAPTER 1
Introduction

The nature of police work exposes police officers to liability risks everyday, resulting in greater chances of them becoming the subjects of civil litigation. Current police liability literature reports that litigation cases involving the police have increased over the past three decades (Archbold & Maguire, 2002; Franklin, 1993; Kappeler, 2001; McCoy, 1987; Novak, Smith & Frank, 2003; Payne, 2002). In turn, the monetary costs associated with lawsuits involving the police have also increased over time. For example, both Los Angeles and New York City paid out over $70 million in settlements for police misconduct from 1991 to 1996 (Human Rights Watch, 1998). On May 22, 2003 the Cincinnati Enquirer reported that the city of Cincinnati would pay out $4.5 million in settlements for 16 lawsuits involving Cincinnati police officers. This settlement will be recorded as the largest legal settlement involving the police in the city's history (The Cincinnati Enquirer, 2003).

Some police managers have recognized this increase in litigation and payouts resulting from litigation, and have begun to take proactive measures to reduce exposure to liability risks. Two of these proactive measures are the employment of police legal advisors and the use of risk management techniques. There is currently no research in the United States on these two measures however. This book presents the findings of the first national study on the use of risk management and police legal advising by law enforcement agencies as part of their efforts to reduce police officer exposure to liability risks.

POLICE ACCOUNTABILITY AND EFFECTIVE POLICE MANAGEMENT TOOLS

Creating a culture of accountability and a high level of professionalism within police organizations can be achieved through various management tools. In a 2001 report written by the U.S. Department of Justice, several policies are recommended to increase police accountability and effective management within police organizations. Some of the suggested practices include: (1) increased supervision over police officers (specifically involving use of force, and search and seizure incidents), (2) acquiring feedback on police services from citizens and community groups, (3) establishing mechanisms where civilians can participate in evaluating police services and programs including civilian review boards or oversight agencies, and (4) implementing information management systems (including early warning systems) (U.S. Department of Justice, 2001).

Risk management and police legal advising easily fit into the list provided by the Department of Justice, as the goal of both approaches encourages increased police professionalism, more effective police management, and greater police accountability.

POLICE LIABILITY

Existing research suggests that police activities that are associated with high exposure to liability risk and that cost police departments large sums of money prompt police administrators to review and alter department policies and practices to avoid future litigation (Alpert & Dunham, 1992; McCoy, 1984). Police chiefs surveyed by McCoy (1984) specifically identified police use of force and auto pursuits as the two areas where policies can be designed to control police officers' actions, and where advanced police training can decrease the chances of litigation. McCoy suggests that police chiefs mentioned these two items because they are likely to result in the most expensive payouts for serious injury in civil litigation cases. The findings of McCoy's study are important because it points out that some police administrators are aware of high-risk liability incidents, and that they also attempt to alter department policies and training to reduce or prevent future litigation involving members of their organizations.

Police managers recognize specific incidents that result in civil litigation against their departments because of large monetary settlements or because of the media attention given to celebrated litigation cases against the police such as the 1991 Rodney King incident in Los Angeles (McCoy, 1984; Cannon, 1997). The incidents that most likely result in litigation include improper use of force (non-lethal and lethal) during arrest, high-speed pursuits, and several other serious allegations of police misconduct (Alpert et al., 2000; del Carmen, 1991; Payne, 2003). In response, law enforcement agencies have attempted to improve police training, police recruitment standards, and department policies and procedures to maintain control over exposure to liability (U.S. Department of Justice, 2001). Police executives are also pushing for national accreditation (Marino, 1998), implementation of community oriented policing programs (Worrall, 1998), and peer counseling programs (Vogt, 1985) to help reduce the chances that their officers will be named as defendants in civil lawsuits.

An important topic that has not been discussed in policing literature is the way that police executives have tried to reduce payouts resulting from litigation by using techniques embraced by legal personnel and risk management assessors. Some law enforcement executives have begun to deal with police liability issues by employing police legal advisors and risk managers within their organizations.

POLICE LEGAL ADVISORS

The role of police legal advisors in law enforcement agencies is to provide a wide range of legal services to all police personnel. For example, legal advisors are often used to examine both existing and newly adopted department policies to ensure that they comply with local, state and federal regulations. They also recommend changes in the standards associated with recruitment and training of all police officers. Legal advisors use their legal expertise to track and analyze past legal cases and settlements involving the police to create preventative measures to combat future legal problems. The scope of police legal advisors duties usually reflects the needs and characteristics of each individual police organization by which they are employed (Caplan, 1967).

Police executives have sought the advice of legal counsel for liability issues since the early 1900s. The New York City Law Library Legal Unit was the first formal legal unit housed within a police department in the United States (Schmidt, 1972). The need for legal advisors within police organizations has increased significantly over time as changes in laws and Supreme Court case decisions have influenced the police role in society. In the 1960s and 1970s, legal advisors were starting to become integrated into police organizations to keep up with the constant changes in law and changes in the procedures used to enforce those laws.

Despite the need for legal advising within law enforcement agencies, the adoption of police legal advisors in the United States has been sluggish over the last four decades. In 1966, the National League of Cities sponsored a national study that revealed that only 14 U.S. police departments employed legal counsel on a full or part-time basis out of the 276 police departments responding to their survey (Bancroft, 1966). To date, there is no current list of law enforcement agencies that employ police legal advisors. Further, the topic of police legal advising has gone virtually untouched by both police scholars and police practitioners since the early 1970s. The national study described in later chapters of this book provides an in-depth look into which law enforcement agencies utilize the services provided by police legal advisors, and also explores the role, function, and perceived impact of police legal advisors on police liability management.

Early literature on police legal advising suggested that the slow pace of the adoption of police legal advisors in the United States could be attributed to several factors. First, the literature reports that there had been resistance from city and county attorneys who proclaim that police organizations that employ police legal advisors would be "doubling up" on legal services (Caplan, 1967; Schmidt, 1972). Therefore, instead of hiring police legal advisors, some law enforcement agencies have continued to utilize their city or county attorney.

Another factor cited in the literature related to the slow adoption of police legal advisors is a lack of resources. As is the case in most public or private organizations, budgetary constraints often hinder police organizations from adopting new, innovative programs. This has reportedly been the case with police legal advisors (Caplan, 1967; IACP, 1998; Schmidt, 1972).

Resistance from police executives who are unfamiliar with the police legal advisor role, more lucrative job opportunities for lawyers in private practices or large law firms, and a lack of formal training for police legal advisors are also factors noted in the earlier literature that are believed to have contributed to the lagged adoption of legal advisors by police agencies (Caplan, 1967; Lorch, 1969). It has been predicted that the level of resistance to police legal advisors may diminish with time because there has been a significant increase in police litigation cases over the past three decades (Franklin, 1993; Kappeler, 1997; McCoy, 1987), which might reflect an increase in the need for more legal advice by police agencies. Employing police legal advisors may be an additional managerial tool for police executives concerned with increasing organizational loss resulting from liability incidents.

RISK MANAGEMENT

Risk management is a management tool that can be used to identify and manage potential risk and liability problems in organizations. In the past, risk management was mostly used as an insurance-based technical tool. Today risk management is viewed as a broad, policy-oriented, managerial technique used by a wide array of organizations (Young, 2000). Organizations adopt risk management practices because of the increase in the threat of litigation, to reduce the risk of harm to both their clients and employees, and to provide a higher quality of services to their clients (Wong & Rakestraw, 1991).

Recently, some law enforcement agencies have implemented risk managers (either in addition to or as a replacement of police legal advisors) to aid in the identification of department policies and procedures that lead to liability-related losses. Similar to legal advisors, risk managers are utilized by police agencies to reduce officer exposure to liability incidents. Risk managers use a variety of insurance-based techniques to assess levels of liability within organizations, and then create various strategies to reduce or manage exposure to the identified risks (Esenberg, 1992).

Risk managers and risk management programs are more underutilized by law enforcement agencies than are police legal advisors. This assessment of the scarce presence of risk management in law enforcement is evident by the lack of published literature and research on the subject in the United States. Ironically, there is a great need for the fiscal management that risk managers provide in some of the largest police departments in the country.

THE LINK BETWEEN POLICE LEGAL ADVISORS AND RISK MANAGEMENT

The national study presented in this book examines the use of police legal advisors and risk management by American law enforcement agencies in an attempt to reduce officer exposure to liability risks. Both risk managers and police legal advisors are included in this study because both groups share common goals and roles within police organizations. Additionally, both groups use similar methods and techniques to accomplish those shared goals.

Police organizations can use police legal advisors and risk managers either separately, together, or in some other unique combination depending on the individual needs of the organization. The duties of risk managers parallel those of police legal advisors because both groups are employed by police organizations for the same reason – to reduce and maintain control over police liability incidents. Both groups use their training to identify, and then examine policies and procedures that often result in litigation (and sometimes monetary payouts) for the police organization. Even with very different professional and educational backgrounds, police legal advisors and risk managers can achieve similar goals when handling police liability incidents.

CONTRIBUTIONS TO THE LITERATURE

This book explores the use of police legal advising and risk management by law enforcement agencies in an effort to reduce police litigation cases, and the costs associated with exposure to liability risks. More specifically, the national study presented in Chapter Four examines: (1) The prevalence of the use of risk management and legal advising in law enforcement agencies in the United States, (2) some of the characteristics and roles of the identified risk management and police legal advising programs in police agencies, (3) some of the factors associated with the adoption of such programs, and (4) the perceived impact of utilizing police legal advising and risk management to handle police liability issues.

The data used in this study is based on three primary data sources: (1) Telephone interviews with police personnel, risk managers, and police legal advisors in 354 U.S. county and municipal law enforcement agencies that employ 200 or more sworn police personnel; (2) a national survey of the municipal and county police departments that reported that they utilize police legal advising and/or risk management in prior telephone interviews; and (3) case study analyses of four police departments that use various combinations of risk management and police legal advising techniques. The research findings presented in this book describe how law enforcement agencies can use such managerial tools to handle police liability and organizational loss resulting from exposure to liability incidents. In addition, the findings of this exploratory study will provide a strong foundation for future empirical assessment of this topic.

CHAPTER 2

Police Liability in the United States

Police liability is of increasing concern to members of the public, police administrators, and individual police officers. Current literature suggests that the management of police liability increases police professionalism, and also contributes to police accountability. This book explores two alternative approaches to liability management: risk management and police legal advising.

A recent report released by the U.S. Department of Justice outlines several ways that police agencies can make organizational changes to promote police integrity, improve police practices and policies, and decrease exposure to liability incidents that often result in litigation. The report suggests alterations in policy and practice in six areas including: (1) use of force, (2) the investigation of complaints and misconduct of officers, (3) promoting police accountability and effective police management, (4) improved police training, (5) ways to practice non-discriminatory policing and data collection on race, and (6) improved standards for recruitment, hiring, and retention of police officers (U.S. Department of Justice, 2001).

Two suggested changes that are not included on the list are the adoption of risk management and police legal advising programs, even though they are closely related to recommendations suggested in the 2001 U.S. Department of Justice report. The premise of this book is to present police legal advisors and risk management as two additional ways that police organizations can increase police accountability, while reducing liability within their organizations.

This chapter provides a discussion of the literature on police liability, as well as a detailed look at the use of police legal advising and risk management by police executives to manage police liability.

THE CURRENT STATE OF POLICE LIABILITY IN AMERICA

Police liability has become one of the most widely discussed topics by police executives, police officers, and police scholars. Police exposure to liability has increased in the past three decades because of significant social, political, and legal changes in the United States. All of these changes, especially the changes in law, have impacted police work. By failing to adjust police policies and procedures to accommodate the changes in law, police executives have seen an increase in litigation and citizen complaints (Beh, 1998; Livingston, 1999). Two indicators of increased police liability are the rising number of civil suits filed against the police, and the monetary loss resulting from those lawsuits.

By varying accounts, the number of civil suits filed against police officers has risen since 1960 (Franklin, 1993; Kappeler, 1997; McCoy, 1987; Payne, 2003). McCoy (1987) found that all of the police chiefs from the 20 largest cities in the United States reported that their departments had been sued in civil cases in the past. Additionally, the total number of federal civil cases filed against police officers under Section 1983 nearly tripled from 1978 to 1996 (Kappeler, 2001). Lawsuits that are filed against police officers under Section 1983 involve any police actions that fall outside of the scope of a police officers official authority, which results in violation of civil rights as defined in the United States Constitution (Kappeler, 2001).

Another indication of the increase in litigation involving the police are the large monetary awards given to citizens that win lawsuits filed against the police. For example, Human Rights Watch (1998) reported that New York City paid out $70 million in settlements for police misconduct lawsuits between 1994 -1996. Similarly, the city of Los Angeles paid $79.2 million in settlements and judgments in civil suits against Los Angeles police officers from 1991-1996. More recently, the Mayor of Los Angeles, Richard Riordan, suggested that "the city set aside 25 years worth of tobacco settlement money – as much as $300 million – to pay for lawsuits anticipated from the city's latest police corruption scandal involving officers in the Rampart district" (Los Angeles Times, 2000). The rising costs resulting from police-related liability incidents indicate that there is a need for additional ways to manage such incidents. The purpose of this book is to suggest the adoption of risk managers and police legal advisors as two additional ways to manage police liability.

POLICE WORK AND EXPOSURE TO RISK

The need for legal advising and risk management in law enforcement becomes apparent when the sources of exposure to liability in police work are examined. First, the nature of police work is inherently dangerous, and regularly exposes officers to liability incidents. Almost all of the basic duties of police work expose police officers to liability on a daily basis (Gallagher, 1990b; Wennerholm, 1985). Additionally, inexperienced police officers working in high crime areas also play a part in police exposure to high-risk liability incidents. Inexperienced officers are sometimes put in situations where they have to make quick decisions with sometimes less than a thousand hours of training in the police academy (Katz, 1998). Lack of experience and limited police academy training, can contribute to the probability that officers will be exposed to potential liability risks.

COMMON LIABILITY INCIDENTS IN POLICE WORK

One aspect of police work that makes it unique to all other professions is the ability of police officers to use lethal and non-lethal force (Bittner, 1970). This unique aspect of police work contributes to police officer exposure to high levels of risk, which could lead to litigation. It has been reported that improper use of lethal and non-lethal force by police officers during arrest, and improper service of due process are two incidents in which damages are most likely sought, and that settlements are paid out to citizens (Blalock, 1974; del Carmen, 1991; Newell et al, 1993).

Liability Assessment and Awareness International (LAAW) (2001) suggests that police executives could manage liability related to use of force through close supervision of patrol officers. The group also suggests that police department policies should be created and maintained to keep the use of force under control. Also, by applying the highest standards to the use of force by police officers, as well as the review process of all misuse of force cases, law enforcement agencies can get a handle on use of force liability incidents (Liability Assessment and Awareness International Inc., 2001). This assertion by the LAAW parallels the findings of most of the research on the use of deadly force, which suggests that policies and mandatory reporting of use of lethal force harnesses police officer behaviors and activities (Culliver & Sigler, 1995; Fyfe, 1979; Fyfe, 1981; Geller & Scott, 1992; Sparger & Giacopassi, 1992).

Another common liability incident that can result in litigation against police officers is false arrest (International Association of Chiefs of Police, 1974; Kappeler, 2001; Schmidt, 1985). Kappeler (2001) defines false arrest as "the unlawful seizure and detention of a person" by a police officer (p. 21). In most cases, false arrest claims consist of those cases where individuals believe that the police did not have probable cause to stop or question them (Kappeler, 2001).

To avoid liability resulting from claims of false arrest, police officers can obtain a warrant prior to making arrests. Securing a search warrant prior to arrest takes the authority of determining probable cause away from police officers, and places the responsibility on judges (Kappeler, 2001). Because making arrests is such a common police action, it is not always possible to obtain a warrant prior to making an arrest, which in turn, exposes police officers to liability.

Another frequent liability incident that often results in payout for police agencies is law enforcement vehicle operation. High-risk liability incidents involving law enforcement vehicles include: high speed pursuits, how and where police vehicles are parked, whether or not emergency lights/equipment is used while police vehicles are parked, where police officers place people and all involved vehicles during the investigation of traffic stops, the misuse or nonuse of vehicle occupant restraints (both officers and passengers in police vehicles), and both major traffic accidents and minor fender benders involving law enforcement vehicles (Liability Assessment and Awareness International, Inc., 2001).

The issue of police liability and risk management for emergency vehicle operations is addressed in an entire chapter of a recently published book, *Police Pursuits: What We Know* (Alpert et al, 2000). Alpert and colleagues discuss several ways to identify and respond to exposure to risks related to emergency vehicle operations within police agencies including: (1) a review of historical loss data, (2) a review of both past and pending lawsuits filed against the police agency, and (3) surveying patrol officers about some of the issues that arise from operating law enforcement vehicles (Alpert et al, 2000, p. 154).

Because the operation of police vehicles is a necessary part of modern policing, identifying and then managing the risks associated with police vehicle operation also becomes a necessary task for police executives.

One of several ways to manage police vehicle liability incidents is to require mandatory reporting of any traffic-related incidents including both major and minor accidents (Liability Assessment and Awareness International Inc, 2001). In addition to mandatory reporting of all traffic infractions, all evidence available after any traffic incidents should be collected and preserved by law enforcement agencies (Liability Assessment and Awareness International Inc, 2001). Incident reports including thorough descriptions of each traffic-related incident, exhaustive lists of evidence collected after traffic-related incidents, and any other important information pertinent to traffic-related incidents should be given to police managers to keep on file in case litigation occurs in the future. All of these steps are believed to help police agencies protect themselves against traffic-related litigation cases.

Police liability can also become an issue when police services are not conducted within defined jurisdictional boundaries. The Liability Assessment and Awareness International, Inc. (2001) assert that roughly 10 percent of law enforcement litigation involves jurisdictional issues. Incidents requiring the use of police services (such as high-speed pursuits, surveillance or investigation, and serving warrants) often require that law enforcement officials involved in those incidents understand jurisdictional boundaries.

Although jurisdictional liability incidents only comprise a small portion of litigation cases against the police, the Liability Assessment and Awareness International, Inc. (2001) suggests several steps that can be taken to reduce those incidents.

First, all police personnel need to be informed of the jurisdictional boundaries, accompanying jurisdictional policies, and any changes in jurisdictional policies as defined by agency directives. This step is important, as jurisdictional boundaries are state law dependent.

Second, it is also important to keep all records and evidence from vehicle-related incidents on file at the police department in case traffic accidents or injuries result from high-speed pursuits that carry over into other jurisdictions (Liability Assessment and Awareness International Inc., 2001).

And third, there should be periodic review of all traffic-related incidents that take place outside of officer jurisdiction by risk managers and/or legal advisors employed by the police department. The results of each review will allow the department to make changes that could impact the frequency of traffic-related incidents outside of the department's jurisdiction (Liability Assessment and Awareness International, Inc., 2001).

Canine unit dog bites are another liability concern for law enforcement managers. The American Civil Liberties Union of Southern California has asked for an investigation of the Los Angeles Police Department K-9 unit practices because of a reported increase in the number of dog bites of citizens. It has been reported "that an average of nearly one person per day is bitten by Los Angeles Police Department canines" and that "more than 900 men, women, and children have been attacked and mauled by these dogs in a 3-year period" (American Civil Liberties Union of Southern California, 1992, p. 21).

The ACLU of Southern California also reports that there is evidence that the LAPD concentrates its use of canine units in predominantly minority-populated neighborhoods of Los Angeles (1992). Statistics included in a June 2000 report by Merrick J. Bobb (Special Counsel to the Los Angeles County Sheriff's Department) corroborate the ACLU's assertion. The statistics in the report suggest that K-9 units may be utilized in minority neighborhoods more often than in non-minority concentrated neighborhoods. With police departments of all sizes implementing K-9 programs, this issue could become more of a liability concern to police agencies in the future.

POLICE LIABILITY ASSESSMENT

There are a variety of liability assessment resources available to law enforcement agencies. Some of those resources are provided by agencies such as the Liability Assessment and Awareness International, Inc., the International Association of Chiefs of Police – Legal Section, and the Public Risk Management Association (PRIMA) which focus on improving police services and police professionalism by reducing police officers' exposure to liability risks.

Public Risk Management Association Liability Assessment Guidelines

The Public Risk Management Association (PRIMA) has published a guide to help law enforcement agencies assess their exposure to liability incidents. The PRIMA Police Liability Assessment Guide (2001) suggests that police managers pay close attention to the following categories during liability assessment:

Law Enforcement Training

- All police officers and police reserve officers should be trained and certified by the State before they have any contact with citizens during regular police activities.

- The basic training in the police academy that is required of all police officers should exceed the minimum standards set by the State.

- All police officers and police reserve officers should be trained and be able to display competency in the areas of using firearms (both on and off duty), impact weapons, shotgun, mace, emergency and pursuit driving, First Aid, defensive tactics, dealing with barricaded subjects, hostage situations, and incidents involving hazardous waste. In addition, legal training should be given to each police officer both before and during their law enforcement career.

- All police officers should be required to go through a Field Training Officer (FTO) program, and should be given "probationary" status for a period of time after FTO training is completed. In addition, the department should maintain records of successful completion of both FTO training, and competency during probationary period.

- All police officers should be required to be re-qualified each year in the use of firearms and other non-lethal weapons, as well as handling other critical tasks.

- All police instructors and trainers should be required to participate in annual or periodic refresher courses to enhance their training abilities.

- Records of all police training and qualifications/re-qualifications for both supervisors and line officers should be formally documented and maintained.

- Law enforcement agencies should require psychological screening of all police recruits, and should provide psychological services to all police personnel thereafter.

Department Policies and Procedures

- All police personnel should be provided with a copy of department policies and procedures. Any changes or updates in policies and procedures should be given to all personnel immediately.

- The law enforcement agency should have clearly stated written policies and procedures for critical tasks including use of force (as well as use of force reports and review of reports), emergency and pursuit driving, off-duty employment and carrying weapons while off-duty, domestic violence, and any situations that involve infectious diseases.

- The agency should also have significant training, and clearly stated policies and procedures for SWAT or tactical units, hostage rescue squads, K-9 Units, and units involved in the handling of bombs or other toxic materials.

Collaborations with Local Legal Counsel

- Law enforcement agencies should have local city attorneys periodically review department policies and procedures to ensure that they reflect current laws that affect police operations.

- Local city attorneys should also be consulted when any new policies or procedures are created by police departments, to make sure that the policies are congruent with formal local and State laws.

- Law enforcement agencies should seek the aid of local city attorneys to train and update police officers on any changes in the law resulting from court decisions or other legislative processes.

- To identify existing risks of liability to the police agency, local city attorneys should conduct periodic reviews of civil suits and payouts from civil litigation to determine potential high-risk situations and police procedures. After any high-risk situations or procedures are identified, both police managers and local legal counsel should collaborate on potential changes that could be made to reduce or eliminate unnecessary risks.

Once a general liability assessment guide or checklist is exhausted, police executives can focus on liability incidents that may be unique to their organization (Barrineau III, 1994). Both past and pending civil suits and citizen complaints filed against the police, and agency records indicating agency loss histories can be used to identify those liability incidents that are unique to each individual law enforcement agency. PRIMA suggests that law enforcement agencies seek the help of legal advisors or insurance risk assessors when assessing agency loss histories.

Gallagher's "six-layered liability protection system"

Liability assessment checklists and guidelines help organizations identify areas of potential exposure to risk. The idea of protecting law enforcement agencies against liability risks while increasing police officer professionalism is the idea that serves as the basis for G. Patrick Gallagher's "six-layered liability protection system" (Gallagher, 1990a, 1992). The six layers that should be covered in law enforcement agencies that Gallagher refers to include: (1) policies and procedures, (2) officer training, (3) supervision, (4) performance management or discipline, (5) continual review and monitoring of identified risks, and (6) revising actions used to counter risks when necessary (1990a, 1992).

Gallagher asserts that if any of the six layers are either excluded or not functioning properly, police agencies are not fully protecting themselves from liability incidents. "All components must be present and interactive. It is the quality of each component and the quality of its interaction with all the others that will forge the highest degree of protection from the system" (Gallagher, 1992, p. 24). The "six-layered" system proposed by Gallagher contains some of the basic components found in liability assessment checklists and guidelines used by a variety of organizations and agencies.

REDUCING POLICE EXPOSURE TO LIABILITY INCIDENTS: RECENT ATTEMPTS

There is debate over whether or not police administrators can make organizational changes or implement innovative programs to reduce lawsuits involving the police. Some scholars suggest that police agencies that utilize innovative programs (such as early warning systems, proactive paramilitary units, and community oriented policing) actually increase their chances of being exposed to liability incidents and citizen complaints (Worrall, 2001).

On the opposite side of the debate, there appears to be some factors that can reduce the probability of police officers becoming involved in litigation cases. Current research indicates that changes made within police organizations such as increased or improved police officer training (Barrineau III, 1994; Blalock, 1974), obtaining accreditation (Marino, 1998), and the use of specific programs, such as community oriented policing (Worrall, 1998) has had an impact on civil suits filed against the police. There is also research that suggests that police officers' fear of being sued also deters some police officers from participating in activities that could result in civil litigation (McCoy, 1984). The following section examines the results of current police liability research, and several methodological issues that impact the results of that body of research.

Approach #1: Community Oriented Policing

Current liability research suggests that the implementation of Community Oriented Policing (COP) programs in police departments has had a positive impact on the number of civil suits against the police. John Worrall (1998) examined the impact of administrative determinants on civil suits filed against the police. Using data from a 1996 survey of 248 police departments and the 1993 Law Enforcement Management and Administrative Statistics (LEMAS) survey, Worrall found that "as departments became committed to community-oriented policing through the adoption of COP policies and programs, lawsuits declined, and quite markedly (1998, p. 307)." This finding suggests that decisions made by police administrators to implement certain programs in their organizations, can have an impact on the number of civil suits filed against them. However, in a 2001 study, Worrall found a mix of effects where community policing had either no effect or a positive effect on civil lawsuits involving the police. Additional research on this issue is needed to further understand the impact of community policing on lawsuits involving police officers.

Approach #2: Accreditation

The Intergovernmental Risk Management Agency (IRMA) is an agency that provides risk management grants to municipal level agencies across the United States. In 1998, IRMA conducted a study to see if there is a difference in the number of liability claims filed against police departments that were accredited by the Commission on Accreditation for Law Enforcement Agencies (CALEA) compared to those agencies that were non-accredited. In addition, IRMA wanted to assess the effectiveness of the risk management services they provide to law enforcement municipality members.

To conduct this study, data from liability claims paid out by police agencies that received IRMA services from 1993-1997 were collected from IRMA underwriting and loss records. An analysis of the IRMA data indicates that accredited police agencies had fewer claims per 100 officers (8.61) compared to non-accredited police agencies (10.28) (Marino, 1998). There was also a significant difference in the severity of the amount of payout resulting from claims that were filed against accredited and non-accredited police agencies. From 1993 through

1997, accredited police agencies that were IRMA members paid out a total of $396,882.76, while non-accredited IRMA police agencies paid out $1,312,089.62 (Marino, 1998). The author concludes that accreditation from CALEA impacts a police agency's ability to better manage liability payouts compared to non-accredited law enforcement agencies.

The results of the IRMA study should be interpreted with caution because of several methodological problems. First, the study does not control for the size of the police agencies included in the sample, the difference in the demands for service placed on each of the police agencies, or demographic differences in the cities where each police agency operates. It is likely that police organizations that are located in urban cities where there are higher police-citizen contact ratios will have increased exposure to high-risk liability incidents. The IRMA study does not control for such factors.

A second problem with the IRMA study is that it is impossible to know if the low number of claims filed against accredited agencies resulted because of accreditation and not some other characteristic of the police agencies (such as management styles, or education and training requirements). For example, some research suggests that police officers that have two or more years of college education receive fewer citizen complaints, are less frequently involved in litigation situations, and have fewer disciplinary problems than their non-college educated counterparts (Carter and Sapp, 1990). This finding casts doubt on the idea that accreditation alone can reduce police involvement in civil litigation cases. The IRMA study does not explore the possibility that other factors could influence the number of liability claims filed against police agencies.

Third, the idea that a police department is more effective because they have all of the policies and programs required by CALEA to be an accredited agency is misleading. Accreditation does not guarantee that there are control mechanisms in place to enforce the required policies that are necessary for accreditation by CALEA. For example, most police departments have policies against sexual harassment of female officers by their male counterparts. Having a sexual harassment policy does not ensure that harassment will not take place in an organization; but the policy can have an impact on harassment if police managers enforce the harassment policy, and if a disciplinary system exists and is properly used whenever harassment has taken place within the organization.

And finally, the study does not use any variables that measure the number of risk management services provided by IRMA to police agencies (such as number of hours of IRMA training). It is impossible to gauge how much IRMA services impact police involvement in civil liability cases without the use of such variables because it is unclear how many IRMA services were provided to each police agency. Thus, to conclude that accreditation alone reduces the number of lawsuits and monetary loss from lawsuits for police-involved liability incidents would be a mistake.

Approach #3: Improved police training

Some literature suggests that increased and improved police training can impact the probability of police officers becoming named as defendants in legal suits. Most of the literature suggests that it is "common sense" that improved training will result in fewer lawsuits, but often does not provide any empirical evidence to support the "common sense" theory.

According to Schultz (1984), improvements in all phases of police training can prove to be beneficial to police officers when it comes to being named defendants in civil suits. George Schrader (1998) also stated, "that documenting firearms training not only reduces liability for the city and department but is an excellent training medium" (p.3). Neither Schultz nor Schrader used empirical evidence to support their assertions on the impact of police training on police liability.

In contrast to Schultz and Schrader's assertions, John Worrall (1998) found that training is not an important factor in determining the probability that civil lawsuits will be filed against police organizations. However, Worrall cautions that the measure he used for the training variable may have been "too simple or crude" to catch the effects of training on the number of civil suits in his study. But because of the lack of research conducted on the impact of police training in nearly all stages of police work, it is still unclear as to its direct or indirect impact on police activities and behaviors.

Approach #4: Police department policies and directives

To date, there are few empirical studies that examine the impact of use of non-lethal force policies and the use of mandatory reporting of use of non-lethal force incidents on civil suits filed against the police. Most of the empirical research has focused on the use of agency policies to regulate the use of deadly force by police officers. In most studies, the implementation of a police department policy on the use of deadly force or the impact of the 1985 Tennessee v. Garner court case decision are assessed to identify the impact of such policies. The results of these studies have overwhelmingly supported the idea that more stringent use of deadly force policies significantly reduces the number of police-involved shootings (Culliver & Sigler, 1995; Fyfe, 1979; Fyfe, 1981; Sparger & Giacopassi, 1992). These studies also reveal that mandatory reporting of any use of firearms by police officers adds to the control and management of the use of deadly force by police officers.

Equally important as having clearly stated policies, is making sure that all police personnel within the organization are familiar with all existing policies. Colletti (1997) suggests that periodic proficiency exams can be given to establish some measurement of understanding of department policies. The results of proficiency exams can easily pinpoint the areas where police officers need further training.

Approach #5: Peer counseling programs

Allegations of police misconduct or misuse of force can sometimes result when police officers are unable to deal with stress or are suffering from job "burn out". Vogt (1985) suggests that police officers form peer-counseling groups to deal with on-the-job stressors and to prevent job "burn-out". There is potential benefit in providing an environment that promotes communication among police officers to discuss on-the-job stressors, as well as ways to deal with that stress. By using peer-counseling groups as a cathartic mechanism to reduce stress, police officers may be involved in fewer conflicts with citizens, thus resulting in fewer complaints or lawsuits filed against them. To date, there is no scientific research to support this claim.

Approach #6: Responding to the fear of litigation

Some police scholars and practitioners believe that there are some police officers that avoid certain police actions that can result in litigation because they fear being named defendants in civil suits filed by citizens (McCoy, 1984). In contrast, there are others that believe that the fear of litigation has little (if any) affect on police actions (Yale Law Journal, 1979). Even though police officer fear of litigation is not a specific approach or type of program used to reduce exposure to risks, there is some literature that suggests that informing police officers of the reality of litigation can impact their decision to initiate certain police actions.

A study conducted by Scogin and Brodsky in 1991 examined the level of "litigaphobia" (litigation + phobia) experienced by individual law enforcement officers. The results of the study indicate that most law enforcement officers moderately worry about work-related lawsuits filed by citizens. Also, 69 percent of police officers report that they take specific actions in their day-to-day work activities to prevent law suits being filed against them, such as "treating people fairly" or "going by the book" (Scogin and Brodsky, 1991, p. 43). And finally, most of the responding officers made statements indicating that they view being sued by citizens as "inevitable and unavoidable" due to the nature of their work. The authors suggest that pre-service and in-service training on police liability and the litigation process would prove beneficial to both the individual police officer and police department.

Candace McCoy (1984) also suggests that the threat of litigation can deter widespread police abuse in police departments. She contends that if police departments were systematically defying constitutional standards, they would be forced to operate under court orders until they began to function legally. McCoy also asserts that "increased procedural review and adequate record-keeping, disciplinary actions, careful police training, and a steady exchange of information between city attorneys and police are all good indicators that police departments indeed take deterrence seriously (1984, p.56)." It is important to note that the author's suggestions were not based on the results of any empirical studies.

In contrast, there is also research that suggests that the threat of civil lawsuits does not deter police officers from participating in unlawful activities. In 1979, student editors of the Yale Law Journal analyzed 149 misconduct cases filed against police officers from 1970-1977. The law students concluded that there was little or no deterrent effect from civil litigation. In most cases, juries sided with police officers, even in cases where there was sufficient evidence pointing to police misconduct or abuse. It was clear in most cases that certain factors (such as the plaintiff's involvement in illegal activity) swayed the jury to side with police officers (Yale Law Journal, 1979). This finding suggests that improper actions by police officers could possibly be overshadowed by the suspect's prior criminal history.

Two alternative approaches that have not been mentioned in police liability literature include the use of police legal advising and risk management by law enforcement agencies. Chapter Three discusses some of the earliest police legal advising and risk management literature, as well as current literature that focus on the use of police legal advising and risk management as police liability management tools.

CHAPTER 3

Police Legal Advising & Risk Management: Alternative Police Liability Management Tools

Some police administrators are beginning to utilize administrative mechanisms to reduce the risk of liability for their organizations with the help of legal and insurance specialists. In general terms, police legal advising takes place when lawyers are employed by police agencies to both manage and prevent legal problems involving police personnel. Legal advising has been slowly adopted by law enforcement agencies since the early 1960s. In contrast, risk management programs are still in the infancy stage of being embraced by police agencies. Risk management programs are adopted from the practices of insurance agencies as an effort to control the amount of unnecessary financial loss in organizations over time. Both approaches are potentially viable options to identify and manage police liability within police organizations.

POLICE LEGAL ADVISORS

The importance of adopting police legal advisors into police organizations was first highlighted in two documents that served as important sources of information for law enforcement agencies in the 1960s. First, O.W. Wilson (1963) discussed the importance of having a police legal advisor within law enforcement agencies in his text, *Police Administration.* The second document that supported the adoption of police legal advising was the *Task Report* written by the President's Commission on Law Enforcement and the Administration of Criminal Justice (1967). The federal government provided resources to fund the position of legal advisors in police departments, which further encouraged the adoption of police legal advisors.

Despite the obvious need for police legal advising, little attention has been given to the use of such people or groups in policing research since the early 1970s.

The first municipal law enforcement agency to adopt a legal unit was the New York City Police Department in 1907. The New York based legal unit was officially titled the "New York City Law Library Legal Unit" (Lorch, 1969). The early duties of the New York City Law Library Legal Unit focused on conducting research on routine police operations including patrol, interrogations, and searches. Essentially, this unit was created to watch over any legal issues that would arise involving New York City police officers. Expected duties and the number of members in the New York City Legal Unit increased significantly by 1970 as the legal needs of the NYPD also broadened (Schmidt, 1972). For a comprehensive history of the New York City Police Department Legal Bureau, see Lorch (1969).

Both substantive and procedural law affects every phase of police work; therefore, police organizations need to have access to full-time, highly skilled legal advisors. It is the police legal advisor that will interpret and adjust police agency policies and directives to keep up with the ever-changing laws that define the police role. In 1967, the need for police legal advising was explicitly stated in the Presidents Commission on Law Enforcement and Administration of Justice's Task Force Report: The Police (1967):

> A major instrument for insuring…increased effectiveness is the introduction of lawyers into the law enforcement process, particularly in the areas of planning and investigation. Even the best policeman and the best police administrator will, at times, need the advice of a lawyer who is knowledgeable in the administrative and criminal law. In fact, the better the office and the department, the more sensitive they will be to the complexity of the law, and the more likely to test their judgments against those of the police legal advisor…. (p. 63).

The National Advisory Commission on Criminal Justice Standards and Goals (1973) also suggested "that every police agency with 200 or more personnel should establish a police legal unit with at least one attorney as a full-time legal advisor" (p. 280). Police executives can hire either full or part-time police legal advisors to make their organizations more legally efficient in training and procedure while at the same time raise the standards of professionalism within their organizations.

Police legal advisors (either alone or with the aid of risk managers) also provide police agencies with advice on ways to maintain a level of fiscal responsibility. "Because the average police chief in the United States presides over the equivalent of a multi-million dollar corporation, it is imperative that the chief demand and get legal advice of a quality commensurate with his or her departments importance. This is all the more crucial given the capacity of police-citizen contacts to generate very significant liability claims" (Geller, 1991, p. 447). In larger cities where there is more exposure to liability incidents for police officers, the advice of a police legal advisor or risk manager could be an important fiscal and management tool for police executives.

Training Programs

To staff a legal unit with properly trained employees or prepare a lawyer with the tools to advise police personnel, it is essential that legal training focuses on liability issues directly related to police work. A program at Northwestern University provided the necessary training for police legal advising in the late 1960s through 1970. The "Police Legal Advisor" (PLA) program began in 1964 as a two-year Masters of Law program and was later changed to a 12-month certification program. In 1970, the Northwestern PLA program became a joint program with the International Association of Chiefs of Police (IACP) for one year. Since 1971, there has not been any formal school for police legal attorneys in the United States (Schmidt, 2001).

Since the early 1970s, the Federal Bureau of Investigations (FBI) has sporadically held "National Law Institute" sessions that cover issues in criminal procedure and labor law. In addition, an association of police legal advisors was formed in 1968, and was later adopted as part of the International Association of Chiefs of Police as the IACP

Legal Officers Section. The IACP Legal Officers Section still meets as part of the IACP annual conference (Schmidt, 2001).[1]

A police internship program at the University of Wisconsin Law School also provided specialized training to law students that had an interest in working as police legal advisors in the 1960s. This program trained law students to understand legal issues that are specifically relevant to police work, and then placed students within law enforcement agencies for hands-on training. The internship program was dissolved six years after it began because of lack of resources to subsidize students that were part of the legal advising program (Goldstein, 2001).[2]

Today, there are no formal police legal advising programs within an academic setting that focus specifically on training law students to become police legal advisors. Some law schools will offer individual courses that deal specifically with legal issues that law enforcement agencies encounter. The International Association of Chiefs of Police (IACP) Legal Section and other independent agencies offer periodic training seminars on police civil liability issues.

In addition to the lack of specialized training for police legal advisors, the role of police legal advisors within police organizations have been given virtually no attention in policing literature. The idea of adopting police legal advisors seems to have diminished just as quickly as it was introduced back in the late 1960s and early 1970s. The topic of police legal advisor often re-emerges in practitioner-oriented publications circulated among police personnel such as *The Police Chief* magazine or the *FBI Bulletin*. For example, a 1998 issue of *The Police Chief* magazine featured an article written by the IACP – Legal Section on the importance of adopting police legal advisors (IACP, 1998). This article contains virtually the same information on

---

[1] Wayne Schmidt is currently the Executive Director of Americans for Effective Law Enforcement, and the Editor of Fire and Police Personnel Reporter newsletter. Schmidt is a graduate of the Northwestern PLA program, and also served as the director of the PLA program from 1968-1973. (Telephone interview, March 2001).

[2] Dr. Herman Goldstein provided historical information on the Police Legal Advising program at the University of Wisconsin Law School in a telephone interview on May 2, 2001.

police legal advisors as was presented by the IACP roughly thirty years ago. Although important, the 1998 IACP article does not contain any new information on police legal advisors that is based on empirical scientific research.

Even more interesting is that police legal advisors within police organizations were adopted at a very slow pace during a time when they were needed the most by police organizations. Since the late 1960s, there have been significant changes in law, and in the way that those laws should be enforced. Because of the changes in law the need for full-time police legal advisors within police agencies presumably should reflect an increased need for specialized legal advice to police organizations.

Types of police legal advisors

In the late 1960s, there was debate over what type of education and professional background legal advisors should have to be effective within police organizations. There are three types of police legal advisors that could be adopted by police organizations: (1) a civilian employee, (2) police officer-lawyer, or (3) prosecutor or city/county attorney. Earlier literature on police legal advising notes both the advantages and disadvantages to all three types of police legal advisors.

<u>Type 1: Civilians as police legal advisors</u>

Some of the legal advising literature reports that the civilian-police legal advisor holds the most promise of all three types of potential police legal advisors (Caplan, 1967). A civilian legal advisor would be someone that has experience practicing law, but does not hold a dual role of police legal advisor and city/county attorney. Civilian legal advisors would have fewer external sources of political pressure when considering changes in department policy within police organizations. Legal advisors that are classified as civilians would also be more open to participating in collaborations with agencies outside of the police department and would most likely consider the needs of agencies and individuals outside of the police organization when making changes that impact the police agency (Caplan, 1967). Moreover, it is suspected that civilian police legal advisors would be more in tune with community needs and community perceptions of the police. However, civilian legal advisors may not have as much experience working with police officers as a police legal advisor with prior law enforcement experience would have acquired while working in the field.

Schmidt (1972) and the National Commission on Criminal Justice Standards and Goals (1973) also recommended that police legal advisors/units be staffed with civilian employees. It is suggested in the literature that patrol officers might be more comfortable coming to a legal advisor if he/she is not a high-ranking police manager within the organization (Schmidt, 1972). In contrast, it has also been suggested that employing legal advisors that have experience in both law enforcement (without any type of rank within the police organization) and legal training would allow a greater degree of comfort to police officers seeking legal advice (Schmidt, 1972). To date, there has not been any empirical research on this particular debate.

Type 2: City attorneys as legal advisors

Early literature on legal advising notes that in some jurisdictions, city or county attorneys will be placed in police legal advising positions either on a full or part-time basis (Caplan, 1967; Schmidt, 1972). The literature also suggests that city attorney-legal advisors may feel pressure to give in to the demands of either the district attorney or police chief (Schmidt, 1972). There is also a possibility that city attorney-legal advisors would be overly sensitive to the policies of district attorneys and comparatively insensitive to possible areas of difference. City attorney-legal advisors may be insensitive to policing that is not geared toward prosecution (Caplan, 1967). A basic problem with utilizing legal services of city attorneys lies in the fact that most do not have in-depth knowledge of day-to-day police operations. Therefore, the utility of legal services provided by city attorney-legal advisors are somewhat limited in scope compared to the other two types of police legal advisors.

The attorney/client relationship is also different between police officers and city attorney-legal advisors compared to the relationship between police officers and civilian legal advisors. For example, if a police officer approaches the police legal advisor (who also happens to be the city attorney), it is still the city attorney's responsibility to take legal action against the officer if he or she admits some type of wrongdoing (Becker, 1994). Therefore, police officers may be hesitant to seek out legal advice from police legal advisors for fear that they could have legal action taken against them.

Another concern of adopting city attorney-legal advisors is the fact that their time is also occupied with legal issues for several other local government agents, leaving limited time for police legal issues (Caplan, 1967; Schmidt, 1972). If there are financial reasons why police departments cannot have an in-house police legal advisor, a city attorney-legal advisor may be the only option available.

Type 3: Police legal advisors with law enforcement experience

A third type of police legal advisor would be advisors that have prior law enforcement experience. One of the benefits of having police legal advisors that have prior law enforcement experience is that they will have firsthand knowledge of police liability issues. Additionally, some police officers may feel more comfortable seeking legal advice from someone that has worked in law enforcement compared to a legal advisor that has no prior law enforcement experience (Becker, 1994).

On the other hand, there is also some concern that legal advisors with policing experience may tailor his/her duties around the good of the police department, resulting in isolation from external agencies and community members (Caplan, 1967). Police legal advisors with prior law enforcement experience may also be less likely to collaborate with outside agencies, or be in tune with concerns of the community (Becker, 1994). Legal advisors with prior law enforcement experience may also face extra pressures from the chief of police when making decisions that will impact changes within the organization.

There are several advantages and disadvantages associated with all three types of police legal advisors. To date, there has not been any systematic study of which type of police legal advisor is the most effective in law enforcement settings. The current study does not examine which type of police legal advisor is better than the others. Instead, this study examines the prevalence of each type of police legal advisor in police agencies across the United States.

Responsibilities of police legal advisors

The responsibilities of police legal advisors are as diverse as the legal needs of both police agencies and individual police officers. There is no standard job description that can be generalized to all police legal advisors. Legal advisors responsibilities will vary based on the size and needs of the police department, as well as the management style and organizational objectives prescribed by the police chief or sheriff (International Association of Chiefs of Police-Legal Officers Section, 1998).

Besides serving the needs that are unique to each law enforcement agency, there are some standard duties that police legal advisors can expect to perform while being employed within a law enforcement agency. The following list of responsibilities is based on suggestions from literature written by Gerald Caplan (1967), the American Bar Association (1973), and the *Guidelines for a Police Legal Unit* written by Wayne Schmidt (1972).

1. Provide legal advice to police personnel

Early literature notes that one of the most important responsibilities placed on legal advisors is to be available to give legal advice to police personnel whenever necessary (Caplan, 1967; Lorch, 1969; Schmidt, 1972). Some of the legal advice given by police legal advisors includes providing legal advice on serving warrant, suggesting ways for patrol officers to prepare for court, and suggesting changes to department policies, training, hiring, and promotion of officers as a way to improve police services (Schmidt, 1972).

Legal advisors need to be available to police personnel at all levels within the police organization, ranging from the chief of police to officers on patrol. In fact, it is important that legal advisors maintain a constant level of contact with patrol officers, because a majority of the legal issues of police organizations begin with incidents that occur daily on the streets (Schmidt, 1972).

It is also important to recognize that legal advice is often given to police personnel before, during, and after police action has taken place (Geller, 1991). The legal advice given to police personnel should reflect the defined goals and objectives of the law enforcement agency. The need for constant availability of the legal advisor to police personnel further emphasizes the importance of having police legal advisors housed within the main police headquarters.

2. Assessing police exposure to risk and crisis management situations

Among other duties, the police legal advisor should also be available to help with the assessment of the level of risk involved in specific police actions (Geller, 1991). Providing potential solutions to handle the identified high-risk incidents would then follow the assessment of risk. Legal advisors within the police organization create potential solutions by collaborating with risk mangers or other professional insurance risk assessors.

Police legal advising is an important tool used to deal with legal issues in high risk or crisis management situations. According to Higginbotham (1994), a legal advisor is helpful with "legal issues that arise in crisis situations which includes dealing with search and seizures, the admissibility of statements used as evidence that were made during the negotiation process, the enforcement of promises made by police negotiators during the negotiation process, the use of any electronic surveillance equipment, any type of use of force used during a crisis situation, and control of access and information given to the media during crisis situations" (p. 27-28).

3. Assist in police training and recruitment

Legal advisors are also an important part of law enforcement recruitment and training. By participating on the planning committee for police academy training, legal advisors ensure that the instruction of important legal matters are conducted properly so that every police cadet is aware of the legal issues they may face in their new career (Schmidt, 1972). Legal advising is also a crucial part of police recruitment, because department recruiting standards are often based on the input of legal counsel within the police department. Schmidt (1972) contends that legal advisors can be valuable for in-service training of experienced officers or when officers are promoted to supervisory positions. Legal advisors describe how the added responsibilities that come along with promotion into supervisory positions also carries additional legal issues that need to be considered.

Legal advisors implement continuous legal training of police officers by distributing periodic legal training bulletins, training memos, or short instruction during the course of roll call (Schmidt, 1972). These continuous training methods are helpful in dispersing information to officers when any changes in policy or directive occur within the police organization.

Participation in the planning, implementation, and training of members and supervisors of specialized units is also a task that legal advisors encounter. For example, police departments often assemble special emergency response teams (SERT) to carry out activities, such as serving high risk warrants and dealing with high risk hostage situations. These specialized units are at a higher level of exposure to liability due to the increased level of danger that comes with the tasks they are required to perform. Legal advisors provide guidance to the members of the unit to ensure that quick decisions can be made to effectively complete the task and to minimize the level of exposure to liability risk as much as possible.

4. Creating, implementing, and reviewing department policies

Another significant duty of police legal advisors mentioned in the literature is the continual review of department publications and directives. This continuous review process allows police organizations to keep abreast of changes and developing trends in the laws that influence their ability to provide effective police services. On the same note, legal advisors also need to translate the "legal ease" of judicial decisions into standard operating procedures within police organizations (Caplan, 1967). It is essential that department policies and procedures are kept current because police organizations can be held legally responsible for the actions (and sometimes inaction) of individual officers.

5. Establishing and maintaining relationships with other agencies

The literature also indicates that some police agencies require that legal advisors maintain working relationships with other agencies both inside and outside of the criminal justice system (Caplan, 1967). Juvenile or correctional agencies, social service agencies, schools, housing and zoning authorities, and community groups are among the various groups that law enforcement officials often collaborate with to enhance police services provided to the community. The IACP (1998) recommends that a "team approach" be taken by police legal advisors when attempting to solve problems that involve the police organization. This team effort and cooperation with other agencies can prevent police departments from becoming alienated from other agencies, as well as the surrounding communities (International Association of Chiefs of Police, 1998).

All of the duties described in the previous sections are basic tasks that police legal advisors encounter in their position. In addition to those basic tasks, some legal advisors also write and submit grant proposals for the adoption of new and innovative programs for police departments, as well as represent police organizations in media events (Becker, 1994). In general, the duties and responsibilities of police legal advisors reflect the needs and organizational characteristics of the law enforcement agencies in which they are employed.

Police legal advisors within the police organizational chart

Early literature suggests that police legal advisors should not be included as an additional part of any existing division or bureau within the police organization (i.e., the Training Division). Instead, Schmidt (1972) suggests that police legal advisors be considered an individual division or unit within the organization, because it will allow police legal advisors to provide a wider range of legal services to all divisions within the police organization. For example, if legal advisors were part of another division, such as the training division, it would narrow the scope of the legal services that are provided to members of the organization. Additionally, Schmidt (1972) and the IACP (1998) suggest that police legal advisors be physically housed within police headquarters. The suggested location would allow police personnel immediate, convenient, and continuous access to legal advice. In addition, the close proximity to the police organization also allows legal advisors to experience daily police operations and procedures firsthand.

Potential sources of resistance against hiring police legal advisors

The idea of employing lawyers to help manage police liability incidents first emerged nearly forty years ago. As indicated in earlier sections of this chapter, only a small fraction of police agencies reported using police legal advisors after the idea first emerged. Early police legal advising literature identifies several potential sources of resistance to the adoption of police legal advisors by law enforcement agencies.

Police legal advising literature from the 1960s and 1970s identifies city or county attorneys as one source of resistance to hiring police legal advisors. Some city attorneys believe that providing legal services to the police is part of their job, and therefore, employing a full-time police legal advisor is unnecessary (Caplan, 1967; Schmidt, 1972). In contrast, the IACP believes that full-time police legal advisors are necessary because city and county attorneys are preoccupied with representing all other local government agencies (1998). Whether or not there is an overlap of legal services provided by city or county attorneys and police legal advisors is still up for debate as the topic has never been fully explored using systematic scientific research.

Another source of resistance for hiring police legal advisors identified in early literature comes from police chiefs or other upper level police managers. The resistance by police managers is based on the idea that there are no benefits of having lawyers without any law enforcement training or experience come into police departments to identify and correct problems in police training or procedures (Caplan, 1967). The literature notes that there can also be resistance if police managers do not fully understand the function or role that police legal advisors play in the organization. For example, some police officials view legal advisors as another police oversight mechanism, similar to an Internal Affairs division or some type of civilian oversight panel.

The literature also cites the legal community as another source of resistance to the adoption of police legal advisors by police departments. Some attorneys that are trained to deal with law enforcement liability issues often have other more prestigious and lucrative job opportunities available to them in either private practice or with large law firms (Caplan, 1967). Schmidt (1972) suggests that one way to overcome this problem would be to define the position of police legal advisor in a way that would highlight the benefits that such positions could bring to police organizations, as well as members of the community. Additionally, Schmidt (1972) suggests that the importance of the police legal advisor position be reflected in both the salary and formal job description of police legal advisors.

Sources of funding available to create, implement, and maintain police legal advisor positions can also become barriers for police agencies (Caplan, 1967; IACP, 1998; Schmidt, 1972). In small or medium-sized police departments, there are often not enough resources available in the budgets to cover new legal advisor positions. Further, it would be even more difficult to justify an in-house legal advisor if the local city or county attorney maintains that they are readily available to advise police departments whenever legal advice is needed.

Dealing with obstacles and resistance

As previously noted, one of the major barriers that law enforcement agencies face when attempting to adopt a police legal advisor is a lack of resources. Schmidt (1972) suggests that one way to deal with scarce resources is to share the costs associated with employing legal advisors with other nearby law enforcement agencies. In some cases where there are several smaller law enforcement agencies, a regional or district police legal advisor could be an economical alternative to each small agency employing their own legal advisor (Becker, 1994; Schmidt, 1972).

The literature also suggests that another economical alternative to a full time police legal advisor would be employing part-time police legal advisors (IACP, 1998; Schmidt, 1972). A reported benefit of employing police legal advisors on a part-time basis is that the costs are more flexible and relatively reasonable compared to the salary of full-time legal advisors (International Association of Chiefs of Police, 1998). The IACP further suggests that if police organizations' budgets cannot afford to implement legal advisors on a full-time basis, they might consider contracting with a legal advisor to provide 24-hour question/answer service or on-call representation at a predetermined hourly rate (1998).

Risk managers and other insurance assessors could also be used as another practical substitute for hiring police legal advisors

(International Associations of Chiefs of Police, 1998). Risk managers and police legal advisors share common goals in that they both have the same interest in seeing that police organizations, as well as individual police officers, operate in the safest manner as possible. In addition, risk managers could turn to city or county attorneys should the need for legal advice arise.

To deal with the resistance of hiring police legal advisors in the past, the literature suggests that some police departments have masked the position of police legal advisor by providing various titles other than police legal advisor. Some of the alternative titles for legal advisor include "research analyst", "research director", "assistant city prosecutor", "assistant to the manager of safety", "general counsel", or "advisor to the chief" (Caplan, 1967; Lorch, 1969).

Prevalence of police legal advisors in the United States

Despite the recommended need for legal advising in law enforcement agencies cited in early literature, the adoption of police legal advisors by law enforcement agencies has been slow. A national study revealed that out of 276 departments responding to a national survey, only 14 departments reported that they employed legal counsel on a full or part-time basis (Bancroft, 1966).

To date, there is not a complete list of law enforcement agencies in the United States that employ police legal advisors or police legal units. An Internet website maintained by Wayne Schmidt of the International Association of Chiefs of Police (IACP) indicates members of the IACP that are employed as police legal advisors in law enforcement agencies across the United States and other countries. The website only includes those police legal advisors that are members of the IACP.

Law enforcement agencies that use police legal advisors have not been surveyed since 1966. The national study presented in this book will provide an up-to-date look at the use of police legal advisors by American law enforcement agencies. The current study will also provide potential explanations for the slow pace of adoption of police legal advisors in the United States since the late 1960s.

The following section will discuss how risk management, similar to police legal advising, is used by some law enforcement agencies to reduce the exposure of law enforcement officials to liability incidents.

More specifically, the following section includes: (1) a definition of risk management, (2) a detailed description of each stage of the risk management process, and (3) case study reports of perceived success of using risk management in law enforcement agencies in the United States. The section concludes by explaining the common goals, roles, and functions shared by both police legal advisors and risk managers within police organizations.

RISK MANAGEMENT AND THE POLICE

Some believe that law enforcement agencies can benefit from employing police legal advisors to aid in the management of police liability. Police legal advisors provide legal guidance to law enforcement personnel before, during, and after liability incidents occur. Similarly, law enforcement agencies have also begun to use the expertise of risk managers to handle the financial aspect of police liability incidents before, during and after liability incidents occur.

What is risk management?

Risk management is a management tool that can be used to identify and control potential risks and liability problems in organizations. In the past twenty years, risk management has been transformed from an insurance-based technical function to a broad, policy-oriented, managerial tool (Young, 2000). Organizations adopt risk management practices due to increasing threats of litigation, to reduce the risk of harm to their clients and themselves, and to provide a higher quality of service to their clients (Wong & Rakestraw, 1991).

Risk management, as defined by Head & Horn (1985) emphasizes the existence of both a decision-making and managerial component. The decision-making component identifies the steps that need to be taken to identify, assess, handle, and monitor risks. The managerial component provides the means to carry out the tasks associated with decisions in handling exposure to risks. Head and Horn (1985) assert that understanding that risk management is based on both decision-making and managerial components makes the process of identifying and managing organization liability easier. Often, the liability problems in organizations are the result of a breakdown in management and supervision over organization members and failure to use adequate decision-making processes (Head & Horn, 1985).

The following terms are frequently used in discussions focused on risk management by both private and public agencies. The Liability Assessment and Awareness International, Inc. (2001) defines the terms as follows:

- Risk Management - a management tool that can be used to identify and manage potential risks and liability problems in organizations or agencies.
- Risk – The degree of likelihood that a loss will occur.
- Loss – Expenditures (monetary or service-related) as a result of an incident.
- Incident – A situation or occurrence that could result in a loss.
- Claim – Any formal notification that an incident has taken place.
- Liability Loss – This occurs when an individual or organization files a lawsuit alleging wrongdoing. A loss is incurred whenever funds are expended as a result of the lawsuit to investigate or defend the suit, or to pay a settlement, judgment or award whether the suit has merit or not.
- Exposure – An exposure is any circumstance, item, or situation that has the potential to result in a loss.

The risk management process

There is not one "best" risk management process that is suggested to be used universally or for specific types of organizations. "No two local governments have exactly the same risks, and the risks change as the jurisdiction and legal climate changes (Wong & Rakestraw, 1991, p. 1)." Risk management process strategies vary depending on the nature of the organization, including management styles and organizational goals (Conrow, 2000). However, there are several basic steps in the process that are applicable to most types of organizations. Those basic steps include: (1) risk planning, (2) risk assessment, (3) application of risk treatment, (4) evaluation of risk treatment, and (5) continuous review of changes of risk liabilities (Ashley & Pearson, 1993; Cragg & Kloman, 1985; Wong & Rakestraw, 1991).

1. Risk Planning

The first step in the risk management process is to create a strategy to carry out all of the necessary steps involved in the implementation of a risk management program. "Risk planning" involves the creation of a risk management plan (RMP) to identify and track organizational risk issues, perform continuous risk assessments to determine how identified risks have changed over time, develop ways to handle identified risks, monitor the performance of risk handling actions, and locate adequate resources to be available throughout the entire process (Cragg & Kloman, 1985, p. 20). The RMP will serve as a "road map" to anyone that is participating in the implementation process.

After the RMP is drafted, responsibilities are delegated to particular individuals or groups based on the various tasks involved in every step of the process. Each step of the risk management process involves different levels of involvement by people both inside and outside of the organization (Ashley & Pearson, 1993). For example, risk control and risk financing decisions within risk management programs within police organizations might include input from police executives, city auditors, police legal advisors, risk managers, local attorneys, citizen review boards, and anyone else that has experience or knowledge of liabilities associated with police work. The various sources of input result in several changes to the RMP as the risk management process progresses.

2. Risk assessment

After the risk management plan has been drafted and revised, the next step is to assess organizational risk. Risk assessment includes two components: (1) risk identification – the process of identifying and documenting all risks associated with the organization, and (2) risk analysis - the process of analyzing each identified risk area or process, isolating the cause of risks, and then determining the effects that the identified risks have on the organization (Cragg & Kloman, 1985). The effectiveness of risk assessment is contingent on the accuracy of risk identification, and pinpointing exactly how those risks impact or affect the organization.

Some of the risk management literature suggests that identifying organizational risk and exposure to liability includes the examination of all property owned by the organization, as well as all of the services provided by the organization.

Most loss exposure can be classified into six broad categories, including: (1) physical property, including buildings, personal property, vehicles, public records, and cash, (2) loss of income, including any disruption in the receipt of fees, charges for service, fines, and budgetary allowances, (3) contingent expenses that include any losses that force state and local government agencies to acquire additional expenses to function as they normally would under normal conditions, (4) all human resources that include losses due to job-related illnesses or injuries to agency workers, (5) any legal liability, that includes any loss resulting from judgment awards and legal costs to defend the organization in legal proceedings, and (6) all perils that include acts of nature or acts of man, such as vandalism, burglary, and human errors that result in organizational loss (Cragg & Kloman, 1985). The preceding list is not an exhaustive list of potential areas of loss for organizations, but it does cover most of the areas where losses occur when members of the organization are exposed to risk.

There are several methods that can be used in the risk identification process. Organizations undergoing risk assessment often use a variation of identification methods including liability assessment checklists; in-depth interviews with organization supervisors; inspections and site visits to organizations; and close examination of any records of incidents, claims, and complaint forms filed within or against the organization over an extended period of time (Young, 2000). Young also notes that current and past budgets, minutes from council or organizational meetings that deal with proposed cutbacks and reforms, and records of property owned or used by the government, also reveals loss exposure that may be overlooked by a casual glance (2000).

The second part of risk assessment is analyzing the impact of financial loss on the organization or "risk analysis". Potential financial loss is often measured in terms of frequency and severity (Young, 2000). Organizations estimate the frequency and severity of their exposure to liability by looking at any federal regulations regarding local government liabilities and immunities, claims histories for the organization over the past three to five years, and sometimes, liability suits filed in nearby communities (Young, 2000). In addition, recent court cases, awards paid out in settlements and other liability cases, and common defense costs in the surrounding region should also be considered when assessing the potential impact of liabilities.

Once a comprehensive list of potential risks has been compiled, the risks are then categorized and ranked according to the level of seriousness they represent to the organization. Potential risks are often categorized in groupings such as "low frequency/low severity", "low frequency/high severity", "high frequency/low severity" and "high frequency/high severity" (Young, 2000). Once risks are identified and then placed into various categories of severity and frequency, an organization makes the determination of which liability areas are of immediate concern.

Organization loss histories often reveal patterns where the most frequent risk incidents are less severe, and the more severe risk incidents are less frequent (Ashley and Pearson, 1993). This assertion is true in law enforcement as more severe incidents (such as use of deadly force) are less frequent, and less severe incidents (such as claims of verbal discourtesies or claims of less serious bodily harm) are more frequent. Risk control efforts become important when dealing with the less severe incidents due to the high frequency of occurrence. The more frequently something occurs (even if it is less severe or minor), the higher the chances that the less severe incident results in a loss for the organization (Ashley & Pearson, 1993). Essentially, this means that organizations should not take the less serious liability incidents lightly, because over time the little incidents add up to a large amount of payouts or organizational loss.

3. Risk treatment/handling

Once the liability risks are identified and categorized according to frequency and severity, the next step is to decide which technique (or combination of techniques) would be most suitable to control risks and to handle the financing of risk incidents (Young, 2000). This step in the risk management process is important, because it will impact the success or failure of the risk management program (Young, 2000). Deciding which control techniques should be used to deal with organizational risks is the first step in the treatment of risk. There are five basic control techniques that can be used either alone or in conjunction with one another to treat liability risks: (1) risk avoidance, (2) prevention of losses, (3) reduction of losses, (4) segregation of resources, and (5) transfer of risk (Ashley and Pearson, 1993).

Risk avoidance is the decision of the organization to not allow their members to participate in high-risk situations (Ashley & Pearson, 1993). By not participating in high-risk incidents, the probability of loss resulting from exposure to risk is eliminated. An example of risk avoidance for law enforcement agencies could include the implementation of a department policy on non-participation in misdemeanor high-speed pursuits (Ashley & Pearson, 1993).

High-speed pursuits are considered a major area of high-risk concern for law enforcement agencies. Upon realizing the high level of risk involved police pursuits, many law enforcement agencies have implemented policies that forbid officers from pursuing fleeing vehicles, or only allow a pursuit to ensue if clearly defined criteria are present (Alpert et al, 2000). For police officers, risk avoidance is not always a salient solution because there are some high-risk situations that cannot be avoided. Police pursuits are just one example of a police activity that could be completely avoided to decrease the probability of financial loss to the organization.

A second control technique, prevention of losses, requires that measures (either changes in policy, training or both) be taken before any exposure to risk occurs. The goal of prevention of loss techniques is to reduce the frequency of the loss-causing activities (Ashley & Pearson, 1993). An example of a prevention of loss technique used in law enforcement might include mandatory training for "high risk" police actions (Ashley & Pearson, 1993). Two examples of using mandatory training as way to prevent losses include the use of proper physical restraints on suspects (such as the use of various "hog-tying" or restraint mechanisms) (American Civil Liberties Union of Southern California, 1995; Commission on the Accreditation of Law Enforcement Agencies, 1999) or training officers to use "verbal judo" to de-escalate conflict situations with citizens before the situations become physical or violent (Thompson, 1983). By changing agency policies or requiring mandatory training of law enforcement personnel in the risk areas that have been identified as major sources of financial loss, organizations could prevent future payouts for high-risk liability incidents (Ashley & Pearson, 1993).

A third control technique, reduction of losses, can be implemented either before or after incidents occur to reduce the probability of losses or to minimize the impact of losses. This type of risk control technique does not completely prevent loss-causing events from occurring, but reduces the chances for financial loss if risk incidents occur (Ashley & Pearson, 1993). In law enforcement, reduction in loss techniques might be as simple as requiring that all occupants in police vehicles wear seat belts at all times (Ashley & Pearson, 1993). Reduction of loss techniques are different from prevention of loss techniques in that some risk situations cannot be completely prevented from happening, but there are ways to reduce the amount of loss that occurs.

A fourth control technique, segregation of resources, requires that the resources of the organization are segregated so that the organization continues to function if severe losses occur. There are two ways that segregation of resources is possible: (1) duplication of resources, and (2) separation of resources (Ashley & Pearson, 1993). Duplication of resources involves creating reserves of resources that are only available for use when the original resource supply is diminished or depleted (Ashley & Pearson, 1993). An example of duplication of resources in law enforcement includes maintaining several extra patrol cars in case other patrol cares are damaged or rendered unusable (Ashley & Pearson, 1993). By having extra vehicles available, the police agency still functions to full capacity if there is a situation where several patrol cars become damaged or unusable at the same time.

Separation of resources is similar to duplication of resources in that an alternative or back-up source of funding is created (Ashley & Pearson, 1993). The major distinction between separation of resources and duplication of resources is that the back-up or reserve resource supply is used daily by the agency. The formation of specialized units would be an example of separation of resources in law enforcement agencies. The implementation of gang suppression units, homicide units, and drug task force units separates police organization resources in that members of specialized units often conduct tasks similar to those officers working on patrol or in the detective division in addition to their specialized tasks. For example, if line officers need back up on calls for service, members of specialized units can be brought on the scene to assist.

Transferring exposure to risks to an outside agency or group is also a risk control technique. By giving up some responsibilities for tasks that can result in losses, organizations can reduce financial losses completely (Ashley & Pearson, 1993). To maximize the benefit of this risk control technique, both legal and financial responsibilities are transferred over to a third party to ensure that no liability will be placed on the agency that is transferring the risk (Ashley & Pearson, 1993).

However, this control technique is not always an option for some organizations, because there are some high-risk tasks that organizations have to handle themselves and cannot transfer to another agency. This would be the case with most police tasks because police officers are given certain powers of authority that other professions are not; therefore, transferring a majority of police duties would be impossible. This control technique is applicable to county or state-based law enforcement agencies that transport or house prisoners. This is one of only a few of law enforcement tasks where risk could be transferred to a third party.

The literature suggests that all five control techniques are designed to be effective when dealing with exposure to risk and liability incidents. The key to successful risk management is choosing the appropriate methods of risk control that meet organizational needs (Ashley & Pearson, 1993).

4. Implementation

This step is important to the risk management process, because it will execute all of the policies and procedures that were created during the planning stage (Cragg & Kloman, 1985). Analysis of loss and exposure to risk alone will not reduce losses for an organization. The success of a risk management program is also contingent on the involvement and level of support by the local government and top officials within an organization (Young, 2000).

The literature notes several ways to ensure that the implementation phase of the risk management process is done successfully. First, it is important to be sure that the basic components of risk management programs are present, and that adequate people and resources are in place for each component (Crouhy et al., 2001). Some of the components that should be included in any risk management program before implementation takes place include (Crouhy et al., 2001):

- An adequate number of risk management staff members that are properly trained in the area of liability concern.

- A risk management committee that consists of all people that has knowledge in liability issues associated with the purpose of individual agencies.

- A risk management policy statement that presents the guidelines for making decisions about controlling finances, and that also exhibits the commitment of the risk management program by the organization.

- A risk management manual that describes and outlines the policies and procedures of the program.

- An annual report that keeps everyone up to date on the progress of the program, and that reviews standard procedures and policies.

- Both written and verbal steps to ensure employee participation in the program through mission statements, assigned staff responsibilities, training programs, employee manuals, staff meetings, publicity, and enforce policies using discipline, if necessary.

5. Program evaluation/risk monitoring

Once a risk management program has been implemented, risk management staff members conduct some type of on-going evaluation (Ashley & Pearson, 1993). The evaluation is accomplished by establishing performance standards, and then determining if the practices utilized are meeting those standards, and if necessary, correcting any ineffective procedures (Ashley & Pearson, 1993).

Results of risk management program evaluations can be measured in dollars, percentages, ratios, or number of losses or claims over a period of time. Activity standards measuring effort is another way to assess whether or not desired goals have been reached (Ashley & Pearson, 1993). An example of measuring activities or effort could include a requirement that a specific number of safety checks and site visits will be conducted over the course of a year, and also keep records to prove that each site visit or safety check was completed. Therefore, it is important that adequate records are maintained by the organization. Without adequate data on liability incidents and organizational losses, it would be impossible to track any changes in liability claims and payouts (Ashley & Pearson, 1993).

The risk management process is not over after all five steps have been completed. The risk management process is continuous, because organizational risks change over time and continuously require re-evaluation (Ashley & Pearson, 1993).

Risk management in the public sector

It has long been a belief that the philosophies and practices of risk management are not applicable to public or municipal agencies (Esenberg, 1992). This is not the case as most municipal agencies function more efficiently with more resources available to them, which can be accomplished by managing available resources using risk management techniques. Zeckhauser & Viscusi (1996) contend that government agencies, including law enforcement agencies, "should undertake the risk reduction efforts that would best promote the welfare of its citizens" (p. 151). Current risk management literature reports that the use of risk management programs in the public sector is among the fastest growing segments of the risk management profession (Esenberg, 1992).

Risk management and the police in America

In May of 2001, the City of Chicago settled a lawsuit involving the shooting of an unarmed suspect by a Chicago police officer for $18 million (New York Times, May 9, 2001). In Baltimore, a jury awarded more than $7 million to a family whose 17-year-old son (unarmed) was fatally shot by a Baltimore Housing Authority police officer (Baltimore

Sun, May 30, 2001). These cases are only two examples of multi-million dollar payouts for improper use of deadly force by police officers in the past few years. The increasing costs resulting from settlements and payouts in police litigation cases, public scrutiny of police work, and increased pressure from public insurance pools to cut losses, are all reasons that some U.S. law enforcement agencies have begun to create and implement risk management programs.

The need for risk management in law enforcement to control the cost of civil litigation is becoming increasingly recognized by both police practitioners and police scholars alike. Walker (2001) reports that "One of the most notable failures of both police departments and other city officials has been their neglect of modern concepts of risk management and in particular, their refusal to examine incidents that result in litigation and seek to correct the underlying problems (p. 100-101)." A discussion on the use of risk management, early warning systems, and citizen oversight as police accountability mechanisms is featured in *Police Accountability: The Role of Citizen Oversight* (Walker, 2001).

The implementation of risk management programs also provides non-monetary benefits to law enforcement agencies. Police executives should also consider how integrity violations of individual officers impact individual officer careers, other officers that work the streets, the entire police organization, and ultimately the relationship between the police and the community. After police managers determine the non-monetary costs of police integrity violations, this information should be incorporated into both internal and external educational and training programs (Gaffigan and McDonald, 1997).

Early Warning Systems as a risk management tool

In recent years, "Early Warning Systems" (EWS) have been adopted by police organizations as a tool to aid in the identification and management of problematic behavior of police officers. Early Warning Systems are computerized programs that track the frequency and pattern of problematic behavior by police officers that often result in citizen complaints, liability claims, or lawsuits filed by citizens. Police executives adopt such programs to enhance the level of police accountability and professionalism within their organizations, as well as part of their effort to improve the relationship with the communities they serve (Walker & Alpert, 2000). Early Warning Systems have been identified as an important accountability mechanism in the "new paradigm of police accountability" (Walker, 2003).

Early Warning Systems are often used as part of risk management efforts within police agencies as they track and assess the risks of individual police officers (Walker & Alpert, 2002). For example, if an officer receives a certain number of citizen complaints within a specified period of time, the Early Warning System will "flag" that officer. Once an officer is identified by the Early Warning System, his/her immediate supervisors are notified, and at that point, need to decide what type of action will be taken to correct the officer's problematic behavior. In some cases informal counseling between the officer and their immediate supervisor is used as a first step in correcting the problem (Walker, 2003). If informal counseling fails, the next step includes a training class with other officers identified by the early warning system, a wide range of disciplinary action taken by police supervisors, and in some cases, dismissal of the problem officer (Walker & Alpert, 2000). The idea behind early intervention systems is to identify and correct the problematic behavior of officers before their behavior leads to a more serious situation that could potentially result in some type of loss for the police agency (monetary or otherwise).

For a comprehensive look at the planning and management of Early Warning Systems within police agencies, refer to *Early Intervention Systems for Law enforcement Agencies: A Planning and Management Guide* by Dr. Samuel Walker at the Office of Community Oriented Policing Services Website (www.cops.usdoj.gov).

Risk managers & police executives: Common interests and goals

Police executives and risk managers have comparable interests and goals when it comes to dealing with liability-related incidents. Police executives want their organizations to have higher standards and greater professionalism. Similarly, risk managers' work toward higher standards and greater professionalism within the organization to reduce the probability of risk. Gallagher (1992) asserts that this relationship can be easily attained at the municipal level in law enforcement compared to the county level because of the variation in roles between chiefs of police and sheriffs. "The police chief is often appointed by the city manager and may be more amenable to cooperative efforts with other top-level managers, whereas the sheriff, an independently elected official, is the highest law enforcement official in the county and understandably less ready to accept overtures from county government (Gallagher, 1992, p. 65-66)."

Obstacles of risk management in law enforcement

Although limited, the existing literature on risk management in law enforcement identifies several obstacles that potentially hinder the implementation of such programs in police agencies including:

1. The idea that policing has traditionally focused on crime fighting without the worry of financial costs (Ceniceros, 1998). With the increase in litigation against police organizations in the past few decades, more police managers are becoming as concerned with fiscal responsibilities as they are with crime fighting efforts. Police agencies need resources to be able to provide quality police services to the public.

2. Limited resources are another problem police agencies face when they attempt to implement risk management programs. Cities with large populations are able to justify their needs for hiring professional risk managers specifically for reducing costs associated with police litigation (Los Angeles County Sheriffs Office, 2000). In contrast, cities with smaller populations have a harder time justifying the need for risk management. Some of the less expensive alternatives to hiring a full-time, professional risk manager include: (1) expanding the duties of safety directors, (2) employing one risk manager to service an area or region that encompasses several small or medium sized cities, or a risk management committee consisting of municipal attorneys, department representatives or managers, and (3) insurance agents or risk assessors could be used on an "as needed" basis (O'Brien and Wilcox, 1985).

3. Another potential problem with implementing risk management programs in police organizations could be measuring the benefit or the impact of risk management programs to justify its existence in

police agencies. The monetary benefits of risk management are easier to quantify and analyze in regard to impact; however, the impact on the level of police professionalism, and the quality of police services provided to the community, are not always as easily identifiable (Young, 2000). Because resources are often limited in police organizations, being able to justify the need for an in-house risk management program could be difficult if there are no outcome measures for non-monetary benefits.

4. The lack of available information on police risk management programs, as well as training geared specifically toward law enforcement agencies, is another obstacle to the adoption of risk management by police agencies. Currently, there are only a few websites on the Internet that provide information on risk management training for law enforcement officials. There are also training seminars offered by individual risk management lecturers (such as G. Patrick Gallagher and Gordon Graham), and several of the professional risk management organizations across the country (including PRIMA). The problem is that some police executives are unaware of the resources, and often have a difficult time locating the implementation and training resources.

All of the previously mentioned obstacles are not based on any type of empirical research. Instead, the obstacles are suggested in the literature written by risk management experts that have aided in the implementation of risk management programs in police organizations across the United States.

Risk management in law enforcement: Recent applications

Based on the testimony of risk management professionals, the reported benefits of using risk management techniques to manage liability in law enforcement agencies become apparent shortly after the program is implemented (Heazeltine, 1986; Katz, 1998). Past evaluations of the Legal Affairs Division in the Los Angeles Police Department and the Maricopa County Sheriffs Office in Arizona report both monetary and non-monetary benefits of their risk management programs.

Legal Affairs Division - Los Angeles Police Department

The Legal Affairs Division of the Los Angeles Police Department was implemented because of the increase in litigation against the police after the Rodney King incident in 1991. The Risk Management Unit was added to the Legal Affairs Division later on in 1996 (Katz, 1998).

The operation of the LAPD Legal Affairs Unit is both preventive and proactive in that measures are taken both before and after incidents occur. Some of the preventive measures used by Legal Affairs include providing legal training to line officers to prevent them from becoming defendants in civil suits, as well as training in the collection and recording of evidence and information after incidents occur just in case any legal action is taken later on (Katz, 1998). This means that police officers are trained to be able to identify incidents that are likely to result in future litigation. Both legal advisors and risk managers within the Legal Affairs Division in Los Angeles reported success in managing litigation involving the Los Angeles Police Department.

More specifically, personnel from the legal affairs and risk management unit reported a 50 percent drop in liability costs (roughly $10 million dollars) between 1993 and 1997 (Katz, 1998). In addition to reducing the costs of civil litigation against Los Angeles police officers, the purpose of the Legal Affairs Division is to get LAPD police personnel more involved in handling civil cases filed against them. Before the creation of the Legal Affairs Division, the Office of the City Attorney handled all civil cases. The problem was that most attorneys did not have a working knowledge of the nature of police work. The Legal Affairs Division utilizes the legal expertise of attorneys trained in law enforcement, along with risk managers that have the ability to identify exposure to risk, and ultimately, reduce the cost of unnecessary payouts (Katz, 1998).

Other sources do not report the same kind of success of the Legal Affairs Division in handling civil suits against Los Angeles police officers. In an article in Business Insurance magazine, Joanne Wojcik reported that the LAPD Legal Affairs Division had in fact reduced payouts from civil litigation against the LAPD in 1993. Wojcik (1994) contends that the decrease would not continue in 1994, because "the LAPD had incurred more losses in the first four months of 1994 than for all of 1993" (p. 20). The article reports that the dramatic decrease in payouts by the LAPD in 1993 was the result of police officers feeling that their actions were being more heavily scrutinized by the public because of the fallout from the Rodney King incident a few years earlier. Wojcik (1994) contends that the short-lived success of the Division was not because of the efforts of the Unit itself; it was the result of increased public scrutiny.

The more recent Rampart Scandal involving Los Angeles police officers also raises questions on the impact of legal and risk management efforts in the Los Angeles Police Department. Chapter 5 of the executive summary report written by the L.A.P.D. regarding the Rampart area corruption incident features a risk management profile of high-risk incidents that took place in that area from 1994-1998. The analysis by the Risk Management Division included an examination of citizen grievances, vehicular pursuits, non-lethal uses of force, officer-involved shootings, and personnel complaints in the Rampart area compared to other neighboring precinct areas (Los Angeles Police Department, 2000, p. 87).

After examining all of the risk management factors, four main areas of concern were highlighted in the LAPD report: (1) lack of supervision over the CRASH unit in the Rampart area; (2) a pattern of an unusually high number of citizens recanting complaints that were filed against police officers in the Rampart area; (3) a pattern of misconduct of officers in the Rampart area, ranging from theft, illegal searches and falsifying reports, and finally; (4) complaints that were filed against Rampart officers were not processed in a timely manner (Los Angeles Police Department, 2000, p. 108).

Based on the Risk Management Division's findings, it is clear that the events that occurred in the Rampart area from 1994-1998 went undetected by L.A.P.D. police managers, as well as the units that were implemented to deal with such issues. As it is clearly stated in the conclusions of the L.A.P.D. report, the Rampart situation was overlooked by the entire police organization.

Risk Management in Maricopa County

The benefits of using risk management in law enforcement agencies was also noted in a 1985 case study of the Maricopa County Sheriff's Department (Heazeltine, 1986). G. Patrick Gallagher of the Institute for Liability Management of Vienna, Virginia spearheaded the application of risk management techniques in Maricopa County.

By using the expertise of the law enforcement personnel, in addition to police legal advisors, and several risk managers, Gallagher was able to identify policies, procedures, training, and previous lawsuits and complaints to identify areas of high liability concern (Heazeltine, 1986). Training was provided for all police supervisors that focused on several areas of liability concern, state tort laws, and federal civil right statutes (Heazelton, 1986). The training of supervisors helped reconfirm the importance of strict supervision over procedures and activities of patrol officers to reduce or eliminate potential liability. After the liability assessment and supervisor training took place, a final report suggesting areas of change (or in some cases elimination of policies and procedures) was drafted and turned over to risk managers and city attorneys to follow-up on all suggestions for change. The entire process in Maricopa County cost the department $36,100 from beginning to end (Heazeltine, 1986).

Heazeltine (1986) also noted the perceived short-term impact that using risk management techniques produced shortly after implementation. Some of the short-term benefits include a closer working relationship between the Sheriffs office and the county attorney's office, an increase in the number of requests for legal advice by deputies, and an overall improvement in accepting responsibility by supervisors and management (Heazeltine, 1986).

Even with a lack of scientific research, the perceived benefits of using risk management hint that this approach could be adopted by law enforcement agencies as alternative way to manage police liability issues. Also lacking in the police liability literature is the examination of the use of police legal advising and risk management in various combinations in police agencies in the United States. The following section discusses the link between police legal advisors and risk managers, as well as some of the differences between the two groups.

The link between risk managers and police legal advisors

Based on the information found in both the risk management and police legal advising literature, police departments can use police legal advisors and risk managers separately, together, or in some other unique combination depending on the individual needs of the organization. The duties of risk managers parallel those of police legal advisors because both groups are employed by police organizations for the same reason – to reduce and maintain control over police liability. Both groups use their training to identify, and then examine policies and procedures that often result in legal problems (and sometimes monetary payouts) for the police organization. Even with very different professional and educational backgrounds, police legal advisors and risk managers can achieve similar goals when handling police liability incidents.

Risk managers and police legal advisors share a common purpose within police organizations: to ensure that the organization and its members provide quality service to the community in a safe, legal, and professional manner, while maintaining financial responsibility over police-involved liability incidents. Gallagher contends that it is absolutely essential that police agencies seek out and utilize legal support staff and services as part of their organization. "What is needed are attorneys who are specialists on police legal and procedural matters who are made available through pools and risk management associations (Gallagher, 1992, p. 23)."

A distinct difference between risk managers and police legal advisors is that risk managers are often more narrowly focused on the financial aspects of police liability. In contrast, police legal advisors are more in tune with the legal aspect of police liability. Despite their differences in training, both groups are equipped with the tools to achieve liability management for most police organizations.

As previously mentioned, law enforcement agencies in the United States have only recently begun to adopt risk management programs. To date, there has not been any research conducted on the use of risk management by law enforcement agencies in the United States. The national study presented in Chapter Four of this book is the first systematic exploration of law enforcement use of risk management in liability management. In addition, the national study updates the use of police legal advisors by police agencies, and explores how both risk managers and police legal advisors are used in combination or alone to manage police liability.

CHAPTER 4

A National Study of Risk Management and Police Legal Advising: Methodology and Theoretical Approach

This chapter describes the first national study of the use of risk management and police legal advising by law enforcement agencies in the United States. The main purpose of the study is to explore the use of risk management and police legal advising by U.S. police agencies in their efforts to manage liability within their organizations. More specifically, this study examines the prevalence of the use of risk management and police legal advising by police agencies, the factors associated with the adoption of such programs, the role of such programs within police organizations, and the perceived impact of risk management and police legal advising programs on police liability management.

QUALITATIVE RESEARCH METHODOLOGY

In social science research, there are several methodological approaches that can be used to examine the behaviors and activities of individuals, groups, and organizations. In most cases, the methodological approach (or combination of methodological approaches) used is based on the specific research questions that are under examination. Social scientists often choose between quantitative, qualitative, or some combination of both types of research methods.

In order to choose the appropriate methodology, it is important to understand the differences between quantitative and qualitative approaches. Some of the main differences include: (1) the logic of qualitative research is often inductive rather than deductive, (2) qualitative research designs are often emergent and flexible, and can change throughout the course of the research process, (3) the qualitative research process is non-linear and non-sequential, (4) samples are smaller in qualitative studies compared to quantitative studies that use larger samples, and (5) qualitative research methods are more appropriate in cases where little is known about a particular topic or problem (Ambert & Adler, 1995; Berg, 2001; Creswell, 1994). These distinct differences in research design result in variations in the presentation of qualitative research findings, and in the evaluation of the reliability and validity of qualitative studies.

The purpose of using qualitative research methods is to learn about how and why people think, behave, or interpret their surroundings as they do (Creswell, 1994). Ultimately, the goal of qualitative research is to turn the data that has been collected into something meaningful and useful (Rossman & Rallis, 1998). When qualitative research methods are utilized, researchers strive for depth and understanding of some phenomenon or problem rather than achieving breadth or generalizability to large populations or groups (Ambert & Adler, 1995). Instead of drawing from a large, representative sample of an entire population, qualitative researchers seek in-depth, intimate information about a smaller number of persons or organizations.

The underlying assumptions of the qualitative paradigm determine the type of data collection methods that can be used in qualitative inquiry. Research methods including open-ended questionnaires, in-depth interviews, ethnographic studies, and participant observation all generate data that describes a social problem or process using the voice of research participants that are directly or indirectly linked to the problem or process (Ambert & Adler, 1995).

The study presented in this chapter utilizes qualitative data collection and analysis techniques, in addition to some basic descriptive statistics (percentages) derived from telephone interviews and survey responses.

RESEARCH QUESTIONS

This study describes how risk management and police legal advising approaches are used to control liability incidents involving police officers. More specifically, this study will explore the following research questions:

1. What is the prevalence of the use of risk managers and police legal advisors in county and municipal law enforcement agencies in the United States?

2. What are some of the factors associated with the adoption of risk management and police legal advising programs by law enforcement agencies?

3. What are some of the characteristics associated with the identified risk management or police legal advising programs?

4. What are some of the roles that risk managers and police legal advisors play within police organizations?

5. According to police legal advisors and risk managers, what is the perceived impact of risk management and police legal advising approaches on department costs related to liability incidents, police professionalism, and accountability within law enforcement agencies?

The examination of these research questions will provide useful information for police executives on the various ways that other law enforcement agencies across the country manage their police liability. Even with an substantial body of literature published on police liability, the issue of how to control or handle police liability resulting in citizen complaints, liability claims, or lawsuits has gone virtually untouched by police scholars.

SAMPLING FRAME, POPULATION, AND RESEARCH SITES

The choice of research populations and research sites that are used in qualitative studies will determine the level of quality and rigor of each study. In qualitative research, "sampling for meaning" often shapes the samples used in each study. Luborsky & Rubinstein (1995) describe the concept of "sampling for meaning" as a technique that attempts to draw a sample that can provide written and/or verbal descriptions directly related to the research topic or problem. The goal of this sampling technique is not to achieve the highest numerical representation of the population; rather it is to acquire rich, detailed information from individuals or groups that have direct and indirect experiences with that particular research topic. Thus, qualitative research is sometimes referred to as "small-N" research (King et al, 1994; Munck, 1998).

There are several things to consider when choosing samples for qualitative inquiry. Some issues to consider include:

- The sampling frame and sample should be based on the overall purpose of the study, as well as clearly stated research questions (Curtis et al, 2000).

- Qualitative samples are often small (compared to samples used in quantitative studies) but generate large amounts of textual data (Miles & Huberman, 1994).

- Qualitative samples are not always pre-specified in the planning stage of research design. Often, samples are selected in a sequential manner or a "rolling process" that takes place during the data collection process. As a result, sample size can vary from one stage of the data collection process to the next (Miles & Huberman, 1994).

- Qualitative samples are "used to make analytic generalizations (applied to wider theory on the basis of how selected cases fit with general constructs), but not statistical generalizations (applied to wider populations on the basis of representative statistical samples) (Curtis et al., 2000, p. 1002)."

- Cases or samples used in qualitative inquiry should meet the criterion of "unit homogeneity". Unit homogeneity is the "assumption that all units with the same value of the explanatory variable have the same expected value of the dependent variable (King et al, 1994, p. 91)." In the current study, unit homogeneity is achieved by requiring that each law enforcement agency included in the sample meet two criteria: (1) the agency must have 200 or more sworn police personnel, and (2) that agency personnel report that they use risk management and/or police legal advising to manage liability in their organizations. These two criteria exclude those agencies that cannot provide direct or indirect experience with using police legal advising and/or risk management to manage police liability.

Each of the five previously mentioned guidelines to qualitative sampling was used in the planning and data collection stages of the national study presented in this book.

Sample of current study

In qualitative research, research populations and research sites are often determined by the specified research questions (Berg, 2001; Crabtree & Miller, 1999; Denzin & Lincoln, 1994; Rossman & Rallis, 1998). Therefore, to study the use of police legal advising and risk management by law enforcement agencies, only law enforcement agencies that use such approaches would be included in the sample and case study research sites.

The literature on police legal advising makes specific suggestions as to which law enforcement agencies should have police legal advisors. O.W. Wilson (1963) hinted at a trend of larger police organizations adopting full-time police legal advisors to handle any legal issues that arise. The National Commission on Criminal Justice Standards and Goals (1973) and the American Bar Association (1967) suggests that police agencies that employ 200 or more officers could easily justify creating positions for police legal advisors.

Similarly, risk management programs would also most likely be used in larger police agencies because of more frequent exposure to risk during police-citizen contacts. Police organizations that have a high number of sworn police officers interacting with citizens will also have a higher probability of exposure to risk incidents that could lead to future litigation.

Guided by suggestions from the literature, all county and municipal law enforcement agencies that employ 200 or more sworn police officers were used for the sampling frame in this study. A list of county and municipal law enforcement agencies employing 200 or more sworn police officers was drawn from the 1999 Law Enforcement Management and Administrative Statistics (LEMAS) report. The 1999 LEMAS report identified a total of 354 county and municipal law enforcement agencies meeting this specific personnel criterion.

Because a triangulated, qualitative methodological approach was used in this study, the sample size varies with each stage of data collection. In the first stage of data collection, all 354 law enforcement agencies with 200 or more sworn police personnel were included in the sampling frame. Representatives from all 354 agencies were contacted by telephone to determine which agencies use risk management and/or police legal advising to deal with police liability issues. Representatives from all 354 law enforcement agencies included in the sampling frame answered interviews questions.

In the second stage of data collection, only those law enforcement agencies that reported any use of police legal advising and/or risk management during initial telephone interviews were included in the sampling frame. Surveys were faxed to 177 of the original 354 law enforcement agencies identified in the LEMAS report.

And finally, in the third step of data collection, four research sites were chosen for case study site visits (Portland, Oregon; Los Angeles, California; Las Vegas, Nevada; and Charlotte-Mecklenburg, North Carolina). These four research sites were chosen because each agency has a unique approach to their use of police legal advising and risk management. The four sites used for case study analyses are described in greater detail in Chapter 6.

Data Collection

Data collection was conducted in a three-step sequential approach. The data collected in the first step of the process determined which agencies would be included in the second step of the data collection process, and so forth.

Step #1: Telephone interviews

The first step of the data collection process began with the identification of law enforcement agencies that use risk management and/or police legal advising to manage police liability. A scan of all 354 county and municipal law enforcement agencies with 200 or more sworn police personnel was conducted by examining police departments' websites to obtain telephone contact information.

Telephone contact was made with police personnel in the administrative offices or internal affairs division at all 354 law enforcement agencies. The telephone interviews inquired about the use of both police legal advising and/or risk management within each police organization. Once it was determined whether or not the agency used risk management and/or police legal advising, agency representatives were informed of the purpose of this study, and were also informed that surveys would be faxed to their agencies within a few weeks.

The purpose of contacting all 354 agencies by phone is to identify the prevalence of the use of risk management and/or police legal advising within police organizations in the United States.

Step #2: National Survey

After using telephone interviews to determine which law enforcement agencies use risk management and/or police legal advising, a cover letter, informed consent form, and survey instrument were faxed directly to police legal advisors and/or risk managers in each agency. The survey instrument contained open-ended questions because little is known about police use of risk management and police legal advising. Devers & Frankel (2000) suggest the use of open-ended survey questions when very little is known about a topic.

Surveys were used to explore the reasons why risk management and/or police legal advising approaches were adopted by the police organizations, what role, purpose, and function risk managers and/or police legal advisors play within each organization, how the use of risk management and/or legal advising has changed each agency, and the perceived impact of risk management and police legal advising on each agency. Additionally, a request for annual or quarterly budget reports was made at the end of the survey instrument to explore the perceived monetary impact of using risk management and/or police legal advising on liability costs.

The data collected from the survey instrument will not be used in any statistical analyses. Instead, the information on the surveys will provide in-depth, descriptive accounts of how law enforcement agencies use police legal advisors and risk managers to control exposure to liability incidents. As with most types of qualitative inquiry, a greater emphasis will be placed on the quality and richness of the survey data, with less emphasis placed on the quantity or response rate of completed surveys (Ambert & Adler, 1995; Berg, 2001; Crabtree & Miller, 1999; Creswell, 1994; Curtis et al., 2000; Denzin & Lincoln, 1994; Devers & Frankel, 2000; Rossman & Rallis, 1998).

Step #3: Case Studies

The third step of the data collection process included case study analyses of four law enforcement agencies that use risk management and police legal advising. Case studies are designed to bring out rich details of research topics that are often missed by other types of data collection techniques (Tellis, 1997). Site visits to each of the four cities provide thick descriptions of the factors influencing the adoption of risk managers and police legal advisors, the way that these management tools are used within each police agency, and the perceptions of risk managers, legal advisors, and police personnel on the impact of risk management and legal advising on police liability. The findings of the cases study analyses provide greater detail of each program than the results of the survey used in the second step of the data collection process.

Gaining access to each case study site was negotiated through several telephone conversations and email correspondences with the supervisors of each risk management and/or police legal unit. The supervisors or "gatekeepers" within each agency was used to help coordinate site visits, and to provide additional resources (such as annual reports and other records) that would provide detailed information specific to each agency. In addition, the "gatekeepers" informed other police & city personnel of the purpose of the study, as well as the planned site visits to each agency prior to its occurrence.

Site visits were conducted in Los Angeles California, Portland Oregon, Las Vegas Nevada, and Charlotte-Mecklenburg North Carolina. These four sites were chosen for case study analyses because of the various combinations of the use of risk managers and police legal advisors in each police agency. The following sections provide a general description of how each research site uses risk management and/or police legal advising, as well as where the units or divisions are physically located in reference to each police agency.

Los Angeles Sheriffs Department – California

The Los Angeles Sheriff's Department uses both risk management and legal advising approaches to control police liability. The Risk Management Bureau is housed within the Los Angeles Sheriffs Department. The Risk Management Bureau consists of specialized units that focus on specific tasks related to risk management. Some of the specialized units include the Civil Litigation Unit, Health and Safety Unit, Risk Impact Unit, Traffic Services Detail Section, Random Drug Testing Program, and the Manuals and Orders Section. The Legal Advisory Unit is housed in a building outside of the Sheriff's Department because of the lack of space in the Sheriff's Department. The Legal Advisory Unit handles all of the legal matters of the Sheriff's Department involving Department employees.

Portland Police Bureau – Oregon

The Portland Police Bureau also uses a combination of both police legal advising and risk management to control liability within their organization. The Police Liability Management Division deals with several liability-related issues including fleet management, and training/policy liability issues. The Police Liability Management Unit is housed within the Portland Police Bureau headquarters. The Police Liability Division also works with the Risk Management Division that provides citywide coverage for Portland. The Risk Management Division is housed outside of the Portland Police Bureau. The Police Liaison, who is also the Deputy City Attorney of Portland, provides legal advice for police personnel. The Police Liaison's office is located within the City Attorney's Offices.

Charlotte Police Department – North Carolina

The Charlotte Police Department is also unique in the way that it uses risk managers and police legal advisors. The Risk Management Division for the city of Charlotte provides risk management services to the Charlotte Police Department. This Division is located within the Charlotte city offices. Recently, the Risk Management Department adopted a Loss Control Team to assist in the handling of police liability claims. All legal advice is provided by the Police Attorneys Office which is included as part of the Charlotte police organizational structure.

Las Vegas Metropolitan Police Department – Las Vegas, Nevada

The Las Vegas Metropolitan Police Department utilizes both risk management and legal advising in their effort to control liability in their organization. The Risk Management Section is part of the Office of Policy and Planning in the Las Vegas Metropolitan Police Department. Although it is officially consider part of the LVMPD, it is physically housed in city hall. The Deputy District Attorney (Attorney of Record for the LVMPD) provides legal services to the LVMPD. A private law firm (Rawlings, Olson, Cannon, Gormley, & Desruisseaux) takes care of all litigation involving personnel of the LVMPD.

After examining the various combinations of risk management and police legal advising in all four research sites, the unique characteristics of each site become clear (see Table 4.1 on the next page). The result of the case study analyses in Chapter Six provides greater detail of the function and role of risk managers and police legal advisors at each research site.

Table 4.1
Case Study Site Matrix

Research Site	Risk Management	Legal Advising
Los Angeles Sheriff's Department (California)	Risk Management Bureau (in-house)	Legal Advisory Unit (outside of police department)
Portland Police Bureau (Oregon)	Police Liability Management Division (in-house) & Risk Management For city of Portland (outside of police department)	Deputy City Attorney Police Liaison (outside of police department)
Charlotte Police Department (North Carolina)	Risk Management Division for the City of Charlotte (outside of police department)	Police Attorneys Office (in-house)
Las Vegas Metropolitan Police Department (Nevada)	Risk Management Section (used exclusively for police, but housed outside of police department)	Deputy District Attorney & Private Law Firm (outside of police department)

Data Management Tools

The use of some type of data management tool (computer-based or otherwise) is essential in data analysis. Data management tools are important because the tools can ensure a higher quality of data; it makes data more accessible and manageable during analysis; it provides documentation of the steps taken during data analysis, and will retain the data for use in future research projects (Huberman & Miles, 1994, p. 428). If all data is collected and then stored with some type of data management tool, it will be easier to reduce the data down to a point where categorization can take place during the analysis.

The analysis for this study was conducted using "Microsoft Access 2000". This computer program allows the response of specific survey questions and field notes to be examined simultaneously, which makes identifying categories and themes that emerge from the textual data much easier.

THEORETICAL PERSPECTIVE

The purpose of this study is not to test the diffusion of innovations theory. Instead, this study will use the diffusion of innovations theory to explain the adoption of police legal advisors and risk managers by law enforcement agencies in the United States. The following sections will explain the basic assumptions of the diffusion of innovations theory, provide a brief history of the application of the theory, and will identify characteristics of organizations, innovations, and the environments outside of organizations that impact the expediency of the adoption of innovative programs and techniques.

Definition of terms and basic assumptions

A basic description of the diffusion of innovations theory would be that it is a social process consisting of people (or groups) within social systems communicating to each other about new ideas as they gradually shape the meaning and usefulness of the innovations (Rogers, 1995). To better understand this theory, Rogers defines each of the key terms associated with this theory (1995, pp. 5-12):

- Diffusion is the process by which innovations are communicated through certain channels over time among members of a social system.

- Innovations are ideas, practices, or objects perceived as new by individuals or groups.

- Social System is a set of interrelated units (individuals or groups) that are engaged in joint problem solving to accomplish common goals.

The four basic elements found in the diffusion of innovations theory include innovations, communication channels, time, and social systems (Rogers, 1994, p. 10). Each of the four elements plays an important role in the adoption of innovations by individuals or groups.

<u>Element #1 – Innovations</u>

Innovations are ideas, practices, or objects perceived as "new" by individuals or groups (Rogers, 1995). Some of the characteristics associated with innovations that influence their rate of adoption include relative advantage, compatibility, complexity, trialability, and observeability (Rogers, 1995).

- Relative advantage is the perceived advantages (economic, social prestige, convenience) that the innovation will produce if adopted by a group or individual. The more perceived advantages created by adopting the innovation; the more quickly the innovation will be adopted (Rogers, 1995).

- Compatibility is how well the innovation parallels the core values, philosophies and practices of an organization or individual. An organization is more likely to adopt an innovation that reflects existing practices and ideologies within the organization so that minimal changes will have to be made if the innovation is ultimately adopted (Rogers, 1995).

- The complexity of the innovation is also an important factor in innovation adoption. If the innovation is easy to understand and easy to use, it will most likely be adopted than would a more complex innovation (Rogers, 1995).

- Trialability refers to the degree to which an innovation can be adopted on a temporary or short-term basis (Rogers, 1995). Innovations that can be adopted temporarily are usually adopted quicker than those that are long term because there is less risk involved in the adoption.

- Observeability includes the observable results or impact of newly adopted innovations (Rogers, 1995). If an innovation can provide dramatic results (in the form of efficiency, advantages, or increased monetary or financial gain) that is easily measured or observed, it is most likely that the innovation will be adopted faster than if the results or impact were less apparent or not easily measured.

Rogers (1995) also identifies a general process that describes how innovation development occurs. The "innovation-development process" can be described in six distinct phases. The identification of a problem or need for innovation is the first phase of the innovation-development process. Once the need or problem is identified, research is conducted on the innovation to see how others have used it, and how (if at all) it has benefited other individuals or groups. The next task is to develop a strategy to put the innovation into motion. Innovations can take the form of programs, techniques, approaches, or policies. Rogers (1995) also asserts that "commercialization" takes place when an individual or group packages innovations in "ready-to-use" forms to be adopted by others. However, not all innovations are "pre-packaged", therefore, the fourth phase of the "innovation-development" process is not a phase that always takes place. Next, innovation diffusion takes place when communication about the innovation occurs between individuals or groups (Rogers, 1995). The adoption of new ideas is often slow in the early stages of the innovation adoption process. Once early adopters of an idea realize and share the benefits of the idea with others, the adoption process increases at a much faster pace (Backer & Rogers, 1998). This slow-to-fast progression is often referred to as the "S-shaped rate of adoption" (Rogers, 1995, p. 40).

The innovation-development process ends with some kind of change resulting from the adoption of the innovation. In some cases, the consequences of adopting the innovation are so subtle or negative that the innovation is never fully implemented. This is often the case with innovations that have a lagged effect or are categorized as a "preventive innovation" where the consequences of the innovation cannot be predicted before the innovation is adopted (Rogers, 1995, p. 217).

Element #2 – Communication Channels

Communication channels are the means by which information is relayed between groups or individuals within social networks. In the diffusion of innovations theory, communication is defined as "the process by which participants create and share information with one another in order to reach a mutual understanding" (Rogers, 1995, p. 17). Communication channels are an important part of the adoption of innovations because any information transmitted from one group or person to the next will influence the probability of adoption.

The level of homophily between individuals or groups also influences the transmission of information about innovations. Rogers (1995) asserts that groups or individuals that share similar interests, social and personal characteristics, attitudes, languages, and problems are more likely to have meaningful communication exchanges compared to individuals or groups that are heterophilous in nature.

Element #3 – Time

The element of time impacts the diffusion of innovations in several ways. First, time is involved in the innovation-decision process beginning with the time that groups first learn of innovations, and ending with the time that an innovation is either adopted or rejected by others. The innovation-decision process can be conceptualized in five steps: (1) knowledge about an innovation is acquired by an individual or group, (2) that knowledge is used by the individual or group to form a positive or negative opinion of the innovation, (3) a decision is made to either adopt or reject the innovation, (4) after the innovation is adopted, it is put to use by an individual or group, and finally, (5) the success or failure of an innovation is confirmed by an individual or group (Rogers, 1995).

There are also specific characteristics of organizations and the external environments surrounding organizations that influence the rate of adoption of innovations. Some of the organizational characteristics that impact the adoption of innovations include organization size, available wealth or resources, various organizational structure and management characteristics (including informality, decentralization, and complexity), span of organizational goals, level of professionalism, strength of leadership within an organization, and the absence of a dominant organizational ideology (Downs, 1976; Mohr, 1969).

The environment surrounding the organization can also impact the rate of innovation adoptions by organizations. For example, Mohr suggests that an "organization may be more likely to innovate when its environment is rapidly changing than when it is steady…and innovation should also be more likely when the social environment to which an organization belongs has norms that favor change…" (1969, p. 112). In this case, the external environment includes social, political, and economic conditions, as well as clientele needs and demands placed on an organization or agency (Mohr, 1969).

Element #4 – Social System

Another element of the diffusion of innovation theory is the social system to which an individual or organization belongs. A more formal definition of a social system is "a defined set of interrelated units that are engaged in joint problem-solving to accomplish a common goal…the members of a social system may be individuals, informal or formal groups, organizations, and/or subsystems" (Rogers, 1995, p. 23). In diffusion of innovation research, a social system represents the boundaries in which innovation diffusion takes place.

The way that social systems are structured impacts the level of innovation adoption that takes place within the social system. For example, if a social system is fragmented or loosely structured the diffusion of innovation will be slower than a social system that is highly structured and interconnected (Roger, 1995). Equally important is the idea that a more structured social system will facilitate more effective and meaningful communication between individuals or groups within the social system.

In conclusion, the four elements of diffusion of innovations theory (social system, time, communication channels, and innovations) all play important roles in understanding, testing, and applying the theory to a wide variety of subjects.

Application of the diffusion of innovations theory

The diffusion of innovations theory has been tested and used to explain the adoption of innovations across a wide range of subjects. In 1977 Everett M. Rogers, Linda Williams, and Rhonda B. West compiled a bibliography of 2,750 publications that either tested or used diffusion of innovations theory to explain some phenomenon. Some of the disciplines that are included in the Rogers et al (1977) bibliography include anthropology, communication, geography, sociology, journalism, public administration, statistics, speech, and industrial engineering. More recently, Musmann and Kennedy (1989) created a bibliographic compilation of publications that focus on the diffusion of innovations theory.

In the last decade, several publications have applied the diffusion of innovations theory to a variety of social and political issues including the adoption of work-site AIDS programs in the United States (Backer & Rogers, 1998), nation-wide health education campaigns (Denard-Goldman, 1994), and policy entrepreneurs and their efforts to promote policy ideas (Mintrom, 1997). Based on the breadth of the literature, it is clear that the diffusion of innovations theory can be used to explain the adoption of innovations across almost any discipline or type of organization.

Diffusion of innovations theory and American policing

One area of study that has not fully utilized the diffusion of innovations theory to explain the adoption of innovations is police studies. To date, there are only a few publications that loosely examine the diffusion of innovations in American policing, with only one study that directly tests components of the diffusion of innovations theory.

One of the earliest studies that examine the diffusion of a police innovation focuses on the growth, extent, and impact of the use of computers by police (Colton, 1972). The International City Management Association (ICMA) sponsored a study on police use of computers in 1971. Based on information provided by surveys and site visits to U.S. police departments, it was revealed that 38.8 percent of police departments reported computer usage (Colton, 1972). Colton also found that large, urban, southern police departments were more likely to report computer use in their agencies compared to other regions across the United States.

In Colton's study, five organizational variables emerged as influential in the success or failure of computer use within police agencies including: (1) the level of involvement and quality of leadership within the agency, (2) involvement of computer use by most officers within the agency, (3) establishment of priorities within the organization, (4) quality of computer systems available and technical staff available to the officers, and (5) a high degree of emphasis placed on human-computer interaction within the police department (Colton, 1972). This study is important because it was one of the first empirical studies to look at how an innovation (in this case, computers) can impact police organizations.

Another study by Skolnick and Bayley (1986) examined innovative policing strategies in six U. S. police departments. This study focused on changes in organizational structure, administrative leadership, and police performance as a result of adopting community policing practices and philosophies. The results of the study indicate that one of the biggest factors impacting positive changes in policing is strong leadership by police chiefs. The theme of strong leadership in relation to the adoption of innovations within police agencies is found in both early and current studies of police organizations.

And most recently, Alexander Weiss (1997) used the diffusion of innovations theory to examine "how information about innovation is communicated among police organizations and the factors that influence adoption of such innovations" (p. 293). More specifically, this study tests a general model of the communication and adoption of innovations in policing containing four major elements (Weiss, 1997, p. 293-294):

1. Cosmopolitanism – is measured by the degree of contact and communication outside of a police organization.

2. Risk Mediation – "the extent to which police organizations seek to reduce their perceived risk of civil liability (Weiss, 1997, p. 293)."

3. Peer Emulation – is measured by the degree to which innovations are influenced by communication with and imitation of other police organizations.

4. Innovativeness – is measured by the number of innovations that a police organization has adopted (including 911 emergency systems, a variety of computerized programs, and problem-oriented policing techniques and programs), as well as how a police agency's perceives its own reputation in the policing community.

Several important findings were revealed after testing Weiss's model containing the previously described elements. In regard to the cosmopolitanism element, Weiss (1997) reports that police executive participation in policy communities would lead directly to the adoption of innovations because they would be provided with information on innovations by others in police organizations, and that participation would lead to peer emulation because there would be increased communication with other police executives (p. 305).

There was also support found for the hypothesis focused on the second element – risk mediation - that "the more risk averse the organization (police), the more likely it would be to engage in peer emulation, and indirectly, be more innovative" (Weiss, 1997, p. 305). Weiss explains this finding by describing how an increase in litigation involving the police impacts how police executives manage their agencies. He uses the example of how some cities are beginning to employ police legal advisors and risk managers to help reduce exposure to risks. This particular finding in Weiss's study accentuates the importance of further research on the use of alternative management tools, such as risk management and police legal advising, to reduce police liability.

Peer emulation (the 3rd element in Weiss's model) between police agencies also contributes to the diffusion of innovations in policing. Weiss (1997) asserts that the "calling around" method is often used by police executives because it allows them to gather information about a particular idea or program quickly, and because the information comes from a source that they view as "legitimate" – other police executives.

And finally, there was also support found for Weiss's assertion "that an organization's innovativeness, viewed as an organizational attribute, is a function of both the adoption of innovations and of an organization's assessment of its innovativeness in respect to its peers (Weiss, 1997, p. 307)." Essentially, the number of innovative programs and ideas used by police organizations influenced their perceptions of their own reputation in the policing community. Weiss's 1997 study is unique because it is the first study to empirically test some of the elements of the diffusion of innovations theory specifically applied to police organizations.

Current Study

Based on the previous description of some of the elements of diffusion of innovations theory, it is possible that the diffusion of innovation theory can help explain the adoption of risk managers and police legal advisors by law enforcement agencies in the United States. As previously mentioned, the current study will not test any of the components of the diffusion of innovations theory. Instead, this study will use this theory to explain the adoption of risk management and police legal advising by law enforcement agencies.

CHAPTER 5

Results of the National Study

This chapter presents the results of a national study on the use of risk management and police legal advising by U.S. law enforcement agencies. The five research questions listed in Chapter Four are addressed individually as the analyses of each data source are reported in each section.

TELEPHONE INTERVIEWS

Telephone interviews were conducted with 354 county and municipal law enforcement agencies to determine the prevalence of the use of risk managers and police legal advisors by police agencies in the United States. The 1999 Law Enforcement Management and Administrative Statistics (LEMAS) report was used to create the list of all law enforcement agencies with 200 or more sworn police personnel. This report identified 354 county and municipal law enforcement agencies. Representatives from each of the 354 agencies were interviewed on how their organization handles police liability issues, as well as which person or group is responsible for any legal matters involving police personnel. Agency representatives participating in the telephone interviews include risk managers, police legal advisors, internal affairs staff, and in some cases, chiefs of police. Telephone interviews are the primary data source used to explore the first research question.

Prevalence of the use of risk management and police legal advising

Based on telephone interviews with all 354 law enforcement agencies, exactly one half (177) of all police agencies reported the use of either police legal advising, risk management, or some combination of both to manage police liability issues. More specifically, 163 of 354 agencies stated that they utilize only police legal advisors, while another 14 agencies reported the use of some combination of legal advisors and risk managers (see Table 5.1 below). No agency reported that they use only risk managers exclusively to manage police liability issues.

Table 5.1
Prevalence of Police Legal Advisors and Risk Managers in United States Law Enforcement Agencies

Only Police Legal Advisors (Used exclusively by police department)	**163**
Only Risk Managers (Used exclusively by police department)	**0**
Use Both Police Legal Advisor & Risk Manager (either in-house or city-wide)	**14**
Other (City/County Attorney, that also serves all local and county agencies)	**175**
Other (Locally contracted private attorney)	**2**
	N=354 agencies

The other half of the police agencies interviewed (177) reported that they rely solely on city/county attorneys to handle liability issues involving law enforcement personnel. As noted in the police legal advising literature from the 1960s and 1970s, city/county attorneys were viewed as a source of resistance to hiring police legal advisors. At that time, some city/county attorneys claim that providing legal services to the police is part of their job, and therefore, employing police legal advisors is unnecessary (Caplan, 1967; Schmidt, 1972).

In the past four decades, there have been significant changes in the legal and social environment in the United States. The evidence of the changes in the legal environment in the United States is reflected in the fact that the police are named as defendants in civil suits filed by citizens more frequently than they were four decades ago (Franklin, 1993; Kappeler, 1997; McCoy, 1987). There have also been significant changes in police procedures because of important court case decisions, including *Miranda v. Arizona (1966), Mapp v. Ohio (1961), and Tennessee v. Garner (1985).*

Another indication of the changes in the legal environment includes the creation of the Special Litigation Section within the Civil Rights Division of the United States Department of Justice. The Special Litigation Section is responsible for enforcing federal civil rights statues regarding civil rights of institutional persons, conduct of law enforcement agencies, access to reproductive health clinics and places of religious worship (United States Department of Justice website, 2002). This Litigation Section enforces the police misconduct provision of the Violent Crime Control and Law Enforcement Act of 1994.

The Department of Justice website notes the impact that the Special Litigation Section has already had on enforcing police misconduct in the United States:

> The Section has already obtained significant relief under its police misconduct authority. For example, in 1997, the Section obtained two consent decrees to remedy systemic misconduct in municipal police departments in Pittsburgh, Pennsylvania and Steubenville, Ohio. The decrees require the police departments to implement widespread reforms, including training, supervising, and disciplining officers and implementing systems to receive, investigate, and respond to civilian complaints of misconduct. The decrees have had a

> widespread impact and are being used as models by other police departments. The Section also has used its police misconduct authority to reform restraint practices in a Louisiana jail and to obtain systemic relief in juvenile correctional facilities. The Section is investigating other systemic problems in law enforcement agencies, including excessive force; false arrest; discriminatory harassment, stops, searches or arrests; and retaliation against persons alleging misconduct.

The decrees obtained by the Special Litigation Section requires that police departments implement widespread reforms including training, supervising, disciplining officers, and implementing systems to investigate and respond to citizen complaints, parallel the risk management and police legal advising efforts that some law enforcement agencies have adopted to manage liability.

Because of these changes in the social and legal environment over time, it would be reasonable to assume that the adoption of in-house police legal advisors and risk managers over the past four decades would reflect the increase in need for specialized legal and risk assessment services to police organization. Survey data in the next section provides additional information on the reasons why some police agencies have adopted police legal advisors and risk managers.

SURVEY DATA

The second data source used in this study is a national survey of county and municipal law enforcement agencies that reported the use of police legal advisors and/or risk managers in initial telephone interviews in the first step of data collection. These interviews revealed that 177 of the 354 law enforcement agencies reported using a police legal advisor, a risk manager, or both in some combination. Surveys were faxed out to all of the agencies a total of three times, and were also accompanied by two rounds of "reminder" letters. A total of 53 surveys (29.94%) were returned out of the 177 agencies that were identified through telephone interviews.

The data from all 53 returned surveys were entered into Microsoft Access for thematic data analysis. Each of the open-ended questions was examined for emerging themes and categories of both similar and contrasting ideas between each of the participating law enforcement agencies. The textual data from the surveys directly responds to research questions 2, 3, 4, and 5. The following sections are organized according to each of the research questions that correspond with the analyzed survey data.

Factors associated with adoption

Date of adoption

The data indicate that the adoption of police legal advisors and risk managers has been occurring at a slow but steady pace from the early 1960s through 2000. Five agencies reported adoption of police legal advisors in the 1960s. Thirteen agencies reported the adoption of such programs in the 1970's, 12 agencies in the 1980s, 18 agencies in the 1990s, and 3 police agencies since 2000. Two agencies did not identify the date of adoption for their programs. It is important to note that the survey data only represents one third of all agencies (53 of 177) that reported using a police legal advisor and/or risk manager in initial telephone interviews.

Reasons for adopting police legal advisors and/or risk managers

A variety of factors were reported by police agencies regarding why they decided to adopt police legal advisors and/or risk managers. The most common factor involved adopting a legal advisor or risk manager out of necessity. Several of the police agencies (14 of 53) reported that an increase in lawsuits (and payouts resulting from those lawsuits) prompted them to implement liability-related programs.

> "There was an increase in third party lawsuits, which made the Sheriff concerned. The sheriff wanted to become more proactive instead of reactive responses that had taken place in the past."

> "We adopted an in-house police legal advisor because of the costs of outside claims management. A private law firm was handling all liability claims for the Sheriff's office. Cost was

> reduced by 50% when the risk management department was established."

> "The chief of police was concerned about risk and liability issues among police managers, and instituted a plan for quality assurance that involves risk management."

A second factor reported in the adoption of risk managers and police legal advisors stems from the changes in the legal and social environment surrounding law enforcement agencies. Some of the agencies reported that the need for full-time legal advice had become necessary because of the complex changes in laws that have occurred in the past three decades.

> "The sheriff realized that as more and more laws were passed, it was becoming difficult to comply with and ensure compliance. The basis for creating the position was to assist deputies in enforcing the law and to aid in complying with law governing our employees."

> "To help officers understand statutes, ordinances, search and seizure, and civil liability issues. Also, forfeiture litigation and legislation."

> "There was a significant need to have in-house council for the police department in order to ensure timely and appropriate responses to law enforcement legal issues."

A third factor for adoption was due to a liability incident resulting in negative publicity by the media. This was the case with some of the agencies responding to the survey, as they reported that several highly publicized police-related incidents prompted the hiring of legal advisors and/or risk managers.

> "The risk management program was implemented when the police department began self-criticism and evaluation in the wake of an incident that resulted in the beating death of a citizen by the police. The police departments top management

> recognized the need for change in the police department's approach to police misconduct and the management of risk."
>
> "We have had legal advisors sporadically for a long time, but have never thought of them as risk managers. There was concern over consent degrees in other cities. Also, there were two large payouts in civil suits over a police shooting and fatal traffic accident."

The first three factors given for the adoption of risk managers and/or police legal advisors can be categorized as reactive. In contrast, the survey data also indicates that only a few police agencies added police legal advisors and/or risk management to improve the quality of police services provided to citizens. Only 3 of the 53 police agencies surveyed mentioned an anticipated improvement in providing better services to citizen by creating a police legal advisor and/or risk manager position within their organizations. Thus, 5 percent of the police agencies that responded to the survey adopted risk managers or police legal advisors in a proactive manner to improve police service to the public.

Persons or groups responsible for adoption

Survey data also revealed that the decision to include additional personnel within a police organization to manage police-related liability incidents derives from a variety of sources. Almost half of the police agencies (25 out of 53) reported that the person responsible for initiating the adoption of a police legal advisor and/or risk manager was the chief of police or sheriff. This finding is especially interesting since early literature identifies police chiefs and sheriffs as one source of resistance to hiring police legal advisors. The literature explains that there can be resistance to adopting such positions if police managers do not fully understand the function or role that police legal advisors will play in the organizations. Some police managers may view legal advisors as a police oversight mechanism, similar to an internal affairs division or some type of civilian oversight panel.

Sixteen of 53 (30%) police agencies reported that it was the initiative of either the city/county attorney alone, or a combination of the city/county attorney and local police chief/sheriff that prompted the adoption of such programs. The early literature also identifies city/county attorneys as another source of resistance to adopting police legal advisors and/or risk managers. Some of the less frequently mentioned people and groups that initiated the adoption of police legal advisors and/or risk managers include county executives, risk managers, city managers, city council members, and county commissioners.

Modeling risk management and police legal advising programs

Often police agencies adopt programs and innovations used by other law enforcement agencies (Weiss, 1997). In the current study, 20% of the surveyed police agencies reported that they modeled their police legal advising and risk management program after one or several other law enforcement agencies programs. One program that was mentioned by several police agencies in survey responses was the Los Angeles Sheriffs Department Risk Management program. The case study analysis in Chapter Six provides a more in-depth look at the organization and operation of the Risk Management program within the Los Angeles Sheriffs Department.

Program evolution

Over half (28 of 53) of the agencies that responded to the survey indicate that their risk management and/or police legal advising program has changed since its inception. The most common change reported was the addition of more personnel to the legal advising/risk management program. Expanding the program includes both the addition of more staff members and changing part-time legal advisor and/or risk manager positions into full-time positions. Several agencies stated that the program had to expand in order to deal with the increase in need of legal and risk assessment services within police agencies.

Another transformation mentioned by 11 of the 28 (39%) agencies was an expansion of responsibilities and duties. In most cases, the additional duties were the result of increases in payouts for litigation or changes in laws.

> "Our program was initiated in 1998. Originally, it was limited to general legal advice, subpoena issues, and coordination of information gathering for the law department defending the claims against the department. In 2000, the program expanded to include all police disciplinary matters including prosecution of charges and advice to the professional standards unit."

> "The police department houses the legal advisor position staffed by the city attorney. This position has taken on roles of preparing departmental roll call training bulletins, legal updates, teaching at the police academy, representing the police department at some court hearings, answering questions by police management regarding civil and job related issues. Due to growing demands, the police department has created a separate legal liaison unit to process all subpoenas, court orders, injunctions, public information requests, etc….."

> "The calculated payouts (from lawsuits against the police department) have become specific to certain types of incidents, such as false arrest. False arrest was categorized into several sub-categories such as civil rights, lack of probable cause, and so forth."

Several agencies reported that their programs have become more elaborate and sophisticated because of the addition of computer systems to help them better manage the documentation and case files associated with liability-related incidents. Computer systems were also credited as a way that police legal advisors and/or risk managers could track citizen complaints and lawsuits filed against their police departments (including both past and pending cases). The computerized tracking system helps identify police procedures and behaviors that most often result in complaints or lawsuits filed against the police by citizens.

<u>Computer technology</u>

Less than half of the agencies surveyed said that they use some kind of computer system to assist them in their work. Several of the agencies that reported that they did not use some kind of computer program in their work noted that another agency within the city or county government used a computer system to keep the records that they needed, and would be available to them upon request.

The most common computer software used by police legal advisors/risk managers responding to the survey is Microsoft Access and Excel. These programs are used to track lawsuits, citizen complaints, and insurance claims filed against their departments. Several legal advisors/risk managers reported that these programs aided in the creation of reports that are often requested by police management and other city or county agents. A few police agencies reported the use of commercial computer program packages, including "Risk Master", "Stars 5.0", and "MT/Imanage".

Several agencies also reported the use of computer programs that were created specifically for the needs of their organization. It was often the case that an officer(s) within the organization that also has computer skills was tasked with the job of building a computer program that parallels the duties of the in-house legal advisor or risk manager.

Characteristics of identified programs

Survey data were also used to explore some of the characteristics associated with the identified police legal advising and risk management programs. Some of those characteristics include where the legal advisor/risk manager is physically housed in relation to the police organization, the training and background of risk managers and police legal advisors, and the extent of collaboration between risk managers/police legal advisors and other agencies outside of the police organization.

Location of police legal advisors and risk managers in police agencies

The physical location of police legal advisors and risk managers is an issue that has been discussed in both past and recent literature. Schmidt (1972) and the IACP (1998) suggest that police legal advisors be physically housed within police headquarters. The close location would allow all police personnel immediate, convenient, and continuous access to legal advice. Survey data reveals that 64% of police legal advisors and/or risk managers maintain offices within police headquarters. Another 28% of the risk managers and/or police legal advisors reported that they maintain two offices: one office within the police department and one office either in the city/county attorneys' offices or an independently owned office.

Education and experience of risk managers and police legal advisors

The education and experience of the risk managers and legal advisors consists of a mix of legal experience, risk management, accounting, insurance assessment/adjustment training, and law enforcement.

Over one third of the police agencies (38%) reported that employees that work with police liability within their organizations have both experience in law enforcement and in practicing law. A recent police legal advising publication notes that the benefits of having police legal advisors that have prior law enforcement experience is that they will have experience and knowledge of police liability issues, and that police officers may feel more comfortable seeking legal advice from someone that has prior law enforcement experience (Becker, 1994).

In contrast, early literature states that police legal advisors with policing experience may tailor his/her duties around the good of the police department, resulting in isolation from external agencies and community members (Caplan, 1967). In addition, early literature also comments that police legal advisors with prior law enforcement experience may also be less likely to collaborate with outside agencies, or be in touch with concerns of the community (Becker, 1994). After analyzing survey data on the background and reported collaboration by police agencies with other agencies, there is no indication that police legal advisors or risk managers that have prior law enforcement experience are less likely to collaborate with other agencies. Of the 30 agencies that reported that they do not collaborate with other agencies, 15 agencies reported having prior law enforcement experience. Of the 23 police agencies that reported collaboration with other agencies, 12 agencies reported that their employees have some prior law enforcement experience.

Another 28% of police agencies reported employing police legal advisors and risk managers with law experience only. Although it has never been empirically tested, it is important to note that some of the early police legal advising literature suggests that the police legal advisor that holds the most promise would be those advisors with experience practicing law, except for the people that have a dual role of police advisor and city/county attorney (Caplan, 1967; National Commission on Criminal Justice Standards and Goals, 1973; Schmidt, 1972).

Fifteen of the 53 (28%) agencies reported that they had training in risk management. The survey respondents described their risk management training as seminars and workshops over a two or three day time period. Most of the speakers at these training seminars are practitioners who have extensive experience in risk management in a variety of organizations other than police organizations. Three of the risk management speakers that were most often noted on the surveys were G. Patrick Gallagher of the Gallagher-Westfall Group, Inc. in Indian Valley, Virginia; Randy Means of Thomas & Means, LLP in Huntersville, North Carolina; and Gordon Graham of Graham Research Associates in Long Beach, California.

Collaboration between risk managers/police legal advisors and other agencies

Further analysis of the survey data indicates that 23 of 53 (43%) risk managers and police legal advisors work in collaboration with a wide variety of agencies outside of the police agency. Some agencies mentioned in survey responses include health departments, claims agents, fiscal affair agencies, risk assessment agencies, insurance agencies, social service agencies, and victims advocate groups.

Of the 23 agencies that reported collaboration with other agencies, 9 (39%) agencies noted the importance of working with insurance-based groups within their communities. Police legal advisors and risk managers described the importance of seeking help from agencies that specialize in handling and managing claims, assessing risks within organizations, and creating strategies to change exposure to liability for police officers. Several legal advisors and risk managers also mentioned that they seek advice from and train with legal advisors/risk managers from surrounding law enforcement agencies.

Relationship with police oversight boards

Police legal advisors and risk managers were also asked about their collaborative efforts with local law enforcement oversight boards. Less than half (41%) of the police agencies surveyed (22 of 53 agencies) reported that some type of law enforcement oversight board exists in their cities. In the cases where police agencies reported the existence of a law enforcement oversight board, there was little evidence of collaboration between the two groups. In fact, over half of the agencies (54%) stated that they have never collaborated with the local oversight board.

Police legal advisors and risk managers that did report some collaboration with the local oversight board usually did so regarding citizen complaints filed against police officers within their organizations. None of the police agencies commented that local law enforcement oversight boards had any input on police liability issues directly related to hiring, training, or police procedures.

Role of risk managers and police legal advisors in police agencies

The current study also explores the role and duties of police legal advisors and risk managers within police organizations. The survey questions focus on the extent to which legal advisors and risk managers influence changes in department policies, police officer training, supervision of police officers, and promotion decisions within police organizations.

Table 5.2 illustrates the results of the survey that focuses specifically on the impact of police legal advisors on police department policies, training, supervision of line officers by police managers, and promotions within police organizations. The most striking finding presented in Table 5.2 is that police legal advisors and risk managers play a significant role in the administration and alteration of department policies, training, and supervision over line officers. In contrast, the table indicates that police legal advisors and risk managers have little to do with the promotion process within police agencies.

Table 5.2
Perceived impact of Police Legal Advisors and Risk Managers on Department Policies, Training, Supervision, and Promotion

	Impact	No Impact
Department Policies	47	6
Police Training	45	8
Supervision of Line Officers	34	19
Promotions	6	47

Changes in department policies

As previously mentioned in Chapter Three, police legal advisors and risk managers maintain and alter department policies and procedures to reduce or prevent police-related liability incidents. This task is one that is constant as there are always changes in laws and the social environment in which the police work. This means that it is the responsibility of police legal advisors and risk managers to keep abreast of any changes that might influence police officers' ability to enforce laws with the least amount of exposure to risk.

A majority of police legal advisors and risk managers that responded to the survey (47 of 53 or 89%) reported that their positions/programs had direct and significant impact on any changes in police department policies. Only 6 out of 53 agencies surveyed reported that they had no impact on department policies. In those cases, the position or program was described as being "too new" to draw any conclusions about its influence or impact on policies and procedures.

The type of department policies that risk managers and police legal advisors reported that they most often influence can be categorized into two groups: (1) police organizational issues, and (2) citizen-related department policies.

The survey data suggests that police legal advisors and risk managers make changes that impact liability costs associated with work-related injuries and motor vehicle incidents involving employees, loss or damage to department property, as well as sexual harassment and discrimination suits filed by employees within law enforcement agencies. There are also separate units or people within police organizations that handle specific employee-related liability incidents, such as fleet managers that handle all motor vehicle related incidents that result in property or financial loss for the organization. The case study analyses presented in Chapter Six provide several examples of people within legal advising and risk management programs whose job is to reduce or prevent unnecessary monetary payouts for claims filed by employees within their organizations. Examples include a fleet manager in the Police Liability Unit in the Portland Police Bureau, and a risk specialist that works specifically with employee-related liability in the Risk Management Unit in the Los Angeles Sheriffs Department.

> "Almost all of the general orders in our policy and procedures manual, which is about 3 inches thick, are reviewed by me. I make many changes. Often the changes involve labor laws to reduce suits against the department by our own employees."

> "There has been change in our work related injuries and motor vehicle accident/incident and loss of property."

Policies that impact people outside of the police organization (such as citizens) are also a major concern of police legal advisors and risk managers. Some of the most common policies mentioned in returned surveys include policies on use of force, field contacts with mentally ill or disabled persons; vehicular pursuits; searches and frisks; property seizures; arrest and custody procedures; and most recently, racial profiling policies.

> "We have made changes to our policies on use of force and police pursuits. Also this position headed up CALEA accreditation and we re-wrote the entire policy manual three times during my tenure."

> "I review or write policies to minimize high risk incidents. Also, I changed the policy so that there is no shooting from moving vehicles, no strip searches without a warrant consent or arrest, and no racial profiling."

> "Our RMS section will occasionally suggest procedural changes to general orders to facilitate timely reporting and tracking. These changes are generally subtle and of little consequence to the daily operation of the sheriffs office. Upon occasion we may be asked to look at specific operational policies to suggest improvement for the sake of reducing a particular type of loss. For example, we were asked to look at the emergency response policy, which required agency units responding to a call to adhere to state law regarding intersections. State law requires the exercise of "due care" when approaching an intersection with a red light or stop sign. We recommended a change requiring out units to come to a full stop under these conditions and ensure all traffic had stopped before proceeding. Our intersection collisions under emergency response mode dropped significantly."

> "Agency attorneys evaluate draft policies for legal sufficiency. For example, the written directive on arrest and search procedures is regularly updated to reflect new state statutes and case law."

The importance of keeping department policies and procedures current to the standards required by local, state, and federal law is a common theme that emerges from the survey data. It is also clear from the survey responses that the maintenance of department policies and procedures is one of the best ways to prevent future litigation for cases involving officers using outdated techniques during field contacts with citizens, (including arrest, search and seizure of property, and physical restraints).

<u>Influence on police officer training</u>

As Table 5.2 indicates, most agencies responding to the survey indicated that police training is a big part of police legal advisors and risk managers role within police organizations. According to several survey respondents, each stage of police training is affected by the work of police legal advisors and risk managers in relation to police officer exposure to liability beginning in the academy and all the way through in-service training.

> "We teach classes at the local and regional training academies to new recruits and within our agency to experienced officers. We also endeavor to keep our officers current on the law through regular issuance of legal bulletins and similar updates."

> "Extensive changes in our Field Training Officer (FTO) program to reflect a variety of state and federal law changes such as pursuits and use of force."

> "Risk Management routinely receives the training schedule for all training (basic to advanced) for the police department. Suggestions are routinely made which are acted upon to change or improve training."

The list of training topics that are covered by police legal advisors and risk managers across all phases of training includes (but is not exclusive to) the following list: incidents related to workmen's compensation and employee injury; defensive driving training; search and seizure of property; vehicular pursuits; racial profiling; civil rights; cultural diversity; sexual harassment training; custody and arrest practices; handling domestic violence situations, and use of force.

The survey data also revealed several creative ways that police legal advisors and risk managers train officers to keep up with the constantly changing laws that also often require a change in procedures. For example, one survey respondent commented that they use streaming videos during roll call to update officers on any important changes that might impact field contact with citizens. Several other survey respondents stated that they distribute legal bulletins via paper or over mobile data terminals. One respondent described how legal advisors and risk managers play a role in the content of training videos that are produced and sometimes distributed to other law enforcement agencies.

Impact on the supervision of patrol grade officer

Over half (64%) of the legal advisors and risk managers stated that they had some level of impact over the supervision of line officers by police managers. Most legal advisors and risk managers commented that they receive additional training tailored to police managers in order to adequately supervise line officers. A common topic of supervisory training mentioned in the surveys includes civil liability-related issues (such as the importance of recording all incidents that could end up in litigation in the future, and how to prepare for trial if you are named as a defendant in a civil liability case). Other training topics include Section 1983 liability, sexual harassment, use of force, search and seizure, racial profiling, forced entries, and recording and protecting evidence. Legal advisors and risk managers also use police supervisors to ensure that all line officers receive, understand, and put into practice any changes in department policy.

In all but two of the returned surveys, police legal advisors and risk managers noted that they impact the supervision of line officers through police managers by providing more supervisory training when there was some change in department policies.

> "Supervisors receive training and education which enhances their ability to provide direction on report writing and completion of contact cards. Training is provided to sergeants, lieutenants, and watch commanders prior to their moving into a new position."

> "Nearly all program changes are reviewed by our office. The office also initially reviews civil suits and disciplinary proceedings. Police supervisors call us 24 hours a day when they encounter legal issues."

> "We train new supervisors proactively and on an ongoing basis. Supervisors often call us from the scenes of potential

liability incidents. We also initiate change upon the review of all forced entries and use of force incidents. It is our job to spot potential problems."

The analysis of the survey data indicates an important relationship among the various duties of police legal advisors and risk managers, specifically with regard to altering or adding to department policies and officer training. Essentially, this means that any changes in department policies could potentially result in changes to department procedures.

Influence on promotions within the organization

Through data analysis, it was revealed that a majority of police legal advisors and risk managers (89%) have no impact on the promotion process. Most survey respondents indicated that promotions within their agencies were based on seniority ranking within the organization, or that promotions are based on state civil service laws that rely on exam scores to determine promotion.

The few police agencies that reported some impact on promotions within their organizations noted that their influence in the promotion process was limited and indirect.

> "Our officers cannot be promoted within two years of a sustained complaint (internal or external complaint). It is my job to track and report complaints"

> "Some of our recommendations include a penalty for officers who are involved in 'at fault' accidents. This could indirectly affect promotions."

> "When there is a test in promotional process, my training of officers could have an impact. I do review procedures to insure fairness, and I also represent the dept in civil service appeals stemming from promotions."

Some of the police legal advisors and risk managers also reported that they review the grammar and content of written portions of exams that are used as part of the promotion process. They examine the questions for legal accuracy, as the questions will change over time as laws and procedures change with time. Other agencies reported that they have been active in negotiations on behalf of the city with police unions in contract modifications regarding the methods used for testing and selection of supervisory officers. Both of these tasks result in an indirect impact on promotions within police organizations.

Nature of police legal advisor/risk manager role: Proactive vs. reactive role

After reviewing the reasons why police agencies have adopted police legal advisors and risk managers, it is clear that there is wide variation in the nature of the police legal advisor/risk manager role. The wide variation in the nature of the legal advisor/risk managers' role within police organizations can best be described using a continuum (see Figure 5.1 below).

Figure 5.1
Proactive-Reactive Continuum

I----------------------------------I----------------------------------I

Proactive | Proactive & Reactive | Reactive

In placing the role of risk managers and police legal advisors on the Proactive and Reactive continuum, proactive positions include those positions implemented, because some person or group became aware of the rising costs related to police exposure to liability, and wanted to prevent future liability problems within their organizations. Police legal advisor and risk manager positions that are reactive in nature are those positions that are created as the result of an incident or series of incidents, resulting in high monetary payouts for the department. The proactive and reactive role includes those agencies that reported that they adopted police legal advisors and risk managers because of monetary loss related to police liability incidents, and also because they became aware of the rising costs of police liability.

In the current study, survey data revealed that 27% (14 of 53) of the law enforcement agencies reported that they adopted a police legal advisor or risk manager because of an increase in litigation involving their employees, as well as the costs associated with police-related liability incidents. These agencies represent the positions that were adopted with a reactive role within the police organization. One agency commented that their role within the police agency could be paralleled with a "banking ATM machine," because it is their responsibility to make monetary payouts in police-involved liability incidents that could otherwise result in lengthy, more expensive litigation.

On the opposite end of the continuum, 40% (21 of 53) of the surveyed police agencies stated that they adopted a police legal advisor or risk manager to serve as a proactive measure against increasing police-related liability incidents. Some agencies commented that they have become concerned about increasing exposure to liability risks by observing other law enforcement agencies. And still other agencies reported that they recognized changes in the surrounding legal and social conditions within their own communities and decided to take a proactive approach to handling police liability.

> "This position was created to respond the rapid growth of the city, more complex legal issues, and to provide easier access to legal assistance."

> "It was created due to an increasing awareness of the liability associated with issues including vehicle accidents, use of force, claims, pursuits."

> "In 1997, the Sheriffs office created a risk management section separate from the county and housed it within the Human Resources Division. It was created to meet the needs of a rapidly growing population. Some of the duties include drafting legal bulletins, responding to requests for information about agency members, conducting forfeiture litigation,

> reviewing contracts, handling nuisance abatement actions, evaluating department policies, teaching instruction blocks, and researching various issues of law."

Police agencies that mentioned both proactive and reactive reasons for why they adopted a police legal advisor or risk managers only comprised 6% (4 of 53) of the agencies surveyed in this study. These agencies noted that there was some precipitating event (such as a large monetary payout for lawsuits) that prompted them to react by adopting a liability position or unit within the police organization, in addition to recognizing the need to take proactive measures with police-related liability issues in their departments. The remaining 27% (14 of 53) of the surveyed agencies provided responses that could not be classified as proactive, reactive, or both proactive and reactive.

Regardless of the nature of the circumstances that surround the adoption of police legal advisors or risk managers, it would be reasonable to assume that some police legal advisors and risk managers eventually take on both proactive and reactive roles within police organizations over time. This assumption is based on the idea that most police legal advisors and risk managers that responded to the survey noted that their current duties in relation to liability within the police organization are both proactive and reactive in nature.

An example of the proactive/reactive dual role over time would be that a majority of the survey respondents reported that their role within the police agency has significant impact on training, policies, and supervision of line officers, because they have to keep up with the constantly changing social and legal environment. By keeping abreast of changes, police legal advisors and risk mangers are proactively preventing future exposure to liability incidents. On the other hand, police legal advisors and risk managers also have to react or respond to liability incidents after they occur. This was the case as some police legal advisors and risk managers reported that they are on-call 24 hours a day, and are often called to the scene when liability becomes an issue for their police department. Future research on the evolution of the role of police legal advisors and risk managers would provide a solid understanding of the proactive and reactive components of their role within law enforcement agencies.

Perceived impact on department costs related to police liability

The survey for the current study also contained questions that inquired about the perceived impact of employing police legal advisors and risk managers within police agencies to manage police liability issues. Again, it is important to note that the perceived impact is based solely on the survey responses of police legal advisors and risk managers, and not on any official financial documents provided by each of the participating law enforcement agencies.

Data analysis revealed that 81% (43 of 53) of the police legal advisors and risk managers surveyed thought that their positions or programs had some impact on the liability-related monetary payouts of their police organizations. Several of these agencies provided testimonial evidence of their impact on financial payouts by their police organizations.

> "Yes, by denying frivolous lawsuits. The Sheriff's office has three in-house attorneys. This alone has reduced our costs by 30%."

> "The number of civil suits within the last six years or so has been significantly reduced. The major part of the fact was at the time we elected a new sheriff who has implemented and reinforced training of supervisors and on-line officers which has greatly reduced the number of incidents giving rise to civil suits."

> "We have been instrumental in early claims resolution saving literally millions of dollars. We are on 24-hour call and roll onto shootings, accidents, and other incidents for early liability assessment. Those are the kind of things that help us save money."

In the cases where police legal advisors or risk managers reported an impact on financial payouts, only 38% reported that they keep official data on the financial impact they have on their police agencies financial payouts. Further, only 30% of those agencies reported that they publish a report either monthly, quarterly, or annually. This finding is surprising given that most law enforcement agencies have to justify having such specialized programs within their organizations. One way to justify the employment of police legal advisors or risk managers within police organizations would be to have records of the financial impact they have on police-related liability. The significance of this finding will be discussed in further detail in Chapter Seven.

Other police legal advisors and risk managers claimed that they do have some impact on financial payouts, but stated that they could not produce evidence of the impact, because it is impossible to quantify incidents or payouts that have been prevented.

> "The police legal advisor is often able to provide "prevent" advice that diminishes the potential for civil action. Additionally, if an event has happened, the police legal advisor becomes involved as soon as possible in the process of obtaining statements, evidence, and preparing for future civil litigation. As an experienced officer, the police legal advisor is also able to interpret police actions as they would apply to civil suits and look for information which an attorney with no prior police experience would be aware of."

> "Proactive claims, as well as earlier and better investigations have helped lead to fewer lawsuits, claims, and infractions. This is true even in the wake of a pending Department of Justice suit against the division."

> "While we can document a marked decrease in collisions during emergency pursuits, we are unable to quantify the number of collisions that have been prevented due to time constraints. Neither our data tracking is not sufficiently sophisticated nor our data of such depth to allow us to be able to document our success at this point. As we mature and as we employ more sophisticated software, we will eventually be able to better demonstrate our victories."

Some police legal advisors and risk managers assumed that their position or program had some impact because of the important duties they are tasked with every day. About 47% of the surveys respondents assume that their input into police training, changes in policies and procedures, and being available to answer any questions from line officers and supervisors will have an impact on the financial loss of their police agencies

> "Our program has significantly reduced payouts by better managing the cases. Prior to our arrival, everything was shipped immediately to an attorney. This method caused our department to pay more for claims because the people handling those claims were making a high hourly wage. By handling everything in-house, we have reduced the initial costs and improved our ability to respond quickly to situations. As a result, minor problems are solved immediately and are prevented from becoming major problems."

> "By reviewing various reports (internal and external) and through discussions I identify potential liability issues and work through training or police suggestions to correct the problem. I operate preventatively and proactively."

The remaining 20% of the police legal advisors or risk mangers that reported that they did not impact monetary payouts gave a variety of reasons for not knowing about the financial impact of their role within their police organizations. Some of the reasons given include that they were just unsure of the impact of their positions, that it would be difficult to make successful claims because prevented liability incidents could not be quantified, or that their programs were "too new", which would make it impossible for them to draw any conclusions about their impact.

CHAPTER 6

BEST PRACTICES & MODEL PROGRAMS

The third data source used in the study presented in Chapter Four are case study site visits to four cities where the police use various combinations of risk management and police legal advising to manage liability within their organizations. The information presented in each of the following sections is based on face-to-face interviews conducted with both risk managers and police legal advisors at each of the sites, and also from a variety of documents and literature provided by risk managers and police legal advisors in each city during each site visit.

The purpose of conducting cases study site visits at each of the four cities was to collect detailed information about the organizational structure of each program, to explore the role of the position in relation to police agencies in each city, and the perceived impact of these programs on managing police liability, professionalism, and accountability from the perspective of risk managers and police legal advisors. The purpose of the case study analyses is not to evaluate the effectiveness of each program.

CHARLOTTE-MECKLENBURG, NORTH CAROLINA

Description of the program

The Charlotte-Mecklenburg Police Department utilizes the services of the Risk Management Division that also serves all other city agencies, Mecklenburg County, and the Charlotte-Mecklenburg Board of Education. Legal advice comes from the Police Attorney's Office housed within the police department.

The Risk Management Division is physically housed within the Finance Department in the city offices. Some of the specialized positions within the Risk Management Division include property and casualty claims workers, workers compensation, insurance management, financial coordination, and risk control.

Recently, the Risk Management Division added a Loss Control Team. The Loss Control Team's main responsibility is to track the history of claims of every city and county agency in the Charlotte-Mecklenburg area. Once a pattern of specific types of liability claims are identified by the Loss Control Team they contact the city or county agency to discuss the identified pattern. The next step is to meet with the agency to come up with a strategy to reduce or eliminate exposure to the identified pattern of risk. The four employees of the Loss Control Team have a variety of training and experience including risk management training, insurance assessment, loss control experience, and one employee has prior law enforcement experience.

The Loss Control Team has employed one individual that works directly with police liability issues. Currently, the Loss Control Team is working with the police department to reduce the number of claims related to traffic accidents. One of the solutions recently implemented to reduce the number of traffic related claims includes advanced training in defensive driving skills. It is hoped that the enhanced defensive driving courses will train the officers to become more aware of traffic situations that could potentially result in financial loss for the department.

The Charlotte-Mecklenburg Police Attorney's Office is housed within the Charlotte-Mecklenburg Police Department. There are five lawyers on staff that handle police-related liability cases. One of the five lawyers holds the title of "Deputy City Attorney". This person serves as the supervisor and manager of the Police Attorney's Office.

Chief Counsel for the Charlotte-Mecklenburg Police Department provides overall supervision and management of Police Attorneys Office including four attorneys and support staff. People working within this office interact with internal and external customers, and the public in general. They also provide legal advice and training to the police department in a variety of areas including basic law enforcement curriculum, police legal issues, and constitutional and personnel law. The Police Attorneys Office also ensures adherence to applicable state and federal employment law practices in hiring, promotion, disciplinary practices, and terminations, analyzes existing departmental policies, and modifies department policies as needed.

The Police Attorneys Office is considered part of the Office of the Chief within the Charlotte-Mecklenburg Police Department. The Deputy City Attorney that manages this office answers directly to the Chief of Police, and is also accountable to the City Attorney. The Police Attorney's Office handles only legal matters that involve the police department. This office does not provide legal coverage to any other city or county agencies in the Charlotte-Mecklenburg area.

Processing claims

The process of handling police-related claims was also discussed during interviews with both the Property and Casualty Claims Manager and the lead Police Attorney. The process of handling claims involving Charlotte-Mecklenburg police personnel is as follows:

1. An incident occurs involving police personnel from the Charlotte-Mecklenburg Police Department.

2. Risk Management can be informed about the incident from a variety of sources including someone from the police department, citizen(s), or media sources. In serious cases (such as police shootings or police pursuits), the Risk Management Division is contacted immediately after the incident occurs. Citizens that file a claim with the city of Charlotte can do so by telephone, the Internet, or by stopping by the division in person.

3. The filed claim is then entered into the risk management database, and is assigned a claim number.

4. Claims assistants send out a letter to the citizen that made the claim explaining that it will be investigated.

5. The Risk Management Division requests a police supervisors report from the police department. Risk management personnel investigate this report and the claim filed by the citizen.

6. Next, Internal Affairs is notified of the claim filed against the officer(s). Internal Affairs then investigates the claim. Next, they then send evidence and investigation report to the Police Attorney's Office. The Police Attorney's Office reviews the case, summarizes the findings, and then researches the appropriate case law if settlements are necessary. They use old cases/claims to help determine the dollar amounts that have been paid out in the past for specific types of claims.

7. The Police Attorney then makes a recommendation to the Risk Management Division to either pursue or drop a claim. The recommendation given by the Police Attorney weighs very heavily in the decision of how claims will be handled.

In some cases, Risk Management will settle claims without the input of the Police Attorney. This is possible because Risk Management keeps track of every claim involving police personnel, and it is sometimes easier in cases where they have dealt with similar claims involving police officers in the past. However, representatives from both Risk Management and the Police Attorney's Office agree that consultation between both groups about claims is important because it keeps both parties informed about the status of claims involving the police. As stated in an interview, "continuous communication between risk management and the police attorney is essential to get the job done right".

There are also cases when Risk Management will send risk assessors out immediately after incidents have occurred to try and settle claims on the spot. "On-the-spot" settlements usually take place in instances where the police department is legally liable for any injuries or property damages to another party. Outside of property damage incidents, "on-the-spot" settlements are somewhat rare. The adjuster is authorized to settle liability incidents for up to \$5,000. This amount can go up to \$12,000 for property damages and \$10,000 for bodily injury if Risk Management supervisors authorize it.

Interviews with Risk Management personnel also revealed that the types of claims that are dealt with most often in regard to the police are auto-related (fleet) incidents. As soon as Risk Management identifies patterns of frequent auto-related claims, innovative strategies are created and implemented to reduce those types of claims.

> "One way that we have worked together to reduce the costs related to fleet is to make changes to the police pursuit policy. Essentially, we made the policy more stringent so that the officers are more cautious when they are making their decision to pursue a suspect that is fleeing by car. Other than that we also have fender-benders and various other incidents with unmarked police vehicles, and motorcycles."

The strategies to reduce or manage police-related claims require that both Risk Management and police personnel track past and pending claims involving police personnel. All claims involving police liability incidents are entered into the risk management computer system. Summary reports are sent out each month to every city department. The claims that are entered into the risk management database are kept separate from any databases on citizen complaints against officers that Internal Affairs might keep because of state laws on confidentiality of police officials.

Risk management and police legal advisors working together

Even though the Risk Management Division is located in a building outside of the police department, both groups work together on a consistent basis. Interviews with both groups revealed that Risk Management and the Police Attorneys Office has contact with each other an average of two to three times per week. The two groups work together to decide how claims should be handled (whether it has been falsely filed or should be let go, overlooked, or dismissed). They also discuss tracked liability claims involving police officers that have resulted in payouts, or that have emerged as a patterned problem over time. The two groups also review police department policies and training standards/issues to make sure that they reflect the guidelines provided by state laws.

Personnel from both the risk management division and the police attorney's office expressed that their jobs are significantly impacted by the efforts of the other group's involvement in managing police liability. The police attorney stated, "we rely on Risk Management to identify 'hot spots' in areas of our work that generate the most claims. They analyze claims and cases in order to point out patterns that emerge from specific procedures we use every day on the job. They also tell us which areas we should consider changing in regard to police training. It is then our job to make the changes and to disperse the information about the changes throughout the police organization." Both groups also agree that they probably could not have the same impact on police-related liability if they did not have help from each other.

Benefits to the community

By working together, the Police Attorney's Office and the Risk Management Division provide several benefits to the citizens in the Charlotte-Mecklenburg area. First, the Risk Management Division identifies potential exposure to risk that can impact both the safety of citizens and police officers. This activity can provide a safer environment for both citizens and police officers. In situations where exposure to risk cannot be avoided, Risk Management can alter police department policies and procedures to reduce the frequency and sometimes the severity of the exposure to risks that could end up as claims filed to their office.

Both groups agree that the alterations made to police department policies and procedures results in improved police services to citizens. Some examples of the changes made to policies and procedures included changes in the procedures that are used in the county jail facilities, changes in evidence protection, property control, and traffic-related losses. It was reported in an interview with Risk Management that "motor vehicles accidents went down by 50% in the last few years because of the changes made to the procedures used in handling city or county motor vehicles." In some cases, additional training in handling motor vehicles was prescribed to some police personnel that had records of incidents that resulted in department losses resulting from traffic-related accidents.

A second benefit to citizens comes from an effort by the Risk Management Division to process claims filed by citizens as efficiently as possible. Risk Management also makes sure that the claims that are filed with their division are processed in a fair manner by conducting thorough investigations of every claim. "Our actions end up saving tax dollars for the citizens in the long run. We work hand-in-hand with the police department to resolve liability matters that involve police officers and citizens as quickly and effectively as possible."

The tasks carried out by the Police Attorney's Office in Charlotte-Mecklenburg also result in benefits to citizens in the community. The Police Attorney's Office assists police officers in carrying out some of the problem-oriented policing activities that they use to provide services to citizens (for example, nuisance abatement incidents). The help of the Police Attorneys Office becomes important in cases where there are complaints that are not criminal in nature, but instead could be handled through existing or newly created ordinances and city codes.

This office also practices an "open door" policy with Charlotte-Mecklenburg police officers by answering questions on criminal law and criminal procedure that the officers might have before they become involved in a situation that could end up as a liability incident. One example would include police officers asking the police attorney questions about the legality of serving search warrants where they are looking for evidence, guns, drugs, and other illegal items in private homes. In these cases, it is crucial that police officers follow the specific details provided on the warrant (such as what areas of the home may be searched, etc..). Being housed within the police department increases the chances that police officers will ask questions before they do something that could result in complaints, liability claims, or litigation with citizens. The Police Attorney's Office believes that this "open-door" policy enhances the quality of police service provided to the citizens of Charlotte-Mecklenburg.

Impact on police professionalism and accountability

By working together, the Risk Management Division and the Police Attorney's Office also believe that they have an impact on the level of police professionalism and accountability. Both groups assert that improved police professionalism and accountability result when changes are made to police department training, policies, and procedures. In most cases the changes that have been made were done so to reduce exposure to liability-related incidents. The Police Attorney stated that this means that police officers become more aware of their actions and behaviors, specifically in instances where exposure to liability is eminent.

> "Professionalism and accountability is enhanced every time that Risk Management recognizes a problem with police procedure, policy, or training and recommends changes to the department. The constant alteration of procedures, policies, and training allows the police officers to give better service to the citizens, and it keeps everyone safe and happy. Risk management can tell the police department what they could be doing better, and then follow up on any changes that they have suggested to the department to ensure that the changes are being made."

Risk Management personnel also believe that their efforts to reduce exposure to risk and liability incidents involving the police have an impact on police professionalism and accountability. By identifying patterns of liability claims that could be reduced or eliminated by making changes to police policy, procedure, and training, Risk Management directly contributes to liability control. An example of this would be identifying the need for more advanced drivers safety and defensive driving classes for police officers in an effort to reduce police-related traffic liability claims.

According to Risk Management, the issue of building trust between the Risk Management Department and Charlotte police officers is also an important part of improving police professionalism in Charlotte.

> "By handling police liability claims in an effective and consistent manner, Risk Management reassures the police officers that they have the support of Risk Management and the City behind them. This support allows the officers to do their jobs without the fear that they will not be supported if they make an error in judgment."

LOS ANGELES COUNTY, CALIFORNIA

Description of program

The Los Angeles Sheriff's Department utilizes a combination of an in-house Risk Management Bureau used exclusively for police liability issues, and a Legal Advisory Unit located outside of the Sheriff's Department that handles only police-related liability cases. The Risk Management Bureau was created in 1993 to provide a department-wide effort in reducing the loss of department resources, to control police liability costs, improve law enforcement services provided to citizens, and to raise police accountability within the Sheriff's Department.

The mission of the Risk Management Bureau describes how it strives to "contribute to providing the highest quality service law enforcement and public safety services by enabling Department employees to perform their duties in a risk-reduced work environment. The Risk Management Bureau will accomplish its mission by: 1) Continually identifying and evaluating activities that have a high risk and liability potential; 2) Aggressively managing personnel health and safety issues, and 3) proactively managing claims and lawsuits, including an immediate response to incidents with a high liability potential (L.A.S.O Risk Management Bureau brochure, 2001)."

The Risk Management Bureau is comprised of several units including the Civil Litigation Unit, Health and Safety, Risk Impact Units, Traffic Services Detail, Random Drug Testing, Wellness programs, and the Manuals and Orders Section.

The Civil Litigation Unit is responsible for managing the Departments civil claims and lawsuits. The primary task of this unit is to reduce the Departments financial liability and exposure to incidents that result in costly litigation. Investigators are on 24-hour call to respond to claims-related incidents that could result in litigation. In some cases, the Civil Litigation Lieutenant can resolve liability incidents on site for up to $2,500. "With this process the unit has reduced the Department's financial exposure compared to previous years. From 1995 to 1997, there has been a 60% reduction in claim settlements. This can be credited to expedited claims for damages such as inmate over detentions and property damage (Los Angeles Sheriff's Department website, 2002)." This Unit is also in charge of a civil litigation-training program for all employees of the Sheriff Department.

The other units within the Risk Management Bureau also have specialized areas in which they strive to reduce costs for the Department. The Health and Safety Unit is responsible for minimizing costs associated with any injuries or illnesses of Department employees. This unit also arranges funeral services for Sheriff's Department personnel. Additionally, this unit is responsible for worker's compensation subrogation.

The Risk Impact Unit coordinates a reporting system for the Department's unit-level risk management plans each quarter. Recently, the Risk Impact Unit created the Sheriff's Critical Issues Forum (SCIF), which is an innovative accountability management approach used to examine areas of liability concern. SCIF deals with more than one hundred topic areas within the categories of crime analysis, risk management and unit fiscal accountability. Police managers at the division level are given the opportunity to present innovative programs that have improved the productivity or responsiveness to liability issues within their divisions.

The Traffic Services Detail is responsible for handling all on-duty employee related traffic incidents involving property damage and/or injuries. This unit is also responsible for providing training that is related to traffic including investigations of traffic scenes and safety issues involving police officer use of motorizes vehicles.

The Manual and Orders Unit maintains and updates the Sheriff's Department's Policy and Procedures Manual. This Unit also preserves a historical library of all of the Department's policy and procedure manuals.

The Random Drug Testing Program is responsible for administering periodic, unannounced, random drug tests throughout the Department. By administering random drug tests, the Random Drug Testing Program will ensure a drug-free work environment. Members of this unit believe that random drug tests of Department employees will increase the public's trust of the law enforcement officials affiliated with the Sheriff's Department. Employees of this program lecture at all training academy classes about the consequences of using drugs either on or off-duty. This unit also provides management level training of police personnel from other agencies that are interested in implementing a random drug-testing program in their agencies.

All of the units that comprise the Risk Management Bureau work in conjunction with the Los Angeles Sheriff's Department Legal Advisory Unit to manage police liability incidents related to the Sheriff's Department's employees. The Legal Advisory Unit is located in a building that is separate from the main Sheriff's headquarters.

The Legal Advisory Unit employs several Deputy County Counsels that are assigned to work with specialized legal issues related to the Sheriff's Department including custody, court services, labor, personnel matters, department records and compliance with state and federal laws, and patrol related issues. Some of the main functions of the Legal Advisory Unit include:

> "Serving as a Department liaison and providing coordination with County Counsel; Interpreting and defining the impact of newly passed legislation on Department Operations; Responding to Department telephonic requests for legal assistance pertaining to law enforcement problems encountered during day-to-day operations; conducting research projects which address Department questions on a variety of law enforcement operations; Assisting Department personnel in the instruction of sworn personnel at Department Advanced Officer Training Programs and Cadet Training; maintaining a legal library for use by Department personnel; and maintaining and updating and distributing a publication of County Ordinances relevant to the Department's law enforcement responsibilities (County of Los Angeles Sheriff's Department Legal Advisory Unit, 1999).

Even though the Legal Advisory Unit and the Risk Management Bureau are two separate entities, they work closely with one another to handle liability issues for the Los Angeles Sheriff's Department. An interview with a representative of the Legal Advisory Bureau revealed that the primary reason that the Legal Advisory Unit is located in a building outside of the main Sheriff's headquarters is because of the large size of the Sheriffs Department. The Los Angeles Sheriff's Department is the largest Sheriff's Department in the United States (Bureau of Justice Statistics, 1999).

Processing claims

Each of the specialized divisions described in the previous section play a unique role in the process of handling liability claims related to the Los Angeles Sheriff's Department. The steps in processing claims is as follows:

1. A claim is filed with the Board of Supervisors within the Sheriff's Department. The Lieutenant of the Civil Litigation Unit is also authorized to accept claims on behalf of the Board of Supervisors. This would include those situations where the Lieutenant of the Civil Litigation Unit shows up on the scene of an incident and attempts to resolve the incident by cutting a check for up to $2,500 to cover any expenses related to the liability incident.

2. After a claim is filed with the Board of Supervisors, it is forwarded on to County Counsel (Legal Advisory Unit). At this point, County Counsel determines if the claim is related to traffic, medical liability division (Risk Management Bureau), or police liability (Civil Litigation Unit).

3. Once County Counsel categorizes the claim and forwards it to the appropriate division, a recommendation is made to either deny the claim or to pay the claim. If the claim is denied, the case will either die or turn into a formal lawsuit (depending on the decision of the party that filed the claim). If the claim is to be paid, the next decision is to determine which source of funds will be used to pay the claim.

4. If it has been determined that the claim will be paid, there are a variety of funds that payment can be taken from including the Contract Cities Liability Trust Fund or the Sheriff's Judgment and Damages Fund. Once the claim is paid, the claims process is officially over.

It is the responsibility of the Risk Management Bureau to track claims and the financial losses resulting from police-related liability incidents. The Civil Litigation Unit (which is part of the Risk

Management Bureau) manages and tracks the claims that end up resulting in civil suits filed against the Sheriff's Department. The Civil Litigation Unit can also expedite the claims process if the costs of the claim is $2,500 or less. And finally, the Legal Advisory Unit takes on the responsibility of researching some of the claims that results in lawsuits against the Department, and also provides legal advice to members of the Sheriff's Department that are named as defendants in civil suits filed against the Department. Each of the divisions plays an important role in the processing of claims that ultimately result in lawsuits against the Sheriff's Department.

Risk management and police legal advisors working together

The unique approach taken by the Los Angeles Sheriff's Department to manage liability issues within their organization incorporates the expertise of both legal advisors and risk managers. Through interviews with employees at the Legal Unit, it was revealed that most of the employees are "cross-trained" to ensure that every case is dealt with in the most effective and efficient manner possible. Some of the members of the Civil Litigation Unit have received training in risk management. It was explained by one legal advisor that, "the program has evolved immensely over time. Today we are better organized as a Unit in regard to our workloads. Having people with multiple talents in multiple types of liability cases (in regard to dealing with certain types of liability cases, such as patrol or custody issues) allows us to spread the workload out among everyone in the department instead of just a few people with limited expertise in a specific area." In this case, a team approach seems necessary in handling the workload of police-related liability cases in the Los Angeles Sheriff's Department.

The Legal Advisory Unit works closely with both the Civil Litigation Unit and the Risk Management Unit in the Sheriff's Department. These two groups discuss strategies about how to handle certain types of cases. For example, the Legal Advisory Unit will often check with the Civil Litigation Unit about specific Department policies and procedures, and also any questions about officer training that may or may not contribute to police-citizen interactions that can result in liability claims or even lawsuits. One of the major responsibilities of the Civil Litigation Unit is to track liability cases with the use of a computerized data management system. The patterns and trends that are generated by the Civil Litigation Unit using the data on claims and lawsuits filed against the Department is extremely useful to the Legal Advisory Unit when they are examining current cases filed against the Department. Members from both the Legal Advisory Unit and the Civil Litigation Unit agreed during interviews that this cooperative effort between the groups is an essential part of their jobs.

The specialized units that are part of the Risk Management Bureau also work with the Legal Advisory Unit. The Risk Impact Unit serves as the "research arm" of the Risk Management Bureau. It is responsible for researching police-related liability incidents in areas both inside and outside of Los Angeles County in order to create strategies to prevent similar incidents from occurring in the Los Angeles area in the future. An example of this would be monitoring how other law enforcement agencies handle volatile situations that expose officers to high levels of risk such as the riots that occurred a few months earlier in Seattle involving the WTO protesters and the Seattle police department, as well as the riots that occurred in Cincinnati Ohio after a police-shooting incident. The idea is that the Los Angeles Sheriffs Department can learn from the actions (or inactions) of other law enforcement agencies in case the situation arises later on in Los Angeles County.

The exchange of information between the Legal Advisory Unit and the Risk Management Bureau is another example of how each group works together in managing liability issues in Los Angeles. An example of this exchange of information would be identified need of improved documentation by police officers and other police personnel. The Legal Advisory Unit and Civil Litigation noticed that the Department was losing a number of use of force cases because officers were not collecting and recording all of the important information necessary to successfully win the case if it would end up in court later on. The lack of documentation resulted in the lack of proof on the part of the accused officer in the courtroom. Together Risk Management, the Civil Litigation Unit, and the Legal Advisory Unit worked together to make changes to the procedures of documenting and reporting incidents that involve any use of force by officers.

Benefits to the community

Employees of the Los Angeles Sheriff's Department identified several ways that the use of both risk management and legal advising can benefit citizens in Los Angeles County. First, both groups mentioned that a reduction in liability incidents would mean a safer environment for both citizens and police officers. By working together to identify patterns of liability in police procedures, training, or policies, both groups agreed that high-risk interactions involving both police officers and citizens could be minimized or eliminated to keep everyone involved safe. A specific example of this would be creating and implementing adequate screening intake tools used in the county jail. By using appropriate in-take tools in the jail, Department personnel can identify inmates who may need specific medical or psychological treatment during their time served in the jail. For example, cases involving the treatment of inmates with diabetes or some form of psychiatric problems were mentioned by several of the Risk Management personnel that were interviewed during the site visit. By identifying problems early on during in-take, problems that could result in injury or in some cases death can be prevented.

A second benefit expressed by Risk Management employees was that a reduction in payouts for liability claims would also mean a reduction in the use of tax dollars to make pay-outs for those incidents. This would provide a financial benefit for citizens of Los Angeles County. The growing expense of liability for the Sheriff's Department is described in the introduction of the "County of Los Angeles Sheriff's Departments Guide to Risk Management" (2001). This guide indicates that the Risk Management Bureau was implemented because of the rising costs of police liability in the Sheriff's Department, and that its overall goal is to reduce the costs associated with liability.

> "The number of cases going to trial in some areas more than doubled, and total liability costs increased over 251% in three years. Between 1985 and 1992, attorney's fees and expenses for auto and general liability cases rose 923% alone. Settlements, court awards, and legal expenses for fiscal year 1991-1992 were over $143 million, up from $53.6 million in fiscal year 1988-1989. Of that $134 million, $61 million (46%) was for legal defense costs alone. Total legal defense

costs for the County of Los Angeles accounted for nearly half of all liability expenditures. These escalating costs demanded alternative solutions for containing costs of tort liability judgments, settlements and litigation. The Department realizes that it will eventually suffer some losses through litigation. At the same time, it is recognized by focusing attention on reducing risks in its daily operations, the Sheriff's Department can become a less costly and more efficient organization (County of Los Angeles Sheriff's Department Guide to Risk Management, 2001, p. A1)."

A third benefit to citizens would be an improved level of police service provided by employees of the Los Angeles Sheriff's Department. Employees of both the Legal Unit and the Risk Management Bureau expressed that there is an overall improvement of the quality of service provided to citizens since the inception of the Risk Management Bureau in 1993. It is believed by both groups that any change in department policies, officer training, and police procedures results in an improvement in service. The continuous tracking of Department losses by the Risk Management Bureau directly impacts any of the changes made throughout the organization. The changes made within the organization are believed to result in improved police services to citizens in Los Angeles County.

Impact on police professionalism and accountability

The improvement of police professionalism and accountability is a main theme that is present throughout the entire contents of the "Guide to Risk Management", which is written and distributed by the Risk Management Bureau in the Los Angeles Sheriff's Department. The risk management plan proposed by the Risk Management Bureau is based on the idea that "Departmental risk management efforts are aimed at improving the quality of our law enforcement service by making it more efficient and effective (Guide to Risk Management, 2001, p. B1)." Part of this effort is to manage risk control efforts at the unit level within the Sheriff's Department. Managing risk control at the unit level is believed to ensure accountability of all of the members working within each unit.

Programs to enhance professionalism and accountability

Two of the risk management programs used by Sheriff's Department employees are additional accountability measures created by the Risk Management Bureau. The first program, Command Accountability Reporting System (CARS), requires that each unit in the Department enter its own data (regarding use of force, collisions, shootings, illnesses, and complaints) into the CARS database system. Once the data is entered into the database system, each unit can compare its own risk issues with other units in the Department. Monthly reports containing data entered by each unit is also used to examine management performance at the unit level. This program allows each unit to be constantly aware of risk issues within their units, and can also allow units with similar risk issues to cooperatively create strategies to reduce or eliminate specific types of risk.

The second risk management program that adds to the culture of accountability within the Sheriff's Department is the Sheriff's Critical Issues Forum (SCIF). This forum meets every month to discuss crime stats, fiscal management, and CARS data base information of every unit. This meeting requires that Divisional leaders including the chief, commanders, and unit commanders come together to discuss the progress of each unit. It requires that unit leaders identify risk-related issues within their units, and also create strategies to reduce exposure to risks specific to the problematic incidents previously identified in SCIF meetings. Both the SCIF and CARS program hold each unit leader accountable for risk related issues that are unique to their divisions.

Department-wide efforts using risk management techniques

In addition to the SCIF and CARS programs, there are several units within the Department (outside of the Risk Management Bureau) that have been identified as having a significant role in risk management efforts. First, the Training Bureau is active in managing Department risks related to the recruitment, hiring, and training of all deputy sheriffs'. This also includes testing each candidate and conducting thorough background investigations. This aspect of risk management is vital to the Department because this Bureau is responsible for adequately training deputy sheriffs' in all potential high risk situations including use of firearms, driving skills, defensive tactics, and understanding Department policy and procedures.

A second bureau within the Department that plays an important role in risk management is the Field Operations Support Services Unit. This unit is responsible for the development and coordination of training for the three field operations regions, and also the detective division. This unit conducts inspections of all training related records, as well as all jail operations records. It is also responsible for examining current patrol techniques, equipment used by deputies, and the development and dispersion of updated training videos. If there were any changes in law that would also require a change in department policy or procedure, this unit would identify and make changes to department policy and procedure to make them compliance with the law.

The Custody Division Training Unit is another unit that contributes to risk management within the Department. This unit is responsible for developing and researching job specific updated (or in-service) training for Department personnel. The enhanced training courses meet state mandated training requirements, and also are believed to enhance the efficiency, professionalism, and effectiveness of all Department personnel.

Accountability Enhancement Committee

In November of 1995, Under Sheriffs and Assistant Sheriffs in the Department sent out a memo to all Division Chiefs outlining plans to enhance accountability within the Los Angeles Sheriff's Department. The memo explained that the Department would create and implement an Accountability Enhancement Committee. The Accountability Enhancement Committee would consist of commanders that will explore various methods of reinforcing accountability within the Department, and will develop guidelines for auditing and reporting that will further enhance accountability. The memo also outlined several broad areas that should be focused on by all Department members in regard to enhancing accountability, managing risks associated with law enforcement activities, and maintaining high levels of service to the public. Some of those areas include use of force management, public complaint process, administrative investigations of personnel, discipline, and performance evaluations. The Accountability

Enhancement Committee is another way that the Los Angeles Sheriff's Department is trying to improve the culture of police accountability and professionalism within its organization.

PORTLAND, OREGON

Description of program

The Portland Police Bureau utilizes three separate groups to manage police liability involving employees of their agency. The three groups include the Police Liability Management Unit, the Risk Management Department for the city of Portland, and a Police Legal Advisor housed within the City Attorney's Office.

The Police Liability Management Unit is part of the Management Services Division in the Portland Police Bureau. This unit's primary responsibility is the management of liability and costs associated with liability incidents involving Portland police officers. More specifically, "the mission of Police Liability Management Unit is to increase citizen's and employee safety while reducing the Police Bureau's civil liability exposure and monetary losses due to civil claims resulting from Police Bureau operations and practices (Portland Police Bureau, 2000, p. 1)."

The Police Liability Management Unit employs a police liability manager, two risk specialists/claims analysts, and a fleet claims specialist. The training and experience of employees of the Police Liability Management Unit are both extensive and diverse. Some of the types of training and experience in this Unit include insurance assessment, investigation, risk and claims analysis, and law enforcement experience. One member of the Police Liability Unit contributed over 25 years of service to the Portland Police Bureau before becoming employed within the Police Liability Management Unit as a civilian employee.

All positions within the Police Liability Management Unit are responsible for any notice of tort claim and/or lawsuit alleging misconduct on the part of Bureau employees, which is filed against the city of Portland and the Bureau of Police. Some of the more specific duties of Police Liability employees include the following:

- Review and analyze tort claims to determine investigative requirements and to form initial opinions as to liability exposure.

- Perform investigative activities, including conducting interviews, site visits, photography when necessary, and obtaining additional relevant documents.

- Review and analyze claim files to ensure an investigation is complete and as thorough as possible to provide a valid judgment as to liability exposure and make effective recommendations.

- Summarize investigations results in written or verbal form to Risk Management/City Attorney along with recommendations.

- Participate in meetings for consultation regarding status, strategies, and degree of liability exposure that may exist in individual claims.

- Consult with Command Staff, supervisors, officers and/or other regarding policies, practices, or procedures, or regarding incidents that may have potential for liability exposures (includes individual counseling and in-service training).

- Review and analyze reports received from involved officers or supervisors who have concerns about liability exposure based on events as they occurred during specific police actions.

- Review and analyze documents received from Risk Management and City Attorney staff related to on-going investigations, requests for additional information and progress of claims that have entered the court process; also attending trials, conferences and hearings.

Another group that is responsible for managing police liability in Portland is the Risk Management Department. Risk Management is part of the Office of Finance and Administration for the City of

Portland. This Department is responsible for managing the liability and costs associated with loss for all city agencies in Portland, including the Portland Police Bureau. Responsibilities with the Risk Management Department can be categorized into several specialized topic areas including Liability, Loss Prevention, and Workers' Compensation.

The Liability Claims Manager works closely with the Police Liability Management Unit in its effort to manage police-related liability incidents. The Liability Claims Manager runs monthly reports that identifies any patterned problems related to police liability. At that point, the Liability Claims Manager brings this pattern to the attention of the Police Liability Management Unit. Alterations can be made to reduce or eliminate the identified liability pattern by making changes to department policies, procedures, and improved police training/re-training.

The Police Legal Advisor is another vital part of managing police liability in Portland. The Police Legal Advisor is part of the Office of City Attorney. Personnel in the Portland Office of City Attorney includes a city attorney, two chief deputy city attorneys, twenty-two staff attorneys, one project manager, six paralegal assistants, nine legal assistants/secretaries, and several people providing administrative support.

The Office of City Attorney is responsible for providing legal services to all city agencies in the city of Portland. Staff Attorneys are assigned to provide specialized legal service to a variety of city agencies, including the Police Bureau. The Attorney assigned to the position of Police Legal Advisor focuses solely on providing legal service to employees of the Portland Police Bureau.

The duties of the Portland Police Legal Advisor are numerous and diverse. The Police Legal Advisor gives pre and post-incident legal advice to the officers involved in any liability-related incidents. This includes answering questions of officers before they take part in situations that will expose them to risk, as well as preparing the officer before he/she goes into court. The Police Legal Advisor also goes to the scenes of more serious incidents that could potentially end up in court. By going to the scene, the Police Legal Advisor can collect important information that could be used in court later on, and can assess the situation to see if similar incidents could be prevented in the future by making changes to policy, procedure or training.

Another duty of the police legal advisor includes the creation and distribution of training bulletins when there are changes in law, policy, or procedures. These training bulletins are dispersed in a variety of ways including placing them in police officer mailboxes, paychecks, and during roll calls. He also teaches at the training academy, and at the advanced training level (police supervisors and managers).

An interview with the Police Legal Advisor revealed that he had prosecutorial experience, but no prior law enforcement experience. He said that he believes that this does not hinder his ability to do a good job. When he first started the job, he went to roll call so that the police officers would get to know who he was and what his purpose was in relation to their jobs. Attending roll call and doing ride-alongs with the officers also helped him learn the day-to-day operations of policing.

Another program used by the Portland Police Bureau to reduce department losses related specifically to traffic is the "Collision Review Board". Once a month, the Board examines all collisions involving police vehicles with other vehicles, objects, or people. This board is also responsible for making recommendations to improve department fleet safety and practices. This board serves as an investigative body, and also as a "checks and balance mechanism" to ensure that police personnel involved in traffic-related incidents are treated fairly.

The Chief of Police appoints the members of the Collision Review Board. The 7-person board is comprised of sworn law enforcement representatives from each of the precincts across the city of Portland. All of them have some experience in handling issues related to auto incidents and liability. The Collision Review Board hears roughly 15-20 auto collision cases per month.

Members of the Collision Review Board get together to review the cases that have occurred over the course of the previous month. The process of hearing cases is as follows:

1. The individual involved in some kind of auto-related incident sits in front of the Board members and tells them their version of what happened involving the damage to the department vehicle.

2. Next, Collision Review Board members ask the individual questions about the incident for clarification, and to learn more specific details about what lead up to the collision.

3. The individual leaves the room while the board members discuss the incident. The board members votes on the incident to determine whether it was "preventable" or "not preventable". They use the criteria established by the National Traffic Safety Council. The guidelines created by this Council ask the question "Did the person do everything possible to avoid the situation that has occurred?"

4. After the vote takes place, Collision Review Board members make recommendations to the individual's supervisor or commander in regard to some kind of discipline. The individual's supervisor can override the recommendation of the Collision Review Board, and determine punishment (if any) on their own. Some of the punishments that individuals can face includes written reprimands, counseling, re-training, days off with and without pay).

Processing claims

Any claim that is filed that involves an employee of the Portland Police Bureau goes through the following process:

1. A claim is filed with the Risk Management Department.

2. A copy of all liability claims that involve Portland Police Bureau employees are sent over to the Police Liability Management Unit.

3. The Assistant Risk Specialist logs the claims into the computer system.

4. Next, risk specialists in the Police Liability Management Unit collect all pertinent information on the claim. The information is collected from police reports (including police supervisor reports) linked to the incident, interviews with all

parties and witnesses involved in the claim, and in some cases, a visit to the scene of the incident for further investigation.

5. Once the investigation is complete, the Police Liability Unit gives the risk adjuster in the Risk Management Department a recommendation for handling the claim. The recommendation is based on any of the information collected during the investigation of the claim, and in some cases, the decision to either pay or reject a claim comes from the handling of similar claims in the past.

6. Risk Management will send out a letter to the person(s) that filed the complaint explaining that their claim has either been "denied" or "paid".

7. The claim will "die" after being rejected by Risk Management, or it will end up in court.

There are two main financial sources that claims filed against Portland police officers can be paid from: (1) the General Fund, and (2) The Law Enforcement Medical Liability Account (LEMLA). The purpose of LEMLA is to provide a source of money "to reimburse medical providers for medical expenses incurred from injuries sustained by someone as a result of law enforcement activity. Injuries related to law enforcement activities includes any injuries sustained prior to booking, citations in lieu of arrest or release instead of booking that occurs during and as a result of efforts by law enforcement officer to restrain or detain, or take or retain custody of the individual. Examples of this would include dog bites sustained during apprehension, gun shot wounds inflicted by officer in attempt to apprehend the individual, and injuries sustained during police pursuits (Law Enforcement Medical Liability Account, 1999, pg 1-3)". Claims are only paid out of the LEMLA account when recovery from the injured party's insurance company fails. LEMLA is established separate from the General Fund. The LEMLA Account is funded solely from assessments added to fines and bail forfeitures, and not from any tax dollars.

Risk management and police legal advisors working together

Interviews with personnel from Risk Management, the Police Liability Management Unit, and the Police Legal Advisor revealed that collaboration efforts between all three groups is the key to effectively managing police liability in Portland.

All three groups agreed that the diversity in the training and goals of all three groups does not pose as a problem when deciding how to handle police-related claims. A Risk Management representative stated that "this is a unique situation because you have three groups that have three different agendas, but it still works out for the most part…there is a sense of balance between the three groups. Risk Management efforts to control police-related liability would not be as effective as it is today if the level of communication between all three groups was not what it is today." He also expressed that "it was not difficult to be accepted by members of the Portland Police Bureau." He said that he "learned more about policing operations as he has been working with the Bureau, and dealing with a wide variety of police-related liability claims over the years." The Risk Management representative also mentioned that he works directly with the Police Legal Advisor as he assists and supports in defense against police-related claims that end up in court.

An interview with the Police Legal Advisor uncovered a perspective similar to that of Risk Management in regard to collaboration between all three groups responsible for managing police liability in Portland. He stated that "my office, the Risk Management Department, and the Police Liability Unit compliment each other because they all have the same goal: the prevention of lawsuits against the Police Bureau."

An example of these groups working together includes representatives from the Police Liability Management Unit and the Police Legal Advisor contributing to lesson plans for various levels of police training focused on police liability. An example of this is a course titled "Civil Liability Based Upon Law Enforcement Activities" that was created and instructed by both the Police Legal Advisor and personnel from the Police Liability Management Unit. The purpose of the class is "to make police officers aware of police activities that may create liability exposure, and to provide methods make defensible police actions in litigation; to make officers more aware of constitutional, statutes, and federal regulatory processes and procedures in civil litigation; and what to do before, during, or after an incident occurs which may create liability exposure."

Another example of the Risk Management Department, the Police Liability Management Unit, and the Police Legal Advisor working together to manage police liability in Portland is creation of the Liability/Loss Control Committee. Liability/Loss Control Committee Team members include representatives from southeast and northeast police precincts, police legal advisor from the city attorney's office, personnel from the training division, two employees from the Risk Management Department, and three reps from the Police Liability Management Unit.

The goals of the Liability/Loss Control Committee includes reducing claim frequency by 10%, reducing claim closure time by 25%, eliminate case backlog, reduce financial exposure by immediately responding to high profile situations, target improvements for police training based on the results of the survey's distributed to Portland Police Officers and claim trends identified by the Risk Management Department, and attempt to increase liability awareness throughout the entire Police Bureau. This Committee is also in the process of creating a "Liability Response Team". This team would be responsible for disposing of menial claims for smaller dollar amounts by carrying a checkbook and "cutting checks" on the scene of the incidents.

Benefits to the community

The management of police liability in Portland results in several benefits in the Portland community. The benefits identified through interviews with representatives from all three groups can be categorized as improved police services provided to citizens, and also financial management over the costs that are associated with claims and lawsuits filed against employees of the Police Bureau. Each of the three groups responsible for police liability management in Portland directly contributes to those benefits.

The Risk Management Department plays an important role in improving the quality of police services that are provided to the citizens of Portland. This is achieved when Risk Management identifies patterns in claims and lawsuits, and then works with the

Police Liability Management Unit and the Police Legal Advisor to make changes to reduce or eliminate exposure to risk situations. A Risk Management representative stated, "once police officers are informed of ways to reduce or eliminate exposure to risk, they can try to make smart decisions every day on the job to avoid becoming part of a claim or lawsuit. We monitor the financial aspect of their (the police) job and try to keep the costs down."

The Police Legal Advisor in Portland expressed similar ideas about the benefits to the citizens of Portland that come from the management and control of police liability.

> "Anything that helps the police officers do their jobs better is a benefit to the citizens of Portland. Better service can be the result of improved and advanced police training, more clearly defined department policies that are also followed up and enforced by police management within the Bureau. All of these things benefit the citizens of Portland in the long run."

The importance of the management of police liability in regard to benefits to the citizens is described in a memo written by a representative of the Police Liability Management Unit. "There is no greater potential financial and public impact for the City than the loss of money and public faith as the result of an allegation of in improper police action. It is incumbent upon the Bureau, the Police Liability Manager, Risk Management, and the City Attorneys Office (Police Legal Advisor) to ensure that the truth about an incident be known. If there is fault (on the part of the Police Bureau) it should be admitted, and if there is no fault, the community should have access to that information."

Impact on police professionalism and accountability

Liability management efforts by the Police Liability Management Unit, the Police Legal Advisor, and personnel from the Risk Management Department contributes to the improvement of police accountability and the level of police professionalism in the Portland Police Bureau. The importance of police professionalism and accountability resulting from liability management is evident as both items are specifically incorporated into the Bureau's goals and objectives. The assumption of having Bureau-wide objectives and goals is that every member of the Bureau will strive to achieve them. Thus, if liability management is part of the Bureau's stated goals and objectives, it is going to have some effect on the individual members of the Bureau that are striving to achieve the Bureau's goals.

The collaborative efforts of the Risk Management Department, the Police Liability Unit, and the Police Legal Advisor directly contribute to several of the objectives and goals outlined in the Portland Police Bureau Community Policing Strategic Plan, 1998-2000:

> GOAL 3 – OBJECTIVE 3.2 – Improve Police Bureau's responsiveness to employee performance; Review and analyze trends of Bureau incidents and losses from resulting liability claims; Develop and implement policies and practices and training to control losses.
>
> GOAL 3 – OBJECTIVE 3.6 – Improve employee training; Provide improved training to all employees; Provide specialized training to meet the needs of specific groups of employees.
>
> GOAL 4 – OBJECTIVE 4.2 – Improve fiscal practices and policies; Ensure that budgeting and fiscal policies are aligned with the Bureau's missions and reflect the community's needs.

Some of the programs and committees that have been implemented to reduce and manage the level of exposure to risk situations also contribute to improved police professionalism and accountability within the Portland Police Bureau. One example would be the Collision Review Board. The Police Bureau requires that all police personnel be held accountable for all auto-related damages and losses, by requiring them to appear in front of the Board. This Board also contributes to increased police professionalism, as it will often require re-training as part of the discipline to those employees that cause damage and financial loss to the organization.

The Liability/Loss Control Committee represents another example of the Bureau's effort to increase police accountability through liability management. As described in an earlier section, this committee has set goals to reduce claim frequency and closure time, eliminate case backlog, reduce financial exposure by immediately responding to high profile situations, target improvements for police training based on the results of the survey's distributed to Portland Police Officers and claim trends identified by the Risk Management Department, and attempt to increase liability awareness throughout the entire Police Bureau. By creating strategies to achieve their goals, the Bureau is reaching toward a higher level of professionalism throughout the entire organization, and is also making people become more accountable for their part in the level of liability claims that result in financial or property loss.

LAS VEGAS, NEVADA

Description of the program

The Las Vegas Metropolitan Police Department (LVMPD) utilizes both risk management and legal advising in their effort to control liability in their organization.

The Risk Management Section is part of the Office of Policy and Planning in the Las Vegas Metropolitan Police Department. Although it is officially consider part of the LVMPD, it is physically housed in city hall. At the time of the site visit, the Risk Management Section consisted of six positions, which includes both sworn law enforcement officials and civilians. A Lieutenant of the LVMPD serves as the supervisor of the Risk Management Division. There are four civilian positions that assist the supervisor in assessing who should handle the various types of cases, the processing of all correspondence, and several other administrative duties. There is also a claims investigator position that is covered by a sworn police officer.

The Deputy District Attorney (Attorney of Record for the LVMPD) provides legal services to the LVMPD. The role of the District Attorney is to defend the police department in lawsuits that deal with police procedure (such as a wrongful death suits, etc). The District Attorney also provides input into any changes that are made to department policies and officer training. A private law firm takes care of litigation involving all personnel of the LVMPD.

To assist in the management of liability associated with police vehicles, the LVMPD created an Accident Review Board. The purpose of this board is to identify, monitor, and make changes to the amount of organizational loss resulting from damages or loss of police vehicles. The Risk Management Supervisor provided a list of the duties of the Accident Review Board. Some of the duties include the following:

- Close accident files after recovery of monies or inactivity.

- Prepare an Accident Review Board Report once a month.

- Enter all LVMPD involved accident into the computer using the "Stars system".

- Set up claims for all LVMPD accidents.

- Act as a liaison between the LVMPD and insurance adjusters, vehicle services division, and citizen insurance companies. This includes faxing copies of requested accident reports to insurance adjusters as requested each week.

- Contact officers and command staff when LVMPD vehicles are not repaired in a timely manner.

- Process subrogations to citizen insurance companies. This includes typing letters and memos, ordering photos of accident scene and vehicles involved in accidents, obtaining insurance information, and sending packet of information to Accounting for collection of monies. Once this is completed, the payments from insurance companies are entered into the computer and the file is closed.

- Process repairs to citizens' vehicles which includes receiving estimates of damage, requesting checks for payment of damages, typing and processing of releases for claimants, and distributing checks for repayment of damages.

The Accident Review Board is an important part of liability management for the Las Vegas Metropolitan Police Department as it identifies patterns of organizational loss involving police vehicles, implements appropriate training and re-training of officers in regard to vehicle safety and operation, and recommends changes to department policies that outline how department vehicles should be operated and cared for by LVMPD personnel.

Processing claims

All liability claims filed with the Las Vegas Metropolitan Police Department are processed using the following procedure:

1. Claims are filed with the Risk Management Division using standardized forms.

2. Information from the liability claim form is entered into the Risk Management database. A hard copy (paper) of the claim is kept on file with the Risk Management Division.

3. Once the data from the form is entered into the computer database, the claim is assigned to the appropriate person for processing. The claim is sent to someone dealing with property claims or claims that are categorized as "non-litigation" cases.

4. Next, all of the reports related to the liability claim are collected for an investigation. The nature of the claim determines who will conduct the investigation. In some cases the Bureau does the investigations, whereas the Risk Management Division handles other types of claims.

5. Once the investigation is completed, a letter is sent out to the person/party responsible for filing the claim. The letter states whether or not the claim will be paid or denied, and also provides a brief description of why the claim will or will not be paid. If the claim will be paid, the person/party filing the claim will be required to sign a release form stating that no further action (legal) will taken in regard to the claim.

6. If the claim is denied and the person/party responsible is not satisfied with this outcome, they have the right to go forward with

legal action. If the claim is paid, and the person/party signs the release upon payment of the claim, the process is over.

A report of all claims is generated every month. The report details the numbers of claims both closed and open, a brief synopsis of any cases in litigation, a total for the money paid out each month, and a running balance of all payouts over the course of a fiscal year.

Risk management and police legal advisors working together

Through interviews with personnel from the LVMPD Risk Management Division, the District Attorney's Office, and the private law firm that handles litigation for the LVMPD, clear and effective communication was mentioned as the key factor to working together effectively. Having regularly scheduled meetings involving personnel from all three groups facilitates this communication.

Each group also mentioned that cooperation from other divisions within the police organization is also needed to maintain an effective liability management team. The Risk Management supervisor identified the Training Division, Internal Affairs Division, and Human Resource Division as valuable resources for information in regard to police liability. These groups are especially important once changes are made to department policies and procedures.

The management of liability in the Las Vegas Metropolitan Police Department is enhanced by the education and experience of the personnel working in the Risk Management Division, the District Attorneys Office, and the lawyers from the private law firm. Each of these groups recognize the importance and necessity of the other groups in order to achieve the ultimate goal - managing the exposure of risk to police officers and the costs resulting from such incidents.

Benefits to the community

The efforts of the Risk Management team, District Attorneys Office, and the lawyers from the private law firm result in several benefits to the citizens of Las Vegas. First, by making changes to police procedures and policies, a higher quality of police service is provided to the citizens. Most of the changes that are made to police procedures revolve around safety issues – for both the citizens and the police officers. This benefit is one that citizens will see most often as they interact with LVM police officers on the streets. Second, the efforts of Risk Management keep the cost of litigation and liability claims down, which results in less money or support needed from the taxpayers. And finally, the degree of trust between police officers and citizens will increase as the citizens notice the level of professionalism that is exerted by LVM police officers.

Impact on police professionalism and accountability

The basic philosophy of the Risk Management Division is that "if something has gone wrong, we need to identify it and then fix it so that it doesn't happen again." Part of the process of "fixing" things that go wrong within the police organization is to acknowledge that there is a problem, and then be accountable for whatever results from the problem.

Accountability and professionalism are enhanced in the LVMPD through the use of two programs. First, the LVMPD utilizes an early intervention system that can identify patterns of officer behaviors and practices that result in the most citizen complaints, liability claims, and lawsuits. This system is one way that LVM police officers are held accountable, and also a way that the organization can monitor the level of services being provided to citizens. A second program that contributes to professionalism and accountability within the LVMPD is the Accident Review Board that was described in a previous section. This board holds every employee within the LVM PD responsible for any damages or loss associated with organization vehicles. If a LVMPD employee is identified as someone who repeatedly causes damages to vehicles, they are offered additional training or retraining to correct the problem. This program holds the employee directly responsible for their actions.

COMPARISON OF FOUR PROGRAMS

After examining each of the case study sites individually, the similarities and differences between the four programs becomes clear. The following section summarizes the similarities and differences between the organizational structures of each program, the procedures used to process claims, the various ways that risk managers and police legal advisors work together, the benefits to the communities, and the perceived impact on police professionalism and accountability according to risk managers and police legal advisors in each of the four case study sites.

Organizational structure and location

Each of the case study sites uses a unique combination of risk management and police legal advising to manage liability within their police agencies (see Figure 6.1 on the following two pages).

As illustrated in Figure 6.1, all four case study sites have both a risk management component to handle the financial aspects of police liability, and a legal advisor or legal unit to handle the legal aspects of police liability. The difference between the programs is that risk managers and legal advisors are physically located both inside and outside of the police department. Early police legal advising literature specifically noted that police legal advisors should be housed within the police agency so that they would be readily available to provide legal advice to police personnel at all times.

Another similarity across all four case study sites is that each program has adopted specialized units beyond risk managers and police legal advisors to assist in managing police liability. For example, the Risk Management Department in Charlotte recently adopted a Loss Control Team that focuses their efforts specifically on police-related liability issues. As noted earlier, the Loss Control Team has been focusing on reducing auto-related losses for the police department. The Risk Management Bureau in Los Angeles has also adopted a Civil Litigation Unit that focuses primarily on handling lawsuits filed against the Sheriff's Department. In Las Vegas an Accident Review Board is used to manage liability related to all department vehicles. And in Portland, they use the Police Liability Management Unit to handle all police-related liability incidents, in addition to the citywide Risk management Department and a Police Legal Advisor from the City Attorneys Office.

In conclusion, each of the four programs shares the same goal, to manage police liability within their agencies. Each agency uses a unique combination of risk management and legal advising to achieve that goal. The unique combinations result from the variety of specialized needs of the community, management styles, and the amount of resources available in each site.

Figure 6.1
Organizational Structure of Case Study Sites

Charlotte, North Carolina

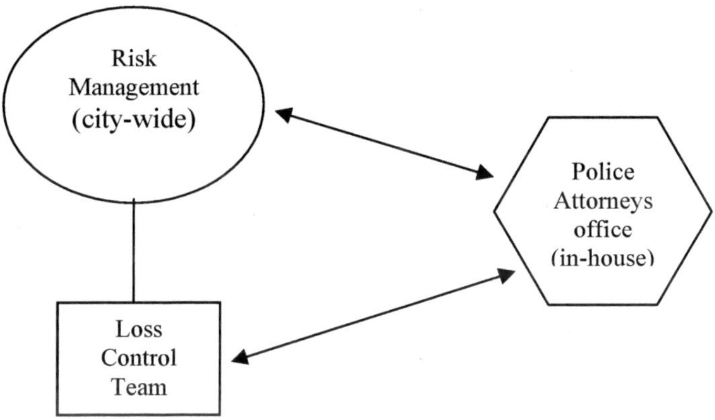

Los Angeles County, California

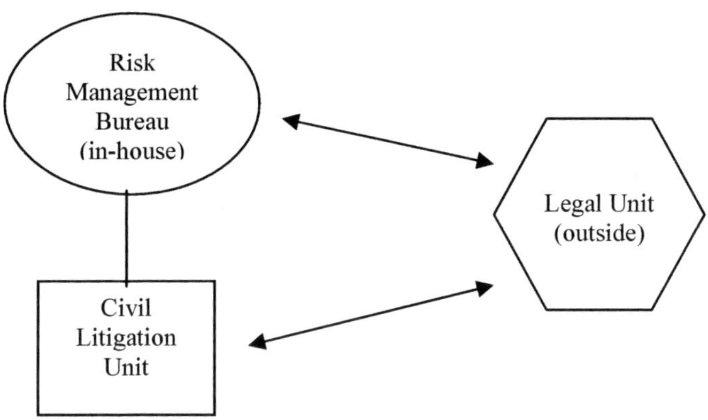

Figure 6.1 (continued)
Organizational Structure of Case Study Sites

Portland, Oregon

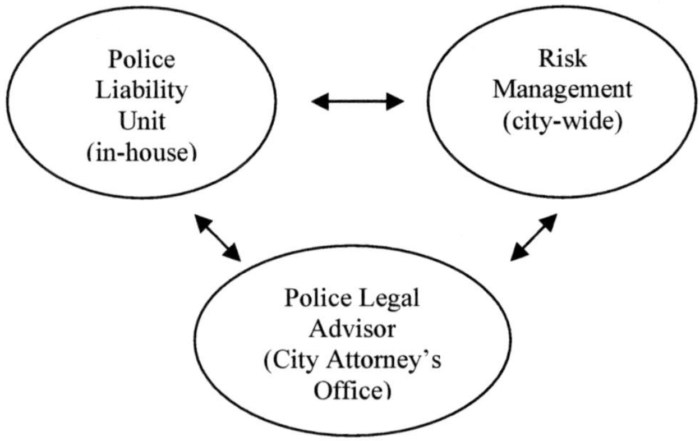

Las Vegas, Nevada

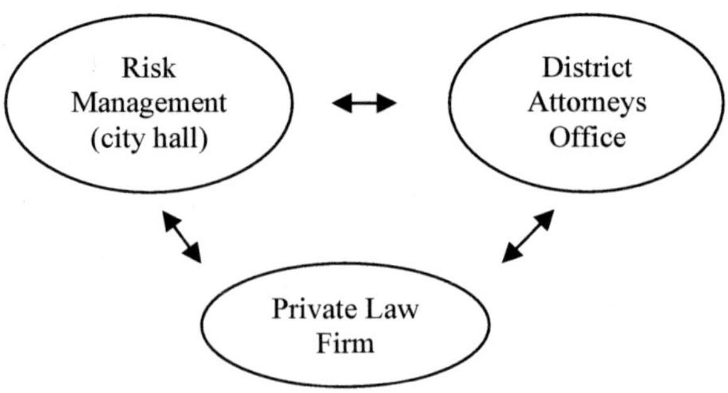

Claims processing

There is also variation in the process of handling claims involving police-related liability incidents. In Charlotte, Portland, and Las Vegas all claims involving police personnel are filed with Risk Management. In Los Angeles, claims are filed with the Board of Directors of the Los Angeles Sheriff's Department. Once claims are filed, an investigation has to take place. In Charlotte and Los Angeles, Risk Management is responsible for investigating all claims. In Portland, the Police Liability Management Unit investigates all claims involving Portland police officers.

The option of an expedited process for handling less serious claims is used in both Los Angeles and Charlotte. Portland is still in the process of creating a Liability Response Team that will be responsible for handling less serious liability incidents on the spot by issuing checks to cover less serious damages and injuries. The main difference in the expedited claims processes of Los Angeles and Charlotte is the dollar amount that can be issued "on-the-spot". For example, in Los Angeles, a member of the Civil Litigation Unit can issue a check for up to $2,500, while a Risk Assessor in Charlotte can issue checks for damage and injuries up to $5,000. In interviews, both agencies believe that the expedited claims process has saved their agencies a significant amount of money.

Working together

Risk managers and legal personnel in all four agencies expressed the importance of working together in order to effectively manage police liability in their cities. More specifically, agents in all four cities reported that frequent and continuous communication is a vital part of working together. This was an especially important thought expressed by risk managers and legal personnel in cities where they are physically located in different buildings from one another.

Another major theme that emerged from the interview data was the importance of information exchange between risk managers and legal personnel. In all four cities, claims information is collected and maintained by one agency (usually risk management), and then is shared on a regular basis with the other agencies that are involved in police liability management. In all four cities, Risk Management personnel are tasked with collecting, managing, and analyzing claim data. They are also responsible for notifying other agents (including police legal advisors) about the identified patterns that emerge from the claims and lawsuit data. At that point, the groups work together to create strategies to reduce or eliminate police officer exposure to the identified risks.

In all four cities, risk managers and legal personnel work together to examine, analyze, and alter changes to police department policy, procedures, and training to make an impact on the level of police liability. There was a consensus among representatives from all four cities that they needed the expertise of the other group (either risk management or legal personnel) in order to be effective at making those changes. Representatives from all four sites also reported that they believe that those changes have impacted liability in their cities.

Benefits to citizens

The case study site visits also provide specific examples of ways that citizens can benefit from police agencies adopting both risk managers and legal advisors to manage liability incidents. Once again, there were similarities and differences in the benefits of using risk management and legal advising mentioned in all four case study sites.

Representatives from all four cases study sites stated that a benefit to citizens would be an improvement in police services that are provided to them. Legal advisors and risk managers in all four sites commented that their efforts result in police officers being more conscientious when they are providing services to citizens. Further, risk managers and legal advisors assert that any changes they make to police training, policies, and procedures will result in some kind of change in the services that are provided to citizens in each city.

A benefit to citizens that was mentioned specifically by Risk Management personnel in Charlotte and Los Angeles was the efficient and effective handling of the claims that are filed against the police. By handling each claim as efficiently as possible, a backlog in claims can be avoided.

> "If a citizen files a claim where they were injured, they will most likely have medical bills and other bills to pay. If the City is clearly at fault in that situation, and the claim is not

handled quickly, the citizen will end up angry and frustrated. To avoid that, we try to keep the turn-around time on each claim reasonable. The turn-around time on a claim will vary according to the special circumstances surrounding the incident, the extent of injury or loss, etc…."

An important factor in handling claims efficiently depends on the resources that are available for staffing. In Portland, the importance of having adequate staffing and resources was part of a discussion on handling backlogged cases. This discussion grew out of one of the stated goals made by the Liability/Loss Control Committee.

Two of the four case study sites also expressed that by monitoring risk exposure in each city, both the citizens and police officers are living and working in a safer environment. An example of this would be how Portland, Los Angeles, Las Vegas, and more recently Charlotte, have implemented programs and committees that focus their efforts on reducing auto-related liability claims. Re-training and changing the ways that police automobiles are handled is believed to result in a decrease in auto-related incidents. This is also believed to result in a decrease in injuries to both citizens and police officers involving auto-related incidents.

Risk managers and legal advisors in all four sites also mentioned the financial benefits to citizens in interviews. Since the goal of risk managers is to reduce frequency of exposure to high-risk situations and to reduce costs associated with exposure to liability incidents, part of the goal is to save money. In all four case study sites, the financial losses of law enforcement agencies are paid either partially or in full from tax dollars. Some sites have alternative funding sources that will cover some types of loss, such as medical bills resulting from injury inflicted by police officers. But in most cities, there is a General Fund that contains money from tax revenue.

Perceived impact on police professionalism and accountability

Each of the case study sites have programs and committees set up with the goal of increasing police accountability and professionalism within each of the law enforcement agencies. Portland has recently adopted the Loss Control Team within the Risk Management Department which has one person that specifically tracks police-related claims (currently auto-related claims). Las Vegas has a similar program that monitors loss resulting from misuse or accidents of motorized vehicles. Los Angeles also has both the Command Accountability Reporting System (CARS) and the Sheriff's Critical Issues Forum (SCIF) in place to make police personnel more aware of the importance of liability management within the Sheriff's Department.

The nature of both the CARS and SCIF programs is to make sure that there is division-level accountability for liability-related incidents involving law enforcement personnel. And finally, Portland has both the Collision Review Board (CRB) and the Liability/Loss Control Committee in place to ensure accountability on a Bureau-wide level, and more accountability for auto-related losses by Bureau employees. By having these kinds of programs in place, each agency is taking extra steps to increase police accountability specifically related to police liability issues.

Interviews with risk managers and legal advisors at all four sites also revealed that police professionalism is enhanced by their efforts in regard to police liability. All four agencies reported that they believe that any changes that they make to police department policies, procedures, and training result in increased professionalism within their police agencies. Representatives from each agency in every case study site also remarked that it would be hard to quantify or measure an increase in police professionalism.

In conclusion, the case study data provides more detailed information about the various ways that each police agency uses both risk management and legal advising in their liability management efforts. The deviation among the different types of programs is easily identifiable when each site is compared to one another. The variation in risk management and police legal advising programs reflects the differences in liability concerns in each police agency, and also the resources available to police agencies to create and implement such programs.

CHAPTER 7

Conclusions, Policy Implications, and Future Research

This chapter provides a discussion of the principal findings of the national study presented in Chapter Four. More specifically, this chapter presents the significance of the use of risk managers and police legal advisors by police agencies, some of the factors associated with the adoption of such positions within police agencies, and the perceived impact of risk managers and police legal advisors on police liability, professionalism, and accountability. This chapter also presents a discussion of the lagged adoption of risk managers and police legal advisors by police agencies since the 1960s in the context of the diffusion of innovation theory. Limitations of this study, and suggestions for future research on the use of risk management and police legal advisors by police agencies are also included at the end of this chapter.

PRINCIPLE RESEARCH FINDINGS

- **Half of all U.S. law enforcement agencies that employ 200+ sworn officers employ a person or group with legal advising and/or risk management experience to manage police liability within their police organizations.**

After making telephone contact with all county and local law enforcement agencies that employ 200 or more sworn police officers, it was discovered that exactly half of all large police agencies (177 of 354) use police legal advising and/or risk management to manage police liability. The other half of the police agencies still relies solely on local city or county attorneys to handle police-related legal issues. This finding identifies the prevalence of the use of such programs by police agencies, but also sparks an interesting discussion about assertions made in early police legal advising literature.

Early literature identifies city and county attorneys as one of several sources of resistance to hiring police legal advisors in police agencies in some U.S. cities. Both Caplan (1967) and Schmidt (1972) noted that city and county attorneys believe that providing legal services to the police is part of their job, and that by hiring police legal advisors they are creating an "overlap" in legal services provided to the police. This "overlap in service" theory proposed four decades ago could explain why half of the largest law enforcement agencies in America still rely solely on their city or county attorneys for legal advice. Additional research on the police agencies that do not employ police legal advisors or risk managers is needed to get a more complete picture of why some agencies do not use such programs.

In contrast to early literature, one third of agencies surveyed in the current study identified city and county attorneys alone, or in combination with police chiefs or sheriffs as the person(s) responsible for initiating the adoption of such programs. This finding casts some doubt on the "overlap in service" theory proposed in earlier literature. It is possible that the changes in the legal environment resulting in an increase in liability claims and civil suits against the police have left city and county attorneys overwhelmed as they also have to provide services to all other city and county agencies. Because of the increase in liability claims and lawsuits, the need for hiring police legal advisors and risk managers to help with police-related liability issues has become necessary because of the changes in the legal environment in which police officers work. In fact, adopting police legal advisors and risk managers out of necessity because of changes in the legal environment was the most common response given by police agencies in survey data used in the present study. Again, future research should focus on the other half of large law enforcement agencies that do not use risk managers and police legal advisors in order to have a better understanding of the reasons why such programs are not used by those agencies.

- **Most law enforcement agencies have implemented police legal advisors and/or risk managers out of necessity in order to respond to the changes in the legal environment.**

Survey data also revealed that most police agencies have adopted police legal advisors and risk managers because they feel that it has become necessary in order to respond to a more complex legal environment. The complexity of the legal environment was most commonly described by (1) an increase in the number of liability claims and lawsuits involving police personnel, (2) an increase in the costs associated with the rising number of liability claims and lawsuits filed against the police, (3) highly publicized police-related liability incidents that have resulted in tarnished images for their agencies, and (4) the changes in law that directly impacts police procedures.

This finding is important because it begs the question of why the adoption of risk managers and police legal advisors by police agencies has been relatively slow considering the reported changes in the legal environment in which police officers work. This point is discussed in greater detail in a later section of this chapter.

- **The chief of police or sheriff is most often responsible for initiating the adoption of risk management and police legal advising programs in law enforcement agencies in the United States.**

Almost half (48%) of the police agencies identified their Chief of Police or Sheriff as the person that initiated the adoption of police legal advisors or risk managers. This finding contradicts assertions made in early literature that identifies police supervisors, including chiefs of police or sheriff's, as a source of resistance to hiring police legal advisors (Caplan, 1967; Schmidt, 1972). Early literature explains that there can be resistance if police managers do not fully understand the function or role that police legal advisors will play within the organization (Caplan, 1967). Some police managers may view police legal advisors as a police oversight mechanism, similar to an internal affairs division. This perception is believed to contribute to the resistance of the hiring of police legal advisors in the early literature.

Results from the present study contradict the idea that police chiefs or sheriff's are major sources of resistance in hiring legal staff to help manage liability within their agencies. In most cases, it was the chief of police or sheriff that recognized an increase in liability claims and lawsuits in their own police agencies or neighboring police agencies, and then sought the expertise of risk managers and/or legal advisors as a solution to the problem. This finding is important because it suggests that police managers are becoming aware of police activities that can be unsafe for both citizens and police officers, and are also taking steps to prevent or reduce those unsafe activities. This finding also suggests that police managers are becoming more concerned with fiscal responsibility within their organizations.

- **Police legal advisors and risk managers work together with police management to alter department policies, police training, and supervision over line officers to manage officer exposure to liability risks.**

Both survey and case study data reveal that police legal advisors and risk managers work closely with police managers to create management strategies to handle police-related liability incidents. Most police managers believe that they could not be as effective handling their liability issues without the assistance of the their police legal advisors or risk managers. It was reported by those same agencies that effective liability management is not possible unless there is some assistance from people with legal and/or risk assessment or insurance experience. Specialized training in law and/or risk assessment is needed in order to identify potential risks that police officers can encounter on the job, identify patterns of risks by examining old liability claims and lawsuits, and be able to keep department policies and procedures in compliance with state and federal laws.

The purpose of adopting police legal advisors and risk managers into law enforcement agencies is to maintain control over police-involved liability incidents, as well as the costs associated with those liability incidents. Police legal advisors and risk managers contribute to liability maintenance by altering department policies and police training to respond to the changes in the legal environment, and also when they identify patterns of police activities that often result in high monetary payouts from liability claims and lawsuits. Some of the police liability literature recognizes the importance of maintaining clear department policies and training (Fyfe, 1998; Newell et al, 1992), but does not specifically suggest the assistance of police legal advisors or risk managers.

In the current study, over 80% of the agencies surveyed report that their risk managers and/or police legal advisors have a significant impact on department policies and training. Some of the examples of changes to department policies and training include changing the use of law enforcement vehicles (including police pursuits and transporting detainees), and the use of physical restraining techniques on people that are taken into custody (including the use of "hog-tying", and placing seatbelt restraints on detainees during transportation). Every time that there is a change in department policy or procedure, there is usually some type of mandatory training or training bulletin issued to all police employees within the organization about those changes. This finding is important because it suggests that training and experience has to go beyond that of police executives in order to have effective police liability management.

- **Police legal advisors and risk managers serve both proactive and reactive roles within law enforcement agencies.**

There is wide variation in the level of reactivity and proactivity in the role of police legal advisors and risk managers in the United States. The reactive nature of their role comes from those instances where officers have already been exposed to liability risks, and as a result, claims or lawsuits have been filed against them. In those situations, police legal advisors and/or risk managers have to determine the best way to handle the financial aspects of the incidents after they have occurred. There are always going to be risks that officers will be exposed to, and that cannot be avoided because of the nature of police work. Due to the inherent risks in police work, there will always be some reactive component in the role of police legal advisors and risk managers.

The proactive nature of the role includes identifying on-the-job risks for police officers, and then creating strategies to reduce or prevent police officer exposure to the identified risks. As a result, police legal advisors and risk managers can make changes to department policies and procedures in an effort to avoid litigation or liability claims filed against them by citizens. Ultimately, the role of a police legal advisor and risk manager is determined by the individual needs of law enforcement agencies. The current study provides examples of this by featuring four case study sites that use police legal advisors and risk managers in ways that reflect the needs of each law enforcement agency.

- **Most risk managers and police legal advisors believe that they have some kind of financial impact on department costs related to police liability incidents.**

A majority (81%) of police legal advisors and risk managers believe that they have some kind of financial impact on police liability within their agencies. The survey data revealed that some police legal advisors and risk managers assumed that their position or program had some impact because of the important duties they are tasked with every day. The survey indicates that 47% of police legal advisors and risk managers assume that their input into police training, changes in policies and procedures, and being available to answer any questions from line officers and supervisors will have an impact on the financial loss of their police agencies. However, very few of these agencies maintain a formal record of this impact.

- **Most risk managers and police legal advisors reported that they do not keep records of their impact on police liability management.**

Only 38% of the police agencies that reported a financial impact on police liability stated that they keep records of their financial impact on liability claims and lawsuits. And of those agencies, only 30% reported that they actually publish reports outlining the financial impact on police-related liability claims and civil suits.

This finding on perceived financial impact is surprising given that most law enforcement agencies have to justify having specialized programs and units within their organizations that cost extra money to operate. One way to justify the employment of police legal advisors and risk managers within police agencies would be to have records of the financial impact they have on police liability. The records could also provide some kind of "proof" that such positions within police organizations are useful and necessary. These records could also help police agencies justify adding additional legal or risk management staff to help control police liability within their agencies.

Survey data also reveals that some police legal advisors and risk managers believe that they cannot measure all of the instances that they save their police agencies money. In most cases, the survey respondents commented on how it is impossible to quantify or measure those liability incidents and civil suits that are prevented because of their efforts. The problem is that those police legal advisors and risk managers neglected to mention the ways that their efforts can be measured and tracked over time to determine their financial impact on police liability incidents.

Three ways that police legal advisors and risk mangers can track their financial impact on police liability within their agencies includes: (1) trend data over a specified length of time, (2) compare liability across agencies by using cross sectional data, and (3) track the rates and trends of specific high risk liability incident categories (such as use of force, false arrest, etc.). Contrary to what was reported by some surveys respondents in the current study, various evaluation research techniques could be used to track the financial impact of risk managers and police legal advisors.

In regard to trend data, some risk managers and police legal advisors in the current study reported that they could track their financial impact by examining cases and liability claims that did not reach the courtroom. Each time that police legal advisors and risk managers settle claims that do not result in lawsuits, they are saving their law enforcement agencies money by avoiding court costs, as well as large monetary settlements that are sometimes awarded to citizens by the court.

Several police legal advisors and risk managers commented that the court costs alone could be very expensive depending on the circumstances surrounding the liability incident (such as those liability incidents that involve serious injury or even loss of life). Survey data from the current study also indicates that in most cases, settlements made outside of the courtroom result in lesser financial losses for police agencies that have been involved in liability incidents. These are examples of the way that trend data can be used to track financial impact.

Police legal advisors and risk managers could also track the number of claims and lawsuits filed against their agencies both before and after they alter department policies, procedures, and training for high-risk situations. If there is a significant decrease in the number of claims and lawsuits associated with a specific type of liability incident after changes have been made to policy, procedures, and training, it would be reasonable to assume that those alterations have at the very least contributed to the decrease in the frequency of a particular type of liability incident.

It is important that law enforcement agencies that have police legal advisors and/or risk managers on staff at least attempt to keep records of their efforts. Since police liability will always be a concern for police agencies, it will be necessary for the people that are tasked with handling police liability incidents to provide some kind of evidence that they are taking steps to manage liability within their agencies. Records would also be a good way to justify hiring additional staff to help with police liability management efforts. And finally, the records could be useful in determining some of the organizational factors that impact the probability that police personnel will be named as defendants in lawsuits.

The Los Angeles Sheriffs Department (LASD) in California provides a good example of how to track and publish the efforts of risk managers and police legal advisors in their effort to manage police liability. In June 1993, Merrick J. Bobb was appointed to be the Special Counsel to the Board of Supervisors. The Special Counsel is responsible for monitoring and reporting the progress of the LASD's efforts to make changes to their use of force against citizens, community sensitivity of deputies, and the handling of complaints filed by citizens against the LASD. Since October 1993, the semi-annual reports written by Merrick Bobb & his staff have detailed the efforts made by the LASD to improve police services provided to citizens, police accountability, and police professionalism.

Each semi-annual report provides information on the number of lawsuits and claims that were filed against the LASD, and also the various programs and training efforts implemented by the LASD to reduce the number of lawsuits and claims involving LASD employees. For example, in the 14th Semiannual Report (October 2001), Merrick Bobb identifies LASD litigation activity from 1992 – 2001. The report identifies the number of lawsuits involving LASD deputies for police malpractice, traffic, general negligence, and personnel cases. The report also indicates that use of force-related judgments and settlements have dropped from $17 million in 1995-1996 to $2.9 million in 2000-2001.

Each of these reports details the efforts of both the Risk Management and Legal Advisory Unit in managing police liability within the LASD. The semi-annual reports are accessible in paper form, and are also available to the public on the Los Angeles County website.

The principal findings discussed in the previous section provides a basic understanding of the prevalence of the use of risk managers and police legal advisors by large law enforcement agencies in the United States, and also provides descriptive information about the adoption, role, and characteristics of such positions within police agencies. These findings indicate that some police managers are taking steps to manage and control police liability incidents involving employees of their police agencies.

A SLOW DIFFUSION OF INNOVATION IN AMERICAN LAW ENFORCEMENT AGENCIES

A recent study by Alexander Weiss (1997) found support for the innovation of diffusion theory among police organizations. Weiss found that the degree of contact outside of police organizations impacts the degree to which police agencies adopt innovations from other police agencies. Weiss also found that an increase in litigation involving the police impacts how police executives manage their agencies. He used the example of how some cities employ police legal advisors and risk managers to help reduce police officer exposure to risks that lead to litigation. Weiss's findings contrast with some of the findings of the current study on the adoption of police legal advisors and risk managers by large law enforcement agencies.

In the current study, the diffusion of innovation theory is used as a way to understand the prevalence of the use of police legal advisor and risk manager positions in large law enforcement agencies in the United States. Even though the study presented in this book does not test any of the components of the diffusion of innovation theory, the findings of the study indicate that the diffusion of police legal advisor and risk manager positions within large police agencies has been slow over the past four decades.

By applying the basic ideas of the diffusion of innovation theory and the findings from Weiss's 1997 study to the current study, we would predict that the adoption of police legal advisors and risk managers by police agencies would have become more common in police agencies since the 1960s. We would assume widespread diffusion of such positions in police agencies because of the following factors within the social system surrounding law enforcement agencies:

- The adoption of such positions were recommended by important national criminal justice commissions including the 1967 President's Commission on Law Enforcement and the Administration of Criminal Justice, and the 1973 National Advisory Commission on Criminal Justice Standards and Goals.

- In 1973, the American Bar Association stated the importance of adopting police legal advisors within police organizations to deal with changes in the legal environment in a publication titled, Standards relating to the urban police function. O.W. Wilson (1963) also discussed the importance of having a police legal advisor within law enforcement agencies in his text, Police Administration. Both pieces of literature note the changes in the legal environment as the primary reason that police legal advisors should be adopted into police agencies.

- The services of police legal advisors and risk managers have become necessary because of the complexity of the legal environment in which police officers work. Some of the changes in the legal environment have resulted from court case outcomes that have changed police procedures (such as *Miranda v. Arizona* (1966), *Mapp v. Ohio* (1961), *Escobedo v. Illinois* (1964), *Tennessee v. Garner* (1985)). In addition, citizens have become more litigious in regard to the police since the 1960s. There is evidence of this in the increased number of lawsuits filed against the police since the 1960s (Franklin, 1993; Kappeler, 1997, 2001; McCoy, 1987), as well as increasing monetary payouts by police agencies for settlements in liability claims and lawsuits.

- Weiss (1997) found that police agencies often borrow innovations and programs from other law enforcement agencies. Additionally, Weiss found that "the more risk averse the organization (police), the more likely it would be to engage in peer emulation, and indirectly, be more innovative" (Weiss, 1997, p. 305). Weiss explains this finding by describing how an increase in litigation involving the police impacts how police executives manage their agencies. He uses the example of how some cities are beginning to employ police legal advisors/units and risk managers to help reduce exposure to risks.

Findings from the current study are not consistent with the diffusion of innovations theory or the findings of the 1997 Weiss study, as only half (177 of 354) of the largest police agencies have adopted police legal advisors and/or risk managers since the 1960s. The diffusion of innovations theory would have predicted that this innovation would have diffused much quicker because of the level of importance that was placed on such positions by groups within the social system, and because of the identified changes in the legal environment in which police officers work (including changes in law and increased litigation involving the police). Additional research on this topic is needed to determine why the other half of the largest law enforcement agencies in the United States does not employ risk managers and/or police legal advisors.

Possible explanations for slow adoption

Some of the findings from the current study and early police legal advising literature provide possible explanations for the slow adoption of risk managers and police legal advisors by police agencies since the 1960s.

Lack of standardized training and resources for positions

One possible reason why police legal advisors and risk managers have not been adopted as quickly by law enforcement agencies in the United States could be the lack of formal training opportunities. Currently, there are no formal police legal advisor training programs that are affiliated with law schools or universities that offer instruction specifically geared toward police liability issues (Goldstein, 2001, and Schmidt, 2001).[3] Throughout the 1960s and 1970s, there were formal legal advising programs offered both at Northwestern University and at the University of Wisconsin Law School. Both programs had dissolved by the mid 1970s because of the dissipation of resources and funding provided for those programs.

Today, there is only limited training available for police legal advisors through professional associations, such as the International Association of Chiefs of Police (IACP) Legal Section, which offer only periodic training seminars on police civil liability issues.[4] Similarly, risk management training specifically directed at law enforcement liability and exposure to risk are only available through seminars presented by professional speakers. Risk Management seminars last anywhere from eight hours, up to two or three days. There is no standardized training that results in some kind of certification or degree in risk management aimed specifically at law enforcement issues. Future research should examine the content of the training that is offered by the professional associations.

---

[3] Telephone interviews with both Herman Goldstein of the University of Wisconsin-Madison, and Wayne Schmidt of the International Association of Chiefs of Police in 2001.

[4] Revealed through telephone interviews with Herman Goldstein and Wayne Schmidt, and also through exhaustive searches on the Internet (specifically websites geared toward law enforcement personnel).

The lack of formal police legal advising and risk management training that results in certification becomes obvious when you attempt to locate such training programs on the Internet. For example, www.officer.com serves as one of the most comprehensive websites for law enforcement practitioners on both a national and international level. This website provides no information on formal risk management and police legal advising training. It would be difficult for police agencies to adopt such programs if training is not easily accessible.

The lag in adoption of police legal advisors and risk managers by police agencies could also be the result of a lack of resources or funding available for such positions. Other law enforcement programs, such as community oriented policing, have government grants readily available for police agencies that are interested in implementing these kinds of programs. Perhaps legal advisors and risk managers would be more common in police agencies if financial resources were available to them to contribute to the costs of adopting such programs.

<u>Lack of information on the role and benefits</u>

A second possible explanation for the lag in adoption of police legal advisors and risk managers by police agencies would be the lack of available information or literature on the topic. If police scholars and practitioners are not researching or writing about police legal advising and risk management, there is not going to be any type of manual or "how-to" guide that explains the benefits of having such programs, or how to proceed in setting up such a program within police agencies. The lack of information available on risk management and police legal advising is apparent as the topic is not discussed in most of the leading textbooks on police administration and management. In the texts where the topic is mentioned, it is usually in relation to the specific types of liability incidents related to police work, not in the context of liability management or risk assessment within police organizations.[5]

---

[5] A scan of the table of contents of ten leading police management and police administration textbooks revealed that risk management and police legal advisors were not mentioned as an important part of modern police management. This observation is important because it reflects the lack of information available for police practitioners.

The lack of available information to police managers also became apparent during initial telephone interviews conducted with police personnel for the current study. Most of the police agencies that already have risk managers or legal advisors in place wanted to know how other police agencies use risk managers and police legal advisors to manage liability within their agencies. Some of the police agencies that do not employ risk managers or police legal advisors were interested in the results of this study in case they decide to adopt a risk manager or legal advisor in the future. The current study serves as the first step at filling the gap in the literature available to both police practitioners and scholars on the use and perceived benefits of risk managers and police legal advisors in police liability management.

"Overlap in services" theory

A third possible explanation for the lag in the adoption of police legal advisors and risk managers is the "overlap in service" theory mentioned in early legal advising literature. Literature from the 1960s and 1970s identifies city or county attorneys as a source of resistance to hiring police legal advisors. The literature explains that some city/county attorneys believe that providing legal services to police agencies is part of their job, and therefore, employing police legal advisors is unnecessary (Caplan, 1967; Schmidt, 1972).

In the current study, telephone interviews revealed that exactly 50 percent of all of the largest law enforcement agencies in the U.S. still rely on their city/county attorneys for legal services. This finding could mean that the half of police agencies that do not employ police legal advisors or risk managers do not because they believe that their local city or county attorney already provides those services to the police. As stated earlier, future research on this topic should explore the reasons why half of the largest police agencies in this country do not use police legal advisors or risk managers to manage their liability issues.

All three of the possible explanations of the slow adoption of police legal advisors and risk managers by police agencies in the past four decades are based on assertions from earlier police legal advising literature, and from some of the findings from the current study. In order to get a better understanding of why some large police agencies have not yet adopted police legal advisors and/or risk managers, additional research is necessary.

CONTRIBUTION TO POLICE LIABILITY LITERATURE

Police scholars and practitioners have not examined the topic of police legal advisors and risk managers in police liability management in several decades. A review of the police liability literature presented in Chapter Two reveals a void in the literature on the use of risk management and police legal advising by police agencies in the United States. In fact, there has never been any empirical exploration of the use of both risk managers and police legal advisors by law enforcement agencies. The study presented in this book serves as the first empirical exploration of the use of both police legal advisors and risk managers by law enforcement agencies to manage police liability.

Descriptive information on the use of police legal advisors is sparse in existing police liability literature. Dating back to 1966, there have been less than ten articles and books that focus specifically on police legal advisors. Of these few books and articles, only one article (Bancroft, 1966) attempts to explore the prevalence of police legal advisors. It is important to note that Bancroft's 1966 study was a general study of police management strategies in which he only included two survey questions on the use of police legal advisors. All other early police legal advising literature is not based on any kind of empirical research or evaluation. The study presented in this book updates the prevalence of the use of police legal advisors by law enforcement agencies, and also provides detailed information on reasons for adoption, some of the roles and characteristics of police legal advisors, and the perceived impact of such programs on police liability, professionalism and accountability.

Literature on the use of risk management by law enforcement agencies is even more scarce than police legal advising literature. To date, there has only been one book and six magazine and journal articles written by professionals that have experience working with risk management in law enforcement agencies. It is important to note that the published books and articles are not based on any data collection or analysis of data from police agencies. The current study is the first of its kind on the use of risk management by police agencies as a police liability management tool. This study serves as the first step in filling the gap in the police liability literature that focuses on the way that police organizations try to manage police liability involving their employees.

IMPLICATIONS FOR PROFESSIONAL PRACTICE AND APPLIED SETTINGS

In addition to filling the void in the academic literature on police liability, the study presented in this book can also serve as an informative resource tool for police managers, city/county attorneys, risk managers, and various other city/county agents that are interested in learning about an alternative way to manage police liability. The present study provides descriptive information on how risk managers and/or police legal advisors are used as liability managers within police organizations, and the perceived impact and benefits of legal advising and risk management programs. This information could be valuable to police managers that are trying to figure out how to deal with police liability incidents. The case studies presented in Chapter Six provide four ways that police legal advisors and risk managers can be used in police liability management efforts.

The findings from this study suggest that adopting risk managers and police legal advisors to manage police liability can contribute to creating a culture of accountability and professionalism within law enforcement agencies, as well as more effective police management. Future research on police legal advisors and risk managers could examine the ways that such positions contribute to the culture of police accountability and professionalism within law enforcement agencies.

LIMITATIONS OF THE PRESENT STUDY AND SUGGESTIONS FOR FUTURE RESEARCH

There are several limitations to the study presented in this book. Several suggestions for future research emerge from the limitations identified in the present study.

First, the perceived impact of police legal advisors and risk managers on the costs resulting from police liability claims and lawsuits, benefits to citizens, police accountability, and police professionalism presented in this study are based solely on the information provided by police legal advisors and risk managers. It is possible that the police legal advisors and risk managers only provided the information that reflected them in a positive light. Future research should evaluate the impact or effectiveness of risk managers and police legal advisors on police liability. Evaluation-based studies could be conducted as longitudinal studies in one or a few sites, or a comparison of several sites could be useful in measuring the effectiveness or impact of such programs in police agencies.

A second limitation of the present study would include the lack of generalizability of the findings from the case study analysis. The original purpose of including case study analyses in this study was to provide three examples of the ways that risk managers and police legal advisors are used in law enforcement agencies to control police liability. The addition of more case study site visits to other police agencies that use risk managers and police legal advisors would strengthen the case study portion of the current study. In addition, the case study portion of this study does not include an evaluation of each program. Future research could focus on evaluations and assessments of the use of police legal advisors and risk managers in each of the case study sites.

A third limitation of the current study would be that the number of returned surveys (53 of 177 or 29.94%) was too low to conduct any type of statistical analysis. Since the present study is exploratory and qualitative in nature, the original purpose of the surveys was to acquire descriptive information about the characteristics, use, role, and perceived impact of police legal advisors and risk managers on police liability. Future research on this topic should attempt to include survey research that uses more than 53 of the 177 agencies that utilize police legal advisors and risk managers. In addition, surveys could be sent out to the other 177 agencies that do not use police legal advisors and/or risk managers in order to compare organizational characteristics of police agencies that use and that do not use such programs in their liability management efforts.

A fourth limitation of the present study is that no information was collected on the reasons why the other half of law enforcement agencies (177 of 354) do not use police legal advisors and risk managers. Future research should include the reasons why the other half of the largest law enforcement agencies in the United States does not employ police legal advisors or risk managers. In addition, future research could also compare the effectiveness of police liability management in law enforcement agencies that use and that do not use the expertise of police legal advisors and risk managers in liability management.

CONCLUSION

The study presented in this book serves as a good starting point for studying the use of police legal advisors and risk managers in an effort to reduce police liability in some of the largest law enforcement agencies in the United States. By contacting some of the largest law enforcement agencies in the country, this study revealed the prevalence of the use of risk managers and police legal advisors in the United States. This study also provides descriptive accounts of the use, perceived impact, and benefits of such programs within four law enforcement agencies. Police liability will continue to be a heavily discussed topic by police scholars and practitioners in the future. Future research on police liability should focus on programs and management techniques that can aid police managers in their efforts to manage and control liability within their agencies.

APPENDIX A

Survey Instrument

The Use of Risk Management (RM) and Legal Advising (LA) Programs by Police Organizations

---

****Please read and respond to each of the following questions. Each question will refer to risk management and legal advising programs with the phrase "RM/LA".**

<u>SECTION I – Origin and history of your program</u>

What year was your risk management/legal-advising (RM/LA) program implemented?

Briefly explain *why* your RM/LA program was implemented. (For example, a controversial incident resulting in civil suit).

Explain *how* your RM/LA program was implemented. (For example, ordinance, initiative of police personnel, executive order, etc.)

Which person or group of people *initiated* the implementation of your RM/LA program? (For example, Mayor, Police Chief, City Attorney, etc.)

Is your RM/LA program modeled after another RM/LA program in another city? If "yes", which program?

Does you RM/LA program use a computer database system? If "yes", please describe the computer system. (For example, names of software packages, etc.)

Has your RM/LA program changed since it was first implemented? If "yes" please briefly explain any changes that have occurred.

SECTION II – Characteristics of the RM/LA program

What is the official title of your RM/LA program?

What is your official title/position within the RM/LA program?

How many people are employed in your RM/LA program? (Including both clerical and professional positions)

What types of training, education or certification do you and others in your department have?
(For example, law degree, risk management training, police training, college degree, etc.)

Is your RM/LA office housed within the police department, or elsewhere?

If "no", please indicate which of the following locations best describes the location of your office:

____ Mayors office
____ Independent office
_____City attorneys' office
_____Other: If other, where?
____

Is your RM/LA program used exclusively for the police department, or does it cover other agencies within the local city government?

If your program serves other agencies, please list the other agencies that your RM/LA program covers.

SECTION III – Role of the RM/LA program

Does your RM/LA program suggest changes to the police department in regard to their **policies** to prevent or reduce civil suits and citizen complaints against the police? If "yes" please provide examples of changes in policies.

Does your RM/LA program suggest changes to the police department in regard to **police officer training** (academy, FTO, or in-service training) to prevent or reduce civil suits and citizen complaints against the police?
If "yes" please provide examples of changes in training.

Does your RM/LA program impact change in the way that **police supervisors** oversee line officers? If "yes" please provide examples of the changes in police supervision over line officers.

Does your RM/LA program impact promotion decisions within the police department? If "yes" please provide examples of changes in promotion. (For example, promotions for those officers that have had none of few complaints or civil suits filed against them, etc…)

SECTION IV – Impact of RM/LA program on police departments, individual police officers, and other local city government agencies

In your opinion, has your RM/LA program reduced the amount of payouts to citizens as the result of civil suits? Discuss how your RM/LA program has reduced police department pay-outs.

What type of data/documentation does your RM/LA program keep to track the impact or progress of your program?

Does your RM/LA publish annual or quarterly reports on its progress? If so, who or departments receive the reports?

Does your RM/LA program collaborate with other local agencies (such as social services, citizen oversight agency, insurance companies, etc….) in an effort to reduce costs of the police department? If "yes", please describe the collaboration with other local agencies.

Is there a civilian oversight agency for the police in your city? If "yes", please explain how your RM/LA program collaborates with the civilian oversight agency.

****If you have any supplemental information, such as annual reports, operations manuals, formal descriptions of your program, etc….please feel free to mail them to Carol Archbold's university address on the cover letter. Any additional information is appreciated.

APPENDIX B

Telephone Interview Questions

1. What person(s) or group is responsible for liability management in your police agency?

2. Does your police agency use risk manager(s) or police legal advisor(s) in its effort to control liability involving police personnel?

3. If risk managers and/or police legal advisors are used by your agency, how do these positions fit into the police organizational structure?

4. Could you provide me the name and phone number of the risk manager and/or police legal advisor employed by your agency?

REFERENCES

Alpert, G.P., and R.G. Dunham. 1992. *Policing Urban America* (2nd ed.) Prospect Heights, Ill: Waveland Press.

Alpert, Geoffrey P., Dennis Jay Kenney, Roger G. Dunham and William C. Smith. 2000. *Police pursuits: What we know.* Washington, D.C.: Police Executive Research Forum.

Ambert, Anne-Marie and Patricia A. Adler. 1995. "Understanding and evaluating qualitative research." *Journal of Marriage and the Family* 57: 879-894.

American Bar Association. 1973. Standards relating to the urban police function. New York, NY: American Bar Association Project on Standards for Criminal Justice.

American Civil Liberties Union of Southern California. 1992. *Analysis and recommendations: Los Angeles Police Department K-9 program.* Los Angeles, Ca: Los Angeles California Police Commission.

Archbold, Carol A. and Edward Maguire. 2002. "Studying Civil Suits Against the Police: A Serendipitous Finding of Sample Selection Bias." *Police Quarterly*, 5, 2: pp. 222-249.

Ashley, Steve and Rod Pearson. 1993. *Fundamentals of risk management.* Eau Claire, WI: Liability Assessment & Awareness International, Inc.

Backer, Thomas E. and Everett M. Rogers. 1998. "Diffusion of innovations theory and work-site AIDS programs." *Journal of Health Communication* 3: 17-29.

Bancroft, Raymond. 1966. "Municipal law enforcement, 1966." *Nation's Cities* 4:15-26.

Baltimore Sun Newspaper. 2001. "Jury finds against officer; $7 million awarded to estate of teen slain by housing policeman." May 30, 2001.

Barrineau III, H.E. 1994. *Civil liability in criminal justice* (2nd edition). Cincinnati, OH: Anderson Publishing Company.

Becker, J.C. 1994. "Chief's Counsel: The role of a legal advisor in the police management team." *The Police Chief* 61:13.

Beh, Hazel Glenn. 1998. "Municipal liability for failure to investigate citizen complaints against police." *Fordham Urban Law Review* 25: 209-254.

Berg, Bruce L. 2001. *Qualitative research methods for the social sciences* (4th Edition). Needham Heights, MA: Allyn & Bacon.

Bittner, Egon. 1970. *The functions of the police in modern society.* Washington, DC: National Institute of Mental Health.

Blalock, Joyce. 1974. *Civil liability of law enforcement officers.* Springfield, IL: Charles C. Thomas Publisher.

Cannon, Lou. 1997. Official negligence: *How Rodney King and the riots changed Los Angeles and the L.A.P.D.* New York, NY: Times Books.

Caplan, Gerald M. 1967. "The police legal advisor." *Journal of Criminal Law, Criminology, and Police Science* 58:303-309.

Ceniceros, Roberto. 1998. "Policing their own risks: Formal risk management growing in law enforcement." *Business Insurance* 32:10-13.

Cincinnati Enquirer. 2003. City settles 16 police suits for $4.5 million. May 22, 2003.

Colletti, Joseph L. 1997. "Risk management: How do they know they know?" *The Journal of California Law Enforcement* 31:16-20.

Colton, Kent W. 1972. *Use of computers by police: Patterns of success and failure.* Washington, DC: Urban Data Service.

Commission on Accreditation for Law Enforcement Agencies, Inc. 1999 *Standards for Law Enforcement Agencies* (4th Edition). Fairfax, VA: Commission on Accreditation for Law Enforcement Agencies, inc.

Conrow, Edmund H. 2000. *Effective risk management: Some keys to success.* Reston, VA: American Institute of Aeronautics and Astronautics, Inc.

Crabtree, Benjamin F. and William L. Miller. 1999. *Doing qualitative Research* (2nd Edition). Thousand Oaks, CA: Sage Publications, Inc.

Cragg, Lauren C. 1985. "Risk management: A developed discipline." In Natalie Wasserman and Dean G. Phelus (eds.) *Risk management today: A how-to guide for local government.* Washington, D.C.: Public Risk and Insurance Management Association and International City Management Association.

Creswell, John W. 1994. *Research design: qualitative & quantitative approaches.* Thousand Oaks, CA: Sage Publications, Inc.

Crouhy, Michel, Dan Galai and Robert Mark. 2001. *Risk management.* New York, NY: McGraw-Hill Publications.

Culliver, Concetta and Robert Sigler. 1995. "Police use of deadly force in Tennessee following Tennessee v. Garner." *Journal of Contemporary Criminal Justice*, 11: 187-195.

Curtis, Sarah, Wil Gesler, Glenn Smith and Sarah Washburn. 2000. "Approaches to sampling and case selection in qualitative research: Examples in the geography of health." *Social Science & Medicine* 50: 1001-1014.

del Carmen, Rolando. 1991. *Civil liabilities in American policing: A text for law enforcement personnel.* Englewood Cliffs, CA: Prentice-Hall, Inc.

Denard-Goldman, Karen. 1994. "Perceptions of innovations as predictors of implementation levels: The diffusion of a nationwide health education campaign." *Health Education Quarterly* 21: 433-446.

Denzin, Norman K. and Yvonna S. Lincoln. 1994. *Handbook of qualitative research.* Thousand Oaks, CA: Sage Publications, Inc.

Devers, Kelly J., and Richard M. Frankel. 2000. "Study Design in Qualitative Research – 2: Sampling and collection techniques." *Education for Health: Change in Learning and Practice*, 12: 263-272.

Downs, Jr. , George W. 1976. *Bureaucracy, innovation, and public policy.* Lexington, Mass: Lexington *Books.*

Esenberg, Robert W. 1992. "Risk management in the public sector." *Risk Management* 39: 72-75.

Frankel, Richard M., and Kelly Devers. 2000. "Qualitative research: A consumer's guide." *Education for health: Change in learning and practice* 13: 113-124, 251-262, 263-269.

Franklin, Carl J. 1993. *The Police Officer's Guide to Civil Liability.* Springfield, Ill: Charles C. Thomas – Publisher.

Fyfe, James J. 1979. "Administrative interventions on police shooting discretion: An empirical examination." *Journal of Criminal Justice*, 7: 309-323.

Fyfe, James J. 1981. "Who shoots? A look at officer race and police shooting." *Journal of Police Science and Administration*, 9: 367-382.

Gallagher, G. Patrick. 1990a. "The six-layered liability protection system for police." *The Police Chief* (June), 40-44.

Gallagher, G. Patrick. 1990b. "Risk management for police administrators." *The Police Chief* (June), 18-29.

Gallagher, G. Patrick. 1992. *Risk management behind the blue curtain: A primer on law enforcement liability.* Arlington, VA: Public Risk Management Association.

Gaffigan, Stephen J. and Phyllis P. McDonald. 1997. *Police integrity: Public service with honor.* Washington, D.C.: National Institute of Justice and the Office of Community Oriented Policing Services.

Geller, William A. 1991. *Local Government Police Management* (3rd edition). Washington, D.C.: The International City Management Association.

Geller, William A. and Michael Scott. 1992. *Deadly force: What we know – a practitioners desk reference on police-involved shootings.* Washington, DC: Police Executive Research Forum.

Goldstein, Herman. 2001. Personal telephone interview, May 2001.

Head, George L. and Stephen Horn II. 1985. *Essentials of the risk management process* (Volume 1). Malvern, PA: Insurance Institute of America, Inc.

Heazeltine, Hal. 1986. "Case study: A risk audit of law enforcement." *Risk Management*, 33, 10:60-63.

Hickman, Matthew J. and Brian A. Reaves. 2001. *Community Policing in Local Police Departments, 1997 and 1999.* United States Department of Justice. Washington, DC: Bureau of Justice Statistics.

Higginbotham, Jeffrey. 1994. "Legal issues in crisis management." *FBI Law Enforcement Bulletin,* 63:27-33.

Huberman A. Michael, and Matthew M. Miles. 1994. "Data management and analysis methods" in *The Handbook of Qualitative Research* by Norman K. Denzin and Yvonna S. Lincoln (eds). Thousand Oaks, CA: Sage Publications, Inc.

Human Rights Watch. 1998. *Shielded from justice: Police brutality and accountability in the United States.* New York, NY: Human Rights Watch.

International Association of Chiefs of Police (Legal Officers Section). 1998. "The police legal advisor: The importance of the advisor's role." *The Police Chief* 65:138-144.

International Association of Chiefs of Police, Inc. 1974. *Survey of police misconduct litigation: 1967-1971*. Evanston, Ill: American for Effective Law Enforcement, Inc.

Kappeler, Victor E. 1997. *Critical issues in police civil liability* (2nd edition). Prospect Heights, IL: Waveland Press, Inc.

Kappeler, Victor E. 2001. *Critical issues in police civil liability* (3rd edition). Prospect Heights, IL: Waveland Press, Inc.

Katz, David M. 1998. "L.A. cops lop $10M off tort costs." *National Underwriter*, 102, 26: 11-12.

King, Gary, Robert Koehane and Sidney Verba. 1994. *Designing social inquiry: Scientific inference in qualitative research.* Princeton: Princeton University Press.

Lersch, Kim Michelle. 2002. *Policing and Misconduct*. Upper Saddle River, NJ: Prentice Hall.

Liability Assessment and Awareness International Inc. 2001. Official website.

Livingston, Debra. 1999. "An essay on accountability." *Buffalo Criminal Law Review* 2: 815-857.

Lorch, Lawrence L. 1969. *The role of the legal advisor in the police department*. Unpublished Masters thesis. New York, NY: John Jay College of Criminal Justice of the City University of New York.

Los Angeles Police Department. 2000. *Board of inquiry into the Rampart area corruption incident public report*. Los Angeles County website.

Los Angeles County Sheriff's Department. 2000. *12th Semiannual Report* by Special Counsel Merrick J. Bobb and Staff. Los Angeles, California.

Los Angeles Times. 2000. "L.A. Mayor suggests tobacco money to pay off lawsuits over corruption." February 17.

Luborsky, Mark R. and Robert L. Rubinstein. 1995. 'Sampling in qualitative research: Rationale, issues, and methods." *Research on Aging* 17: 89-114.

Marino, Frank J. 1998. *Risk report*. Intergovernmental Risk Management Agency. Fairfax, VA: Commission on Accreditation for Law Enforcement Agencies.

McCoy, C. 1984. "Lawsuits against Police: What impact do they really have?" *Criminal Law Bulletin*, pg. 49-56.

McCoy, C. 1987. "Legal Liability: Not a Crisis." *Crime Control Digest*, pg. 1.

Miles, M.B., and A.M. Huberman. 1994. *Qualitative data analysis: An expanded sourcebook* (2nd edition). Newbury Park, CA: Sage Publications.

Mintrom, Michael. 1997. "Policy entrepreneurs and the diffusion of innovation." *American Journal of Political Science* 41: 738-771.

Mohr, Lawrence B. 1969. "Determinants of innovations in organizations." *The American Political Science Review* 63: 111-126.

Munck, Gerardo L. 1998. "Canons of research design in qualitative analysis." *Studies in Comparative International Development* 33:18-46.

Mussman, K. and W. Kennedy. 1989. *Diffusion of innovations: A select bibliography*. New York, NY: Greenwood Press.

National Advisory Commission on Criminal Justice Standards & Goals. 1973. *Police.* Washington, D.C.: United States Government Printing Office.

Newell, Charldean, Janay Pollock and Jerry Tweedy. 1993. *Financial aspects of police liability. International City/County Management Association Baseline Report.* International City/County Management Association 24: 1-8.

New York Times. 2001. "National briefing Midwest: Illinois $18 million settlement in shooting." May 9, 2001.

O'Brien, L.E. and Duane E. Wilcox. 1985. "Risk management organization and administration." In Natalie Wasserman and Dean G. Phelus (eds.) *Risk management today: A how-to guide for local government.* Washington, D.C.: Public Risk and Insurance Management Association and International City Management Association.

Payne, Dennis M. 2002. *Police Liability: Lawsuits against the police.* Durham, NC: Carolina Academic Press.

Presidents Commission on Law Enforcement & Administration of Justice. 1967. *Task force report: The police*. Washington, D.C.: United States Government Printing Office.

Public Risk Management Association. 2001. *PRIMA-file Online: Police Liability Assessment Guide*. PRIMA website.

Reaves, Brian and Timothy Hart. 1999. *Law Enforcement Management and Administrative Statistics, 1999: Data for Individual State and Local Agencies with 100 or More Officers*. Bureau of Justice Statistics. United States Department of Justice.

Reaves, Brian and Matthew Hickman. 2001. *Sheriffs' Office, 1999*. Bureau of Justice Statistics Report. United States Department of Justice.

Rogers, Everett M., Linda Williams, and Rhonda B. West. 1998. *Bibliography of the diffusion of innovations*. Monticello, Ill: Council of Planning of Librarians.

Rogers, Everett M. 1995. *Diffusion of innovations* (4th edition). New York, NY: The Free Press.

Rossman, Gretchen B. and Sharon F. Rallis. 1998. *Learning in the field: An introduction to qualitative research.* Thousand Oaks, CA: Sage Publications.

Schrader, Lt. George E. 1988. "Firearms Training/Civil Liability: Is your training documentation sufficient?" *FBI Law Enforcement Bulletin*, June, p. 1-3.

Schmidt, Wayne W. 1972. *Guidelines for a police legal unit.* Gaithersburg, MD: Police Legal Center - International Association of Chiefs of Police, Inc.

Schmidt, Wayne W. 1985. "Section 1983 and the changing face of police management." In William A. Geller (ed.) *Police leadership in America: Crisis and opportunity* (pp.226-236). Chicago, IL: American Bar Foundation.

Schmidt, Wayne W. 2001. Personal telephone interview, March 2001.

Schultz, Donald O. 1984. *The Police as the Defendant*. Springfield, Ill: Charles C. Thomas – Publisher.

Scogin, Forrest and Stanley L. Brodsky. 1991. "Fear of Litigation among Law Enforcement Officers." *American Journal of Police*, Vol. X, No. 1.

Skolnick, Jerome, and David Bayley. 1986. *The new blue line: Police innovations in six American cities.* New York, NY: Free Press.

Sparger, Jerry R. and David J. Giacopassi. 1992. "Memphis revisited: A reexamination of police shootings after the Garner decision." *Justice Quarterly*, Vol. 9, No. 2, p. 211-225.

Tellis, Winston. 1997. "Application of a case study methodology." *The Qualitative Report* 3, 3 September.

Thompson, George J. 1983. *Verbal Judo: Words for street survival.* Springfield, Ill: Charles C. Thomas Publishing.

United States Department of Justice. 2001. *Principles for promoting police integrity: Examples of promising police practices and policies*. Washington, DC: U.S. Department of Justice.

United States Department of Justice. 2002. Official Website.

Vogt, Robert C. 1985. "Police liability suits." In Natalie Wasserman and Dean G. Phelus (eds.) *Risk management today: A how-to guide for local government.* Washington, D.C.: Public Risk and Insurance Management Association and International City Management Association.

Walker, Samuel. 2001 *Police Accountability: The Role of Citizen Oversight*. Belmont, Ca: Wadsworth Publishing.

Walker, Samuel. 2001. *Early Warning Systems: Responding to the problem police officer.* National Institute of Justice Research in Brief. Washington, DC: United States Department of Justice.

Walker, Samuel. 2003. "The new paradigm of police accountability: The U.S. Justice Department "Pattern or practice" suits in context." *Saint Louis University Public Law Review*, 22, 1: 1-52.

Walker, Samuel. 2003. *Early Intervention Systems for Law Enforcement Agencies: A Planning and Management Guide*. The Office of Community Oriented Policing Services.

Weiss, Alexander. 1997. "The communication of innovation in American policing." *Policing: An International Journal of Police Strategies & Management* 20:292-310.

Wennerholm, Robert W. 1985. "Officer survival recommendations: New civil liability concerns." In Natalie Wasserman and Dean G. Phelus (eds.) *Risk management today: A how-to guide for local government.* Washington, D.C.: Public Risk and Insurance Management Association and International City Management Association.

Wilson, O.W. 1963. *Police Administration* (2nd Edition) New York, NY: McGraw-Hill Publishing.

Wojcik, Joanne. 1994. "Liability lawsuits rise again for LAPD." *Business Insurance* 28: 20-22.

Wong, Kwok-Sze Richard and Kathleen M. Rakestraw. 1991. *The A, B, C's of risk management*. Washington, D.C.: International City/County Management Association.

Worrall, John. 1998. "Administrative determinants of civil liability lawsuits against municipal police departments: An exploratory analysis." *Crime and Delinquency* 44: 295-314.

Worrall, John. 2001. *Civil lawsuits, citizen complaints, and policing innovations*. New York, NY: LFB Scholarly Publishing LLC.

Yale Law Journal. 1979. "Suing the police in federal court." *The Yale Law Journal* 88:781-824.

Young, Peter C. 2000. *Risk management: A comprehensive approach.* Washington, D.C.: International City/County Management Association

Zeckhauser, Richard J. and W. Kip Viscusi. 1996. "The risk management dilemma." In Howard Kunreuther and Paul Slovic (eds.) *Challenges in risk assessment and risk management. The Annals of the American Academy of Political and Social Science.* Thousand Oaks, CA: Sage Publications.

INDEX